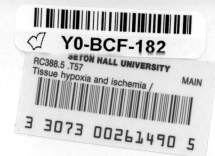

TISSUE HYPOXIA
AND ISCHEMIA

ADVANCES IN EXPERIMENTAL MEDICINE AND BIOLOGY

Recent Volumes in this Series

TISSUE HYPOXIA AND ISCHEMIA

Edited by

Martin Reivich, Ronald Coburn, Sukhamay Lahiri, and Britton Chance

University of Pennsylvania, Philadelphia

PLENUM PRESS • NEW YORK AND LONDON

Library of Congress Cataloging in Publication Data

Main entry under title:

Tissue hypoxia and ischemia.

(Advances in experimental medicine and biology; v. 78)
Proceedings of a symposium held at the Annenberg Center of the University of
Pennsylvania Aug. 13-14, 1976; sponsored by the Respiratory Physiology Group,
Dept. of Physiology, School of Medicine, University of Pennsylvania, and others.
Includes index.
1. Cerebral ischemia—Congresses. 2. Oxygen in the body—Congresses. 3. Chemo-
receptors—Congresses. 4. Vascular smooth muscle—Congresses. I. Reivich, Martin.
II. Pennsylvania. University. Respiratory Physiology Group. III. Series [DNLM: 1.
Anoxia—Metabolism. 2. Ischemia, Transient—Metabolism. S991t v. 78 1976]
RC388.5.T57 ᴹᴱ for SC.   611'.01   76-53008
ISBN 0-306-39078-7

Proceedings of a symposium on Tissue Hypoxia and Ischemia held at the Annenberg Center
of the University of Pennsylvania, August 13–14, 1976

© 1977 Plenum Press, New York
A Division of Plenum Publishing Corporation
227 West 17th Street, New York, N.Y. 10011

Sponsors

The Respiratory Physiology Group
Department of Physiology
School of Medicine
University of Pennsylvania

Cardiopulmonary Section
Department of Medicine
School of Medicine
University of Pennsylvania

Johnson Research Foundation
University of Pennsylvania

Cerebrovascular Research Center
School of Medicine
University of Pennsylvania

Head Injury Center
School of Medicine
University of Pennsylvania

Institute for Environmental Medicine
School of Medicine
University of Pennsylvania

International Society of Oxygen Transport to Tissue

This symposium was supported by Ayerst Laboratory

Preface

This monograph contains the proceedings of a symposium entitled, "Tissue Hypoxia and Ischemia," which was held at the Annenberg Center of the University of Pennsylvania on August 13 and 14, 1976. The symposium was jointly sponsored by the following groups at the University of Pennsylvania: the Respiratory Physiology Group of the Department of Physiology, the Cardiopulmonary Section of the Department of Medicine, the Johnson Research Foundation, the Cerebrovascular Research Center of the Department of Neurology, the Head Injury Center of the Department of Neurosurgery, the Institute for Environmental Medicine, and the International Society on Oxygen Transport to Tissues.

Its purpose was to promote an interdisciplinary discussion of oxygen sensors in various tissues and their mechanism of action as well as to examine the deleterious effects of hypoxia and ischemia with special reference to the brain.

There were four sessions, one on the biochemistry of physiologic oxygen sensors, two on the mechanism of oxygen sensing in tissues and one on the circulatory and metabolic aspects of cerebral hypoxia and ischemia.

In the first session, conceptual problems concerning what constitutes a molecular oxygen sensor and the transduction process were considered. In addition, the oxygen sensing characteristics of microsomal enzymes were discussed as well as microsomal oxygenase reactions, in particular those in which cytochrome P-450 plays a central role. The role of hydrogen peroxide formation in oxidation-reduction reactions involving the microsomes was explored. Other molecules which were considered as possible oxygen sensors were monoxygenases, myoglobin and hemoglobin. The reactions and kinetics of these oxygenated hemeproteins were examined. There was also discussion of the peroxisomal enzymes; catalase and three oxidases (urate, L-α-hydroxyacid and D-aminoacid oxidases) with emphasis on their

properties which are important under physiologic conditions.
Mitochondrial production of superoxide radicals and hydrogen
peroxide, the oxygen dependence of this production and the
physiologic relevance of these substances at the cellular level
were considered.

The second session dealt with the mechanism of oxygen
sensing. Data concerning the bioelectric activity of chemoreceptors and the effect of acetylcholine release on chemoreceptor function was presented. Oxygen tension sensors of
vascular smooth muscle were examined and a hypothesis to
explain the production of oxygen dependent mechanical tension
in vascular smooth muscle was put forth. Evidence was presented
that the effect of hypoxia may be mediated by a mechanism other
than inhibition of aerobic energy production. The mechanism of
oxygen induced contraction of the ductus arteriosus and the roles
of ATP, calcium ion and prostaglandins in this system were discussed. The sensing of oxygen tension in the pulmonary circulation and the circulatory effects of tissue oxygen sensors,
particularly in regard to coronary blood flow, were considered.
The adenosine hypothesis for the regulation of blood flow in
cardiac and skeletal muscle was critically examined.

In the third session the examination of the mechanism of
oxygen sensing in tissues was continued. The oxygen linked
response of the carotid chemoreceptors and the interaction of
hypoxic and hypercapnic stimuli were discussed. Data from microelectrode studies of the effects of changes in oxygen and carbon
dioxide tension, temperature and osmolarity on carotid body
cells were presented and the mechanism by which the chemoreceptors sense changes in arterial oxygen and carbon dioxide
tension were examined. The role of catecholamines and cyclic AMP
in the chemoreception process of the carotid body was considered.

The fourth session was concerned with the circulatory and
metabolic aspects of cerebral hypoxia and ischemia. The characteristic metabolic features of hypoxic hypoxia both at normal and
reduced perfusion pressures as well as of incomplete and complete
ischemia and how these metabolic changes relate to irreversible
neuronal damage was discussed. Data demonstrating the presence
of increased energy consumption and glucose metabolism in the
brain following ischemia of transient duration was presented.
Regional changes in energy metabolism and glycolysis in incomplete ischemia were also considered. The effects of ischemia
of the cerebral cortex on other regions of the brain and spinal
cord were examined in regard to cyclic nucleotide levels. The
changes in tissue PO_2, ion fluxes and redox state produced by
cerebral hypoxia and ischemia were discussed. Consideration was
given to intracellular events possibly marking irreversible

injury following ischemia. The cerebral hemodynamic and metabolic alterations that occur in patients with cerebrovascular accidents and in animal models of strokes were examined. The effects of hypovolemic shock on cerebral blood flow and its regulation as well as on brain metabolism and mitochondrial function were discussed.

The organizing committee would like to express its appreciation to all those who participated in this symposium and helped make it a most successful one. We would also like to thank Ayerst Laboratory which generously provided support for this symposium.

The Organizing Committee

Contents

CIRCULATORY AND METABOLIC ASPECTS OF CEREBRAL HYPOXIA-ISCHEMIA
Chairman: M. Reivich

The Biochemistry of
Physiologic Oxygen Sensors

Chairman: B. Chance

WHAT IS A MOLECULAR OXYGEN SENSOR?   WHAT IS A TRANSDUCTION PROCESS?

Frans F. Jobsis

Department of Physiology and Pharmacology

Duke University, Durham, North Carolina   27710

The task set for me by the organizing committee is simultaneously difficult, simple and intimidating. Difficult because of the need to look for order in a nebulous meeting ground of physiology and biochemistry. Simple because of a relative lack of solid information. And intimidating because of the importance of the topic and this audience of distinguished investigators of the topic assembled here before me.

In these brief remarks I will look for some order in the physiology of responses to hypoxia, then discuss a number of molecular candidates for the sensing of oxygen and finally add some brief speculations on transduction processes. Since I must deal mainly with generalities, it is difficult to properly ascribe the development of these areas of science to individual investigators. In addition, the contributors to this symposium are exactly those who are most active in this area. Thus these Proceedings will give the equitable accounting. Only the experimental data to be shown will be referenced. They are taken from the work of colleagues working closely with me and since I must face them every day this is wise and prudent, aside from being proper and correct.

Let me start with pointing out a puzzle. The effects of PCO_2 and pH have been found to be much more clear cut and dominant in physiological regulation and adaptation than those of PO_2. This holds true at all levels: cellular, organ and for the entire, integrated system constituting the organism. Chemoreceptor cells react more sensitively to PCO_2 and pH, so does the microvascular system and so does the central regulation of respiration. This is a puzzle since it appears to go against our principles of good

3

engineering. When we design a feedback system for the maintenance of a given condition, we tend to measure that parameter rather than a distant one signifying malfunction of the system. We measure room temperature in a thermostat system rather than the amount of heat lost through the walls. In a furnace we regulate air and fuel flow on information about the flame rather than about the smoke. Nevertheless, there is information in the quality of the smoke that may signify incomplete combustion and it would be quite possible to adjust the air flow into the system after malfunction occurs as signified by an increase in carbon monoxide production.

I would like to pose that regulation by PCO_2 and/or pH may well be an emergency system that implements the most powerful physiological responses. Under more normal functional conditions, however, other systems more directly concerned with oxygen make the more subtle and perhaps precise adjustments. In the past we have probably concentrated on PCO_2 and pH because the effects are so dramatic. It is proper, therefore, that this conference promises to concentrate more on oxygen itself. It is, however, not excluded that a transduction mechanism, common to all, unites the three parameters. I will return to this speculation at the very end of my remarks.

Different sensors have different tasks. Somewhat arbitrarily we might recognize three classes, distinguished by the O_2 concentration to be maintained. The arterial chemoreceptors provide information utilized by the system to maintain a P_aO_2 in the range of 100 torr. Local tissue concentrations are maintained at pressures from 50 down to perhaps a dozen torr. I would tend to look for these receptors in the vascular system of each organ, probably at the micro scale, i.e. arterioles, capillaries and venules. Finally at the cellular or even the mitochondrial level the biochemists urge us to consider the range of one torr or less since cytochrome oxidase (cytochrome $\underline{a}, a_3$) has an oxygen affinity in that range when studied in vitro. This classification of ranges does not preclude common molecular mechanisms. We only know that on the integrated level the results differ. But if they do happen to work through a common molecular mechanism, it will be our task to elucidate the physiological or morphological entities and variations that produce the distinctions.

Not surprisingly the regulating systems differ in complexity and number of elements in the feedback loop. On the one end of the scale there are those cells that regulate their function directly by ambient oxygen. The ductus arteriosus is perhaps the best studied example. As Dr. Fay will discuss, this smooth muscle tissue reacts directly to oxygen without intervention of neuronal elements or any other external messenger system. On the other end of the scale, the carotid body produces signals that are transmitted over long and complex pathways before the effector motor system is reached. This

provides the opportunity for further influences by inhibition and
facilitation on the information flow. There are also systems of
intermediate complexity. In our search for molecular systems that
sense oxygen we must be careful not to be confused by these complex-
ities at the multicellular level. In our task to describe physiological function, however, they should be at the center of our
attention.

Candidates for molecular sensors

We can try to enumerate or at least classify a number of
cellular compounds or enzymes that might be involved in the sensing
of oxygen. Here I am truly treading on thin ice since these systems
have mainly been studied in vitro, most often in isolation from
other cellular components.

Transfer of information to the cell and from cell to cell is
considered to involve the membrane and neurotransmitters. At
least this is the case for the time realm in which adjustment to
PO_2 variation occurs. The long term adjustments provided by the
endocrine systems are probably not directly relevant to our topic.

Thus, it is logical to consider possible direct effects of
oxygen on membranes and their constituents. Changes in structure
could easily lead to permeability effects and these in turn to
membrane potential differences, excitability and perhaps to action
potentials. A chemical mechanism in the form of oxidation of structural lipids or lipo-proteins could easily be envisioned. However,
at the risk of showing much ignorance, I must state that no observations of such effects and their excitability consequences have
come to my attention; certainly not if we consider the limits that
the time scale and the need for rapid reversibility impose. In the
carotid body, for example, the studies of Dr. Eyzaquirre (presented
later in this symposium) have failed to turn up such results. Thus
at this point in time, I would generalize that oxygen sensing by
means of direct effects of oxygen on membrane constituents is not
a likely mechanism.[1]

Neurotransmitter production involves enzymes of the general
class of oxygenases and mixed function oxidases. Their apparent
K_m's for O_2 (O_2 concentration for half maximal enzymatic activity)
are in the range of $10^{-5}M$ (approx. 12 mm Hg or 1.5% of one atmosphere of O_2). This value is extremely relevant to the task at

---

[1] The observations by Dr. Chalazonitis, presented later in this
symposium, immediately gainsayed this generalization. The ubiquity
of the system he describes must, however, still be tested for other,
especially vertebrate systems from which most other data have been
obtained.

hand, i.e. maintaining a tissue PO2 in the 10 to 50 torr range.
Again, however, the time relations of these processes are much
slower than those that would be expected for immediate transfer of
information. They are more likely to come into play in the long
term maintenance of transmitter concentrations. O2 modulation of
their release does not appear to occur in the time scale of seconds.

Here I want to digress for a moment to point out that intercellular information exchange also takes place by means of other
messengers whose concentration or release are only indirectly
affected by O2 lack or scarcity. Release of metabolic products
from anaerobically enhanced pathways, such as lactate, pyruvate
and also H^+, falls in this category. Other examples are the release
of intracellular K^+ and of adenosine during depletion of high energy
phosphate production and stores caused by hypoxia or anoxia. When
proposed as candidates for local PO2 regulators, all these "transmitters" are generally considered to act on vascular smooth muscle
adjacent to their site of release. I want to point out, however,
that they are mainly released in higher than normal concentrations
in emergency situations. The O2 provision system has broken down.
The cells are at the end of their rope. Draconian measures must
be taken. The vascular smooth muscles are paralyzed and flaccid.
Local bloodflow rises dramatically and often excessively, leading
to luxury perfusion--a misnomer indeed. Further consideration in
the context of molecular oxygen sensing is not warranted. More
properly these "transmitters" should be considered under the rubric
of transduction processes. But even then I would demur. These
systems tend to come into play after failure of the O2 provision.
They are unlikely to provide signals matching O2 supply to O_2
demand during normoxic tissue PO2 conditions.[2] This is probably a
highly personal and minority point of view. Nevertheless, I am
willing to debate it albeit with some timidity in view of the intimidating assembly of knowledge and expertise in this auditorium.

Let me turn now from the edge of the cell to the interior.
Aside from the Pasteur reaction which is mediated partially by a
direct effect of O2 on phosphofructokinase and which is probably
again part of the glycolytic emergency system, the main candidates
for molecular oxygen sensors are the O2 utilizing enzymes themselves.
These might conveniently, though somewhat arbitrarily, be subdivided
into cytochrome c oxidase (alias cyt a, a_3 or oxygen reductase) and
all the others.

---

[2] In his presentation in the symposium Dr. Berne pointed out that
the adenosine system may well be operative in the matching of O2
supply to demand during variations in work load without the occurrence of cellular ~P deficiency. This is a most elucidating and
liberating finding since, as pointed out later on in my presentation
the greatest deficiency in our present knowledge lies exactly there.

To start with the latter we have the oxygenases and mixed function oxidases, already mentioned above, which appear to be mainly involved in slower reactions than the time scale we are considering. Then there is P_{450}, the microsomal enzyme found in great abundance in the liver. Because of its limited distribution among organs this enzyme is a most unlikely candidate. In addition no hint exists about possible control functions on the microvasculature of the reaction products generated by the microsomal system. This may well indicate nothing but ignorance on my part and the presentation by Dr. Estabrook may well show it to be of the grossest sort, yet I can not arrive at a better conclusion. The same is true for superoxide dismutase, peroxidase, catalase and the autocatalytic flavoproteins. All these enzymes are an integral part of the enzymatic machinery of many cells but most appear to be mainly occupied with the task of limiting the harmful oxidizing tendencies of oxygen such as radical formation and the production of hydrogenperoxide. Once more I may well have to retract my opinion as later speakers in this symposium discuss these systems, but to me, at this point in time, they seem unlikely candidates. Which leaves me with cytochrome a,a₃.

Cytochrome oxidase handles by far the main bulk of the O_2 used in the cell and as the terminal oxidase of the respiratory chain is directly involved in cellular energy provision by oxidative phosphorylation. Interference with this system would bring the direst consequences. A signal pertaining directly to the adequacy of the O_2 supply to this enzyme would appear very relevant indeed.

However, there are a few stumbling blocks. The affinity of purified reduced cytochrome oxidase for O_2 has been determined to be extremely great. Pressures in the range of a fraction of a torr suffice for full activity in vitro, as will probably be emphasized by Dr. Chance in the lecture immediately following mine. This produces a problem in our search for molecular oxygen sensing. The difference between the PO_2 required for full activity and for the half maximal rate is smaller yet, perhaps 20 to 40 millitorr. A minor increase in energy demands would suddenly produce the needed signal and precipitate an immediate crisis for the cells involved. In addition, in a tissue there would only be a very narrow zone where oxygen lack would be graded. This feast-to-famine situation might possibly serve as an on-off alarm switch signalling emergency, but it could not serve as a generator for graded, quantitative information. Thus the properties of a system with such a very low apparent K_m for oxygen would make it an unlikely candidate for O_2 sensing. It would only come into play at a point where energy metabolism is thoroughly harmed.

Over the last years, however, we have turned up evidence that

this may not be the actual situation in a number of tissues. In
fact only in excised amphibian skeletal muscle and in perfused
mammalian liver has evidence been revealed that cyt a,a_3 has such
a very high O_2 affinity and reacts to increased demands for oxidative phosphorylation in agreement with the in vitro studies on
isolated mitochondria. In this preparation cyt a is better than
96% and a_3 better than 99% oxidized under all conditions except
when the PO_2 drops below 0.05 torr. In all other tissues that we
have studied the respiratory chain and cyt a,a_3 are much more
highly reduced at normal and raised O_2 pressures. This signifies
a much higher O_2 concentration required for saturation with O_2
(expressed as a higher P_{50} for cyt a,a_3) and implies directly a
much higher apparent K_m or lowered affinity of the reduced form
for oxygen. Most strikingly this occurs in tissues in which a
large part of the energy is expended in active transport of ions.
In addition the reduction levels of cyt a,a_3 and the other members
of the respiratory chain vary with the rate of transport in ways
that do not agree with the behavior of the respiratory chain of
isolated mitochondria during variations in rate of oxidative
phosphorylation when ADP levels are manipulated. Let me illustrate
these points with a few examples.

When the gastric mucosa of a bullfrog is stripped from the
muscularis and mounted in an Ussing chamber made of clear lucite,
H^+ production, voltage, short circuit current and the reduction
state of the respiratory chain can be monitored for many hours.
The last parameter is measured spectrophotometrically by means of
instruments specially designed by Britton Chance for highly scat-
tering samples. After such a preparation is allowed to equilibrate
overnight at a low temperature (< 10° C), acid secretion will not
occur when returned to room temperature. Addition of a secretagogue
such as theophylline or histamine and a substrate, pyruvate for
example, will then stimulate H^+ secretion. The full rate will be
obtained in 20 to 40 minutes and will be maintained for most of
the rest of the day. At the start the respiratory chain is found
to be mainly oxidized, cyt a,a_3 completely so, much as is the case
for isolated mitochondria in vitro. During the period of rising
H^+ secretion rate the chain will become more reduced until the
cytochromes attain a reduction level of 20 to 40% of the total
(Fig. 1). All members show this behavior. Variations in secretion
rate are accompanied by changes in this reduction level. Most
notably, the application of a counter potential (mucosa positive),
which inhibits the electrogenic secretion of H^+ and also inhibits
O_2 consumption, will induce an immediate further reduction of the
chain including a,a_3 (Fig. 2). Clearly the high reduction level
does not signify an anoxic core but appears to be a necessary
condition for acid secretion (2). Similar observations have been
made in the midgut of the silkworm and the tobacco hornworm during
the process of K^+ transport (3) and in other transport tissues
(unpublished).

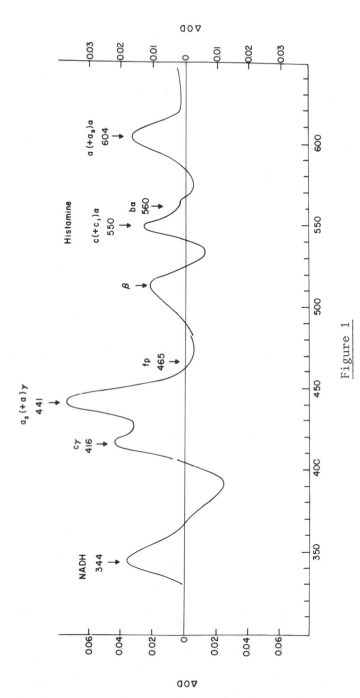

Figure 1

Spectrum of the reduction of the respiratory chain in the gastric mucosa. The reduction takes place concomitant with the stimulation of acid secretion by the addition of histamine and pyruvate to the serosal side. Abscisse; wavelength scale in mμ. Ordinate: change in optical density from the previous non-secreting state. (From Hersey and Jobsis (1), reprinted with permission from Biochem. Biophys. Res. Comm.)

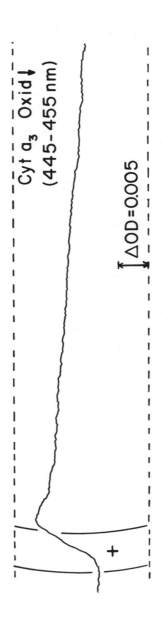

Figure 2

Reduction of cytochrome a_3 by the application of a 180 mV counter potential for 30 seconds between the two ordinates. The mucosal surface was made positive in relation to the serosal side. Bullfrog, 18° C (Previously unpublished data of F.F. Jobsis).

These observations are not limited to transport epithelia. The cerebral cortex also exhibits a high reduction level of the chain. Recent observations with hyperbaric O_2 at 4 atmospheres shows cyt $\underline{a},\underline{a}_3$ in the intact cortex to be extremely highly reduced under normoxic conditions (4). This state is sensitive to the rate of neuronal activity as shown by observations on the responses of NADH and cyt $\underline{a},\underline{a}_3$ to increased activity evoked by local stimulation as is shown in Fig. 3 (5). In fact there exists an excellent correlation between the kinetics of the extracellular K^+ and the oxidation of $\underline{a},\underline{a}_3$ in these responses. When mitochondria in a cuvette are stimulated to higher rates of oxidative phosphorylation by addition of ADP, cyt $\underline{a},\underline{a}_3$ responds with a small reduction. However, in vivo increased oxidative metabolism produces instead an oxidation of all respiratory chain members including cytochrome $\underline{a},\underline{a}_3$ (6).

Even more remarkably, the steady state redox level of $\underline{a},\underline{a}_3$ in the cerebral cortex is sensitive to the ambient tissue PO_2. This is shown by respiring the cat or the rabbit on 100% O_2 or, even better, on 95% O_2 plus 5% CO_2 (Fig. 4) (7). The fact that the redox state of cytochrome $\underline{a},\underline{a}_3$ responds to the relatively small changes in tissue PO_2 that are the results of changes in F_iO_2 indicates that an ample, graded range is available if cytochrome $\underline{a},\underline{a}_3$ were the molecular oxygen sensor.

As for evidence that cytochrome oxidase may in fact be the molecular oxygen sensor, very little is available. The most direct correlation has been observed in the carotid body. When the PO_2 of the perfusate to an excised body is dropped, a continuous increase in cytochrome $\underline{a},\underline{a}_3$ reduction level is observed. The absolute absence of O_2 produces a sudden further reduction (Fig. 5). We have concluded that two populations of $\underline{a},\underline{a}_3$ exist: one with the low affinity for O_2 observed in transport tissues, the other with extremely high affinity found in vitro, i.e., a low apparent K_m for O_2 (8). The change in reduction level of the former fraction with changes in PO_2 parallels satisfactorily the discharge rate from the chemoreceptors observed in the sinus nerve.

Therefore I want to emphasize the idea that cytochrome $\underline{a},\underline{a}_3$ does exhibit the proper, graded sensitivity to tissue PO_2. Some direct evidence is available that $\underline{a},\underline{a}_3$ may be intimately involved in the oxygen sensing process in the carotid body. Possibly this is also the case in the ductus arteriosus at the other end of the complexity scale as will be discussed by Dr. Fay. The same may be true for other tissues in which $\underline{a},\underline{a}_3$ in the blood vessel musculature or in the tissue cells themselves may function similarly. In my mind cytochrome $\underline{a},\underline{a}_3$ is the prime candidate as the molecular oxygen sensor for the sensitive matching of O_2 supply to O_2 demand in the normoxic range.

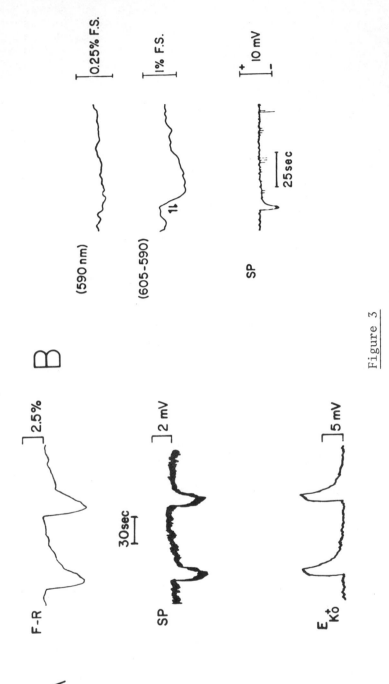

Figure 3

Responses of NADH (A) and cytochrome a,a$_3$ (B) to 2 seconds trains of stimuli applied in the field of observation on the suprosylvian gyrus of preparations of two cats. Downward deflection denote oxidations. SP - steady potential. EK^+_o-extracellular K$^+$ measurements with K$^+$ sensitive electrodes directly below the field of observation. (From Rosenthal and LaManna (5), reprinted with permission of Professional Information Library.)

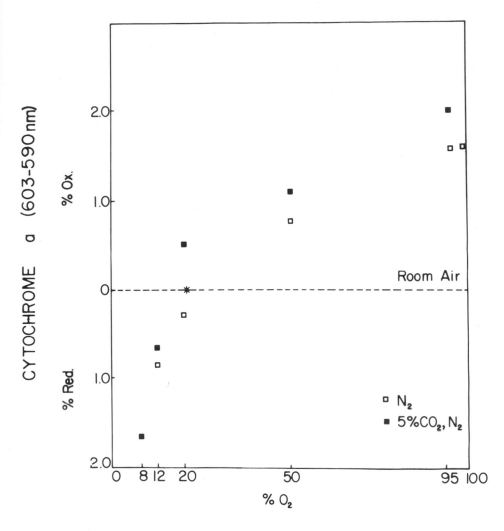

<u>Figure 4</u>

Oxidation and reduction of the steady state redox level of cyto-
chrome $\underline{a}, \underline{a_3}$ by manipulation of O_2 and for CO_2 the respired gas
mixture. Observations on the cerebral cortex of an awake, unse-
dated rabbit provided with a chronically implanted cranial window.
Abscissa: F_iO_2 . Ordinate: change in optical signal expressed as
percent of the total reflected light intensity. In terms of total
cytochrome $\underline{a}, \underline{a_3}$ these numbers should be multiplied by approximately
2 to obtain % changes in cytochrome content. (From Rosenthal et
al (7), reprinted with permission from Brain Research.)

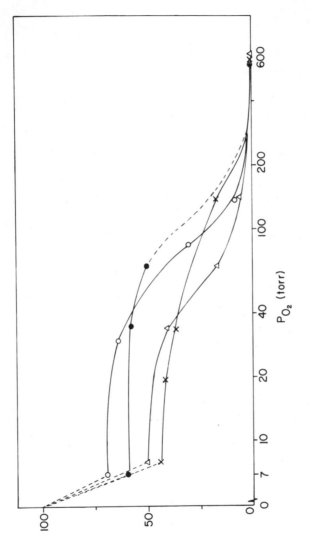

Figure 5

Reduction of cytochrome a,a₃ (445-465 nm) with decreasing PO_2 in the perfusate supplying an excised cat's carotid body. The final reduction was achieved by complete extraction of O_2 by the addition of $Na_2S_2O_4$ to the perfusate. (From Mills and Jobsis (8), reprinted with permission from J. Neurophysiol.)

Parameters of transduction processes

A number of steps must take place between the molecular sensing of O_2 and the reaction of the effector system. These can properly be designated the transduction process. From an a priori point of view a cell membrane is the most likely candidate for the ultimate effector element of the system, the goal of the transduction process. The blood vessel wall would be the target organ for tissue homeostasis. The afferent nerve endings of the carotid body could best be considered as the terminus of transduction in central control systems. I will limit my brief speculations to the processes aimed at transmitting information to these two targets.

Again I want to make a distinction between emergency systems and the more delicate adjustments of tissue PO_2 during normal functional loads. When challenged with hypoxia, increases in blood flow can take place in the cerebral cortex or the myocardium, for example, before measurable decreases in high energy phosphate compounds can be detected. The evidence for this will surely be discussed at length in the last session of this meeting. At more extreme degrees of O_2 deprivation, however, high energy stores become depleted while perfusion rates increase even more dramatically. In the latter case increased adenosine production and release occurs and mediates the dilation of the blood vessels; anaerobic glycolysis with consequences for tissue pH does the same. This situation does not primarily interest me at the moment. The continuous adjustment of O_2 provision to need may perhaps be mediated by the same system but not necessarily so. For good reasons, much more attention has been paid to the extreme situation but I believe it is high time to focus on regulation during more normoxic conditions. Since I have tried to make a case for cytochrome a,a_3 as the molecular O_2 sensor in such conditions, I will emphasize the possible consequences of increased or decreased activity of this enzyme.

The striking synchrony between respiratory chain reactions and transport processes, illustrated before, and many other more peripheral observations has led me to the working hypothesis that the turnover of the respiratory chain is closely coupled to ion transport. This notion is not new. It has been brought forward time and again, with Lundegardh, Conway and Chalanozitis perhaps the best known and most active proponents. Much has changed in our concepts about the respiratory chain since first they advocated their hypotheses, most importantly the launching of Mitchel's chemi-osmotic theory of oxidative phosphorylation. And much has stayed the same in the general reluctance of the biochemical community to embrace the idea of a redox pump, to use Conway's term. This is not the time or place to give the evidence and my reasoning

for accepting a variation of the redox pump concept as my working
hypothesis. Let it suffice for me to say that I look upon the
consequences for ion transport of changes in turnover of the respiratory chain and most specifically of cytochrome a,a_3 as the
main step in the transduction process for the precise matching of
O_2 supply to demand.

   Which ions should be considered? I believe there are three,
Ca^{++}, K^+ and H^+ that could serve as candidates. It is well known
that Ca^{++} transport in and out of mitochondria is closely coupled
to the energy state of the respiratory chain and since this ion
has such widespread biological effects it should be considered.
Loss of Ca^{++} from intramitochondrial stores occurs only, however,
when electron transport is severely limited by a fall in the
ambient PO_2 well below 0.05 torr. It is one of the last functions
of the respiratory chain to be lost with encroaching anoxia and,
therefore, occurs in the realm of what I have called the emergency
state. In addition there are three arguments against calcium
effects playing a role in the transduction process. It is not
certain that release of mitochondrial Ca^{++} results rapidly in
release from the cell. Ca^{++} has a constrictive effect on the microvasculature. And, finally, it tends to stabilize nerve membranes
rather than lower their threshold. I believe it is safe, therefore,
to eliminate calcium as an important contributor to the transduction
process.

   The fact that extracellular K^+ levels and respiratory chain
activity are so closely bound together, for instance in the
cerebral cortex as just one example, raises the question whether
this ion might be the main messenger in the transduction process.
If a slight inhibition of the cytochrome a,a_3 turnover rate,
signalled by the first changes in a,a_3 reduction level with mild
decreases in tissue PO_2, interferes with K^+ reabsorption, local
concentrations might rise sufficiently to lower the membrane
potential of adjacent nerve endings below threshold. In fact we
launched a theory of chemoreception of O_2 incorporating this idea
(8). For direct O_2 sensing and microvascular regulation the pros-
pects for this idea are not as promising. Elevated extracellular
K^+ would, of course, lead to smooth muscle contraction rather than
relaxation. In order to consider K^+ as the mediator in the transduction process, it would be necessary to interpose a neuronal
system of some complexity between the sensing and ultimate effector
systems. There is evidence, however, that autoregulation does not
require neuronal participation. In addition there is some evidence
against this hypothesis from direct, experimental applications of
K^+ to the microvascular bed. Thus K^+ is pretty well ruled out as
the mediator in the local transduction process, but it remains a
viable possibility in the chemoreceptor system. Aesthetically
this is unsatisfying but further studies may find it to be the case.

Finally then, the hydrogen ion relations must be considered. There are at least three observations that have generated my interest. Intra- to extramitochondrial H^+ shifts are part and parcel of the operation of the respiratory chain and oxidative phosphorylation. Intimate involvement of the respiratory chain in acid secretion by the gastric mucosa has been described. Thirdly, extensive effects of pH and/or PCO_2 have been described or are implied in carotid body and microvascular physiology. Whether these effects are mediated by H^+ directly or through the CO_2-bicarbonate system is relatively immaterial at this point but would become of prime importance in any detailed follow up of the notion. This will surely receive considerable attention in the second and especially the third session of this workshop. I hasten to say that I do not have a detailed mechanism of this transduction process in mind and I look forward to a great learning experience today and tomorrow. From my personal point of view, however, the possibility of H^+ as the mediator in the transduction process is extremely attractive since it would provide a common mechanism for normoxic regulation and in the more extreme hypoxic or anoxic states.

Much of the experimental research leading to the conclusions quoted in this presentation were supported by NIH grants HL 17391, NS 10384, AM 17876. Aside from my collaborators quoted in the text, I also want to acknowledge the important contribution of all the students and fellows supported on our Neuroscience training grants (NIMH 1T01 MH 08394, 2T01 MH 12333) whose critical but interested attitude to my notions has provided much appreciated stimulation of my intellectual transduction processes.

References

1. Hersey, S.J. and Jobsis, F.F.: Redox changes in the respiratory chain related to acid secretion by the intact gastric mucosa. Biochem. Biophys. Res. Comm. 36:243-250, 1969.

2. Hersey, S.J. and High, W.L.: Effect of unstirred layers on oxygenation of frog gastric mucosa. Am. J. Physiol., 223:903-909, 1972.

3. Mandel, L.J., Moffett, D. and Jobsis, F.F.: Redox state of respiratory chain enzymes and potassium transport in silkworm mid-gut. Biochem. Biophys. Acta., 408:123-134, 1975.

4. Hempel, F.G., Jobsis, F.F., LaManna, J.C., Rosenthal, M. and Saltzman, H.A.: Oxidation of cerebral cytochrome a,a_3 by oxygen plus carbon dioxide at hyperbaric pressures. Submitted to J. Appl. Physiol.

5. Rosenthal, M. and LaManna, J.C.: Oxidative metabolism and
    electrophysiological activity in the intact central nervous
    system. In: Oxygen and Physiological Function. F.F. Jobsis,
    Ed. Professional Information Library, Dallas, 1976.

6. Moffett, D. and Jobsis, F.F.: Response of toad brain respir-
    atory chain enzymes to ouabain, elevated potassium and elec-
    trical stimulus. Brain Re. In press, 1976.

7. Rosenthal, M., LaManna, J.C., Jobsis, F.F., Levasseur, J.E.,
    Kontos, H.A. and Patterson, J.L.: Effects of respiratory
    gases on cytochrome a in intact cerebral cortex. Is there a
    critical PO_2? Brain Res., 108:143-154, 1976.

8. Mills, E. and Jobsis, F.F.: Mitochondrial respiratory chain
    of carotid body and chemoreceptor response to changes in
    oxygen tension. J. Neurophysiol., 35:405-428, 1972.

THE OXYGEN SENSING CHARACTERISTICS OF MICROSOMAL ENZYMES[*]

Ronald W. Estabrook and Jurgen Werringloer
Department of Biochemistry
University of Texas Health Science Center
Dallas, Texas 75235

The endoplasmic reticulum (microsomal fraction) of many types of tissues contains an electron transport system composed of hemoproteins and flavoproteins which function in the oxygen dependent transformation of a wide variety of natural and foreign chemicals. Although less well characterized than the mitochondrial respiratory chain, microsomal oxygenase reactions, in particular those in which cytochrome P-450 plays a central role, have attracted a great deal of attention recently because of the potential harmful effects of formed epoxide products as causative agents for chemical carcinogenesis as well as the function of this electron transport system for the detoxification of a variety of drugs as related to the pharmacologic effectiveness of these chemicals. The purpose of the present paper is to provide a brief overview of our current knowledge of the oxidative reactions catalyzed by microsomes and to identify a few areas of current interest related to the reaction of oxygen with the unique hemoprotein, cytochrome P-450. The details of many of these reactions have been discussed at recent symposia (1-4).

The microsomal electron transport complex. Microsomes as isolated from liver homogenates contain at least two hemoproteins, cytochrome b_5 and P-450, as well as three flavoproteins. One possible

*Supported in part by a grant (NIGMS - 16488) from the National Institutes of Health of the USPHS.

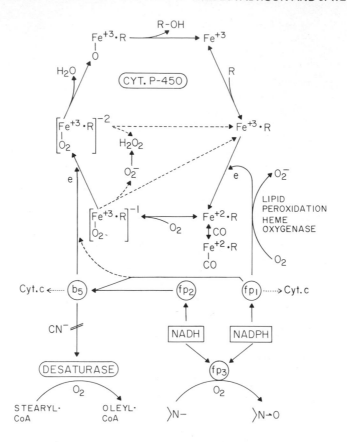

Figure 1.   Schematic representation of microsomal electron
            transport reactions.

representation of the interrelationship of these electron transport carriers in the transfer of reducing equivalents from NADH
or NADPH for the activation of oxygen associated with the oxidative conversion of different substrates is shown in Figure 1.
Basically four types of reactions are presented.

     (a) The NADPH dependent flavoprotein (fp_1) catalyzes the re-
duction of cytochrome P-450. The details of this reaction will
be discussed in greater detail below. In addition the oxidative
degradation of unsaturated fatty acids, presumably involving a
substrate peroxide intermediate (5,6), occurs during an oxygen
dependent oxidation of the reduced form of this flavoprotein (fp_1).
Current evidence indicates (7,8) that the resultant superoxide
anion, O_2^- or singlet oxygen derived from the superoxide anion,
initiates these reactions of lipid peroxidation. A similar

mechanism also may be responsible for the cleavage of the porphyrin ring in the degradative breakdown of heme to bile pigments and carbon monoxide - a reaction generally termed heme oxygenase (9,10).

(b) The oxygen dependent desaturation of fatty acyl CoA compounds occurs via a recently isolated (11) iron containing protein (the so-called cyanide sensitive factor) working in concert (12,13) with cytochrome b_5 reduced by the NADH reactive flavoprotein (fp_2) (NADH-cytochrome b_5 reductase) or the NADPH dependent flavoprotein (fp_1) (NADPH-cytochrome P-450 reductase).

(c) The flavoprotein (fp_3) catalyzed oxidation of tertiary amines may give rise to potentially harmful N-oxide compounds. Zeigler and his coworkers (14,15) have purified and characterized this flavoprotein which reacts with either NADH or NADPH. Of interest are recent results (16) which suggest that the same flavoprotein (fp_3) functions in an oxygen dependent oxidation of sulfhydryl groups for the formation of disulfide bonds.

(d) Most thoroughly studied are mixed function oxidation reactions where a family of hemoproteins, termed cytochromes' P-450, function in the oxidative degradation of a wide variety of lipophilic compounds ranging from steroids and polycyclic hydrocarbons to a vast array of pharmacologically active drugs. For these reactions one atom of molecular oxygen is incorporated into the product concomitant with the oxidation of reduced pyridine nucleotide.

The cyclic function of cytochrome P-450 (Figure 1) can be divided into at least six reaction steps although additional uncharacterized intermediates may yet be shown to be participants in the reaction sequence. Briefly our current knowledge suggests the following series of reactions for cytochrome P-450.

1. The reversible interaction of a molecule of substrate (R) with the ferric form of the hemoprotein. The association of substrate in the proximity of the heme iron results in a spectral perturbation reflecting the transition from the low spin to the high spin form of the hemoprotein.
2. The enzymatic reduction of the substrate complex of the ferric hemoprotein by reducing equivalents transferred from NADPH via the flavoprotein (fp_1), NADPH-cytochrome P-450 reductase.
3. The reduced hemoprotein can readily react with carbon monoxide to form a spectrally identifiable complex with an absorbance band maximum at about 450 nm, hence the name cytochrome P-450. Alternatively the reduced hemoprotein can react with oxygen to form a ternary complex of substrate, oxygen, and cytochrome

P-450. This complex, oxycytochrome P-450, may
dissociate giving rise to a superoxide anion while
regenerating the ferric hemoprotein.

4. Less well understood and more controversial is the
further reduction of oxycytochrome P-450, either
by reduced cytochrome b_5 or the reduced flavoprotein
(fp_1) giving rise to the equivalent of a peroxide
anion adduct for the ferric hemoprotein. This complex may also dissociate resulting in the formation
of hydrogen peroxide and the ferric hemoprotein.

5. In a reaction analogous to the formation of Complex
I of peroxidase, water is presumably abstracted
and an "oxene" is formed which can readily carry-out
an electrophilic attack on the substrate (R)
molecule resulting in hydroxylation of the substrate.

6. The hydroxylated product (ROH) dissociates from
cytochrome P-450 reestablishing the low spin form of
the ferric hemoprotein.

Many of the reaction intermediates proposed require further
experimental verification - therefore the scheme described above
should be considered merely as a working hypothesis.

Quantitative Considerations. The content of microsomal cytochromes
in liver is nearly double that of the mitochondrial cytochromes.
More interesting is the observation (17-19) that treatment of animals with a variety of drugs, such as phenobarbital, results in a
pronounced increase (Figure 2) in the content of cytochrome P-450
per gram of liver. Indeed, the high concentrations of cytochrome
P-450 (0.15 mM) in liver after induction with various drugs has
led to the suggestion (20) that it may function in a myoglobin-
like capacity for the transfer and storage of oxygen. However,
the ability of oxygen to interact with cytochrome P-450 appears
restricted to the reduced hemoprotein and this reaction rapidly
results in the oxidation of the reduced pigment.

After treatment of animals with phenobarbital the liver contains approximately ten times the concentration of cytochrome P-450
when compared to mitochondrial cytochrome c. This increase in
content of cytochrome P-450 results from a rapid synthesis of new
protein associated with the endoplasmic reticulum. It is of interest
to consider that as much as 20 percent of the protein of microsomes
can be attributed to a single class of hemoprotein (cytochrome
P-450) of molecular weight approximately 50,000.

The membrane bound nature of microsomal electron transfer proteins places unique restrictions on the mode of interaction of
these carriers during the reactions of mixed function oxidation or
fatty acid desaturation. As shown in Table I, the stoichiometry

Table I

Content of Microsomal Electron Transport Components

	nmole per mg protein	Ratio
Flavoproteins		
NADPH – Cytochrome c reductase	0.06	1
NADH – Cytochrome b5 reductase	0.015	0.25
Hemoproteins		
Cytochrome b5	0.56	9
Cytochrome P-450	2.1	35

Rat liver microsomes from phenobarbital treated animals were examined spectrophotometrically for the determination of hemoprotein concentration.   The content of flavoproteins was determined by kinetic measurements and compared to purified reductases.

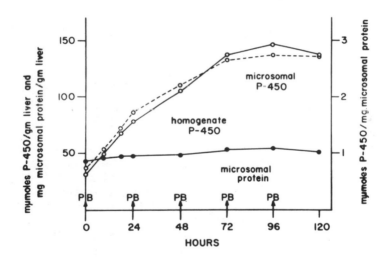

Figure 2.   Changes in the liver content of cytochrome P-450 after treatment with phenobarbital. Male rats were injected intraperitoneally with phenobarbital (50 mg per kg body weight) every twenty four hours as indicated by the arrows. Six rats were sacrificed every 24 hours and the content of cytochrome P-450, in the combined liver homogenate as well as microsomes isolated by differential centrifugation of the homogenate, was determined spectrophotometrically as described elsewhere (21).

of approximately 30 to 40 molecules of cytochrome P-450 per molecule
of flavoprotein reductase undoubtably mollifies the types of interactions which might occur. This had led to a number of interesting
speculations (22-24) on the topology of these proteins as they reside within the mileu of the membrane. Of course, one cannot exclude the potential role of membrane fluidity as a means of accounting for the types of interactions occurring.

Studies by Sholz and Thurman (25,26) as well as Sies et al
(27,28) using the perfused liver have shown that the microsomal
electron transport system as it functions in the mixed-function

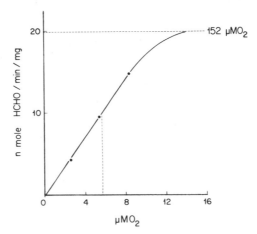

Figure 3.   Effect of oxygen concentration on the rate of micro-
            somal mixed-function oxidation of ethylmorphine. Rat
            liver microsomes from phenobarbital treated animals
            (2.2 nmole cytochrome P-450 per mg protein) were di-
            luted to a protein concentration of 1 mg per ml in a
            reaction medium containing 50 mM tris-chloride buffer,
            pH 7.5, 150 mM KCl, 10 mM $MgCl_2$, 5 mM ethylmorphine,
            5 mM sodium isocitrate, and 5 I.U. of isocitrate de-
            hydrogenase. The reaction was initiated by the addi-
            tion of 0.2 mM NADPH. The sample was vigorously stir-
            red in a vessel constructed to give maximal surface
            exposure of the sample as well as permit the rapid
            flow of gas mixtures of varying oxygen content. Ali-
            quots were removed every 30 seconds during the first
            5 minutes of the reaction at each oxygen concentration.
            The rate of product (formaldehyde) formation was
            determined colorometrically using the Nash reagent (33).

oxidation of drugs, such as aminopyrine, may contribute as much as
25 percent to the overall oxygen uptake of this tissue. A calculated turnover number of 15 to 20 per minute per molecule of
cytochrome P-450 in the perfused liver experiments is consistent
with results obtained using isolated liver microsomes suggesting
that the observed stimulation of oxygen utilization on challenging
the perfused liver with a metabolizable drug results in the nearly
maximal capacity for the contribution of this system to the oxidative metabolism of this tissue.

Oxygen affinity of mixed function oxidation reactions. The influence of varying oxygen concentrations on the rate of cytochrome
P-450 function during mixed-function oxidation reactions is of direct interest to the role of the microsomal electron transport system as an "oxygen sensor" for cellular function. We have recently
returned to reexamine this problem using isolated rat liver microsomes as they catalyze the N-demethylation of ethylmorphine. For
these experiments rapidly stirred samples were incubated in special
reaction vessels equipped for the removal of aliquots to determine
the rate of product formation concomitant with the rapid superfusion
of the sample by gas mixtures containing varying concentrations of
oxygen. As illustrated in Figure 3, half-maximal rates of metabolism
are obtained when the oxygen concentration is approximately 0.4
percent, i.e. 5 μM O_2 or 3 torr. This result confirms our earlier
studies (29) where the effect of varying concentrations of oxygen
on the rate of aminopyrine demethylation by liver microsomes was
determined (a K_m for oxygen of approximately 4 μM was observed)
and kinetic experiments (30) where the effect of varying concentration of oxygen on the extent of oxidation of reduced cytochrome
P-450 of adrenal cortex mitochondria was measured. These experiments
plus studies by Staudinger et al (31) as well as Kiese (32) all
demonstrate the relatively high affinity for oxygen of the
microsomal electron transport system involving cytochrome P-450.

Hydrogen peroxide formation. Recently interest has been rekindled
in the associated formation of hydrogen peroxide during the oxidation of NADPH by liver microsomes. As shown in Figure 4, hydrogen peroxide is rapidly generated concomitant with oxygen reduction and NADPH oxidation with approximately 50 percent of the
reducing equivalents directed toward hydrogen peroxide formation
(34). For such experiments necessary precautions must be taken
to insure the inhibition of adventitious catalase and the enzymatic
destruction of reduced pyridine nucleotide by an active pyro-
phosphatase associated with rat liver microsomes.

Knowledge of the mechanism of hydrogen peroxide generation
may serve as the necessary key to unlock the mystery of "active
oxygen" proposed for a form of oxygen (35) required for insertion
into the substrate molecule during cytochrome P-450 catalyzed

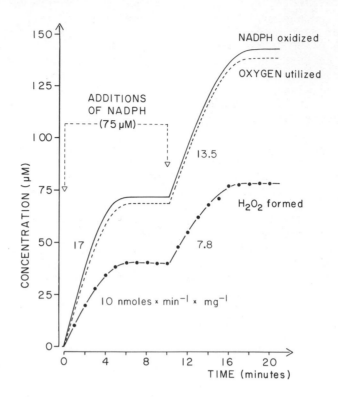

Figure 4.   The determination of hydrogen peroxide formation,
             oxygen utilization, and NADPH oxidation by rat liver
             microsomes. Three types of experiments were carried
             out under identical conditions. Liver microsomes
             from phenobarbital treated male rats were diluted
             to 1 mg of protein per ml in a reaction mixture
             containing 50 mM tris-chloride buffer, pH 7.5,
             150 mM KCl, 10 mM $MgCl_2$ 1 mM sodium azide and 2 mM
             of 5'AMP. The reaction was initiated by the addition
             of 75 μM NADPH. Oxygen utilization was determined
             polarographically; NADPH oxidation was measured
             spectrophotometrically at 340 nm using an Aminco
             DW 2 spectrophotometer in the split-beam mode.
             The concentration of hydrogen peroxide formed was
             determined colorometrically using ferrous ammonium
             sulfate and potassium thiocyanate as described by
             Hildebrandt and Roots (40).

mixed-function oxidation reactions. Further an understanding of
hydrogen peroxide formation during NADPH oxidation may resolve the
controversy (36) of a unique alcohol metabolizing system proposed
(37-39) to reside within the microsomal fraction of liver. As an
aside, it is appropriate to report that studies in our laboratory
do not favor the hypothesis that a special MEOS system exists in
liver microsomes prepared from rats pretreated with phenobarbital,
that is when suitable precautions are taken to insure the inhibition
of adventitious catalase no oxidation of methanol to formaldehyde
can be detected during NADPH oxidation by these rat liver microsomes.

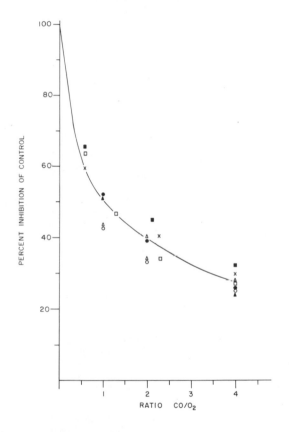

Figure 5. The inhibition by carbon monoxide of the generation of hydrogen peroxide or the N-demethylation of ethylmorphine during NADPH oxidation by rat liver microsomes. A series of experiments were carried out using various gas mixtures of carbon monoxide, oxygen, and nitrogen with the concentration of oxygen maintained at 20 percent following the procedure described in Figure 3. The concentration of hydrogen peroxide formed was determined as described in Figure 4.

The source of hydrogen peroxide. Reactions catalyzed by cytochrome
P-450 are generally characterized by a sensitivity of the reaction
to inhibition by carbon monoxide (41). As illustrated in Figure 5,
studies carried out to evaluate the CO sensitivity of hydrogen peroxide formation and companion studies to determine the CO inhibition
of a known cytochrome P-450 catalyzed reaction, the N-demethylation
of ethylmorphine, indicate that the two types of reactions are in-
distinguishable when compared at various ratios of carbon monoxide

and oxygen. This is presumptive evidence for the conclusion that hydrogen peroxide is generated during the cyclic function of cytochrome P-450.

Examination of the proposed scheme (Figure 1) for cytochrome P-450 interaction with oxygen reveals at least two possible sites for the generation of hydrogen peroxide. The first would be via dissociation of a superoxide anion from the one electron reduced state of the ternary complex of cytochrome P-450, oxygen, and substrate. The resultant dismutation of the superoxide anion would lead directly to hydrogen peroxide. A second mechanism would involve the protonation and dissociation of the peroxide anion associ-

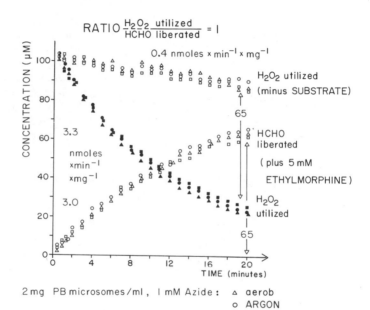

Figure 6.   The hydrogen peroxide dependent N-demethylation of ethylmorphine as catalyzed by liver microsomes. Rat liver microsomes from phenobarbital treated animals were diluted to 2 mg protein per ml in a reaction mixture containing 50 mM tris-chloride buffer, pH 7.5, 150 mM KCl, 10 mM $MgCl_2$, 1 mM sodium azide and 5 mM ethylmorphine where indicated. The reaction was initiated by the addition of 100 µM hydrogen peroxide. The changes in concentration of hydrogen peroxide utilized and formaldehyde formed were determined colorometrically as described in Figures 3 and 4.

ated with the proposed <u>two</u> <u>electron</u> reduced state of the ternary
complex of cytochrome P-450, oxygen, and substrate. Studies in
our laboratory (42), based on the absence of a synergistic effect
of NADH during the NADPH dependent formation of hydrogen peroxide,
suggest that the dissociation of superoxide anion from oxycytochrome
P-450 is the more favored reaction.

<u>Peroxidatic reactions catalyzed by microsomal cytochrome P-450.</u>
The addition of organic peroxides to liver microsomes results in
the oxidative conversion of a number of different organic substrates
(43). Hrycay and O'Brien (44-46) have provided evidence that cytochrome P-450 can function as a peroxidase - these observations suggest that "active oxygen" formed during cytochrome P-450 function
may be analogous to complex I of peroxidase. Indeed studies in
our laboratory (47) have demonstrated the formation of optical
spectral changes during the reaction of peroxides with cytochrome

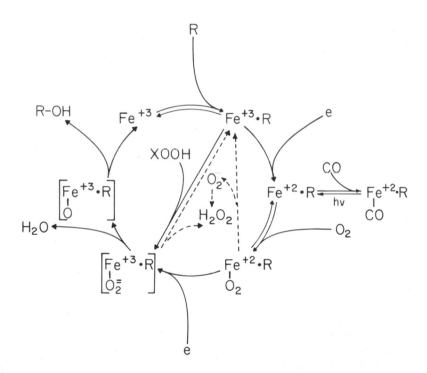

Figure 7.   Schematic representation of cytochrome P-450 function
            during substrate hydroxylation reactions including
            the proposed pathways for the generation and utiliza-
            tion of hydrogen peroxide.

P-450 as well as the generation of a free radical signal, detectable
by electron paramagnetic resonance spectrometry, remarkably similar
to that observed by Yonetani and Schleyer (48) during the function
of cytochrome c peroxidase. Considerable interest currently
centers on this peroxidatic function of cytochrome P-450. As shown
in Figure 6, hydrogen peroxide can initiate the N-demethylation
of ethylmorphine in the presence of liver microsomes. This
reaction occurs aerobically as well as anaerobically and is not
inhibited by carbon monoxide unless NADPH is added to the reaction
mixture. It should be noted that a stoichiometry of one mole of
hydrogen peroxide utilized per mole of product (formaldehyde)
formed is observed. Such studies strongly support the possible
role of an oxenoid species of oxygen playing a central role in
the function of cytochrome P-450 during substrate hydroxylation
reactions.

Summary

     The microsomal electron transport complex, in particular
the segment associated with cytochrome P-450 function, is
both qualitatively and quantitatively an important contributor
to the cellular respiration of tissues such as liver. Although
our knowledge is still limited, it is apparent that oxygen plays
a pivitol role in dictating the mode of substrate hydroxylation
or the generation of hydrogen peroxide. As illustrated in Figure
7, current evidence suggests that hydrogen peroxide is formed
by the dismutation of the superoxide anion resulting from
the dissociation of oxycytochrome P-450. Of interest are recent
studies demonstrating the ability of hydrogen peroxide to initiate
a cytochrome P-450 dependent peroxidatic reaction competent for
supporting substrate hydroxylation. The fact that the function of
cytochrome P-450 is sensitive to changes in oxygen tension esta-
blishes its role as an "oxygen sensor" for cellular metabolism.

References

   1.   Oxidases and Related Redox Systems, edited by T. E. King, H.
        S. Mason and M. Morrison. University Park Press, Baltimore,
        Md., 1973.

   2.   Microsomes and Drug Oxidations, edited by R. W. Estabrook, J.
        Gillette, and K. Leibman, The Williams and Wilkins Company,
        Baltimore, Md., 1973.

   3.   Biological Hydroxylation Mechanisms, edited by G. S. Boyd and
        R. M. S. Smellie, Academic Press, London, 1972.

4. Proceedings of The Third International Symposium on Microsomes
    and Drug Oxidations, edited by V. Ullrich, A. G. Hildebrandt,
    R. W. Estabrook, and A. Conney, Pergamon Press, Oxford, in
    press.

5. Hochstein, P. and Ernster, L., ADP-activated lipid peroxida-
    tion coupled to the TPNH system of microsomes. Biochem.
    Biophys. Res. Commun. 12: 338-394, 1963.

6. Tam, B. K. and McCay, P. B., Reduced triphosphopyridine
    nucleotide oxidase - catalyzed alterations of membrane
    phospholipids, III Transient formation of phospholipid
    peroxides. J. Biol. Chem. 245: 2295-2300, 1970.

7. Pederson, T. C. and Aust, S. D., The mechanism of liver
    microsomal lipid peroxidation. Biochim. Biophys. Acta
    385: 323-341, 1975.

8. Kellogg, E. W. and Fridovich, I., Superoxide, hydrogen
    peroxide, and singlet oxygen in lipid peroxidation by a
    xanthine oxidase system. J. Biol. Chem. 250: 8812-8817,
    1975.

9. Schmid, R. and McDonagh, A. F., The enzymatic formation of
    bilirubin. Annals of the New York Academy of Sciences, 244:
    533-552, 1975.

10. Masters, B. S. S. and Schacter, B. A., The catalysis of heme
    degradation by purified NADPH - cytochrome c reductase in
    the absence of other microsomal proteins. Annals of Clinical
    Research, Vol. 8, suppl. 17: 18-27, 1976.

11. Strittmatter, P., Spatz, L., Corcoran, D., Rogers, M. J.,
    Setlow, B., and Redline, R., Purification and properties
    of rat liver microsomal stearyl Coenzyme A desaturase.
    Proc. Natl. Acad. Sci. (USA), 71: 4565-4569, 1974.

12. Holloway, P. W., A requirement for three protein components
    in microsomal stearyl Coenzyme A desaturation. Biochemistry:
    10, 1556-1560, 1971.

13. Oshino, N., Imai, Y., and Sato, R., A function of cytochrome
    b_5 in fatty acid desaturation by rat liver microsomes. J.
    Biochem. (Tokyo): 69, 155-168, 1971.

14. Ziegler, D. M. and Mitchell, C. H., Microsomal Oxidase IV:
    Properties of a mixed function amine oxidase isolated from
    pig liver microsomes. Archives of Biochem. Biophys. 150:
    116-125, 1972.

15. Kadlubar, F. F. and Ziegler, D. M., Properties of a NADH-dependent N-hydroxy amine reductase isolated from pig liver microsomes. Archives of Biochem. Biophys. 162: 83-92, 1974.

16. Ziegler, D. M., Hyslop, R. M., and Poulsen, L. L., Sulfur containing substrates for the microsomal dimethylaniline monooxygenase (N-oxide forming). Hoppe-Seyler's Z. Physiol. Chem. 357: 1067, 1976.

17. Remmer, H. and Merker, H. J. Effect of drugs on the formation of smooth endoplasmic reticulum and drug metabolizing enzymes. Annals of the New York Acad. Sci. 123: 79-97, 1965.

18. Conney, A. H. Pharmacological implications of microsomal enzyme induction. Pharmacol. Rev. 19: 317-366, 1967.

19. Estabrook, R. W., Franklin, M. R., Cohen, B., Shigematsu, A., and Hildebrandt, A. G. Biochemical and genetic factors influencing drug metabolism: The influence of hepatic microsomal mixed function oxidation reactions on cellular metabolic control. Metabolism 2: 187-199, 1971.

20. Longmuir, I. S., Sun, S., and Soucie, W., Possible role of cytochrome P-450 as a tissue oxygen carrier. In Oxidases and Related Redox Systems, edited by T. E. King, H. S. Mason, and M. Morrison, University Park Press, Baltimore, Md., 1973, Vol. 2, pgs. 451-455.

21. Estabrook, R. W., Peterson, J., Baron, J. and Hildebrandt, A., The spectrophotometric measurement of turbid suspensions of cytochromes associated with drug metabolism. In Methods in Pharmacology, Volume 2, Physical Methods, edited by C. F. Chignell, Appleton-Century-Crofts, New York, 1972, pgs. 303-350.

22. Rogers, M. J. and Strittmatter, P., Evidence for random distribution and translational movement of cytochrome b_5 in endoplasmic reticulum. J. Biol. Chem. 249: 895-900, 1974.

23. Peterson, J. A., Ebel, R. E., O'Keeffe, D. H., Matsubara, T., and Estabrook, R. W., Temperature dependence of cytochrome P-450 reduction. A model for NADPH-cytochrome P-450 reductase: cytochrome P-450 interaction. J. Biol. Chem. 251: 4010-4016, 1975.

24. Yang, C. S. and Strickhart, F. S., Interactions between solubilized cytochrome P-450 and hepatic microsomes. J. Biol. Chem. 250: 7968-7972, 1975.

25. Thurman, R. G. and Scholz, R., Mixed function oxidation in perfused rat liver. The effect of aminopyrine on oxygen uptake. Eur. J. Biochem. 10: 459-467, 1969.

26. Thurman, R. G. and Scholz, R. Interactions of mixed-function oxidation with biosynthetic processes. 2. Inhibition of lipogenesis by aminopyrine in perfused rat liver. Eur. J. Biochem. 38: 73-78, 1973.

27. Sies, H. and Brauser, B., Interaction of mixed function oxidase with its substrates and associated redox transitions of cytochrome P-450 and pyridine nucleotides in perfused liver. Eur. J. Biochem. 15: 531-540, 1970.

28. Brauser, B., Sies, H. and Bucher, Th., Action of amobarbital on microsomal and mitochondrial respiratory state in perfused rat liver with and without phenobarbital induction. FEBS Letters, 2: 170-176, 1969.

29. Estabrook, R. W., Hildebrandt, A., Remmer, H., Schenkman, J. B., Rosenthal, O., and Cooper, D. Y. The role of cytochrome P-450 in microsomal mixed function oxidation reactions. In Biochemie des Sauerstoffs, edited by B. Hess and Hj. Staudinger, 19. Colloquium der Gesellschaft fur Biologische Chemie. Springer-Verlag, Berlin, 1968, pgs. 142-177.

30. Ullrich, V., Cohen, B., Cooper, D. Y., and Estabrook, R. W. Reactions of hemoprotein P-450. In Structure and Function of Cytochromes, edited by K. Okunuki, M. D. Kamen, and I. Sekuzu, University of Tokyo Press, Tokyo, and University Park Press, Baltimore, Maryland, 1968, pgs. 649-655.

31. Staudinger, Hj., Kerekjarto, B., Ullrich, V. and Zubrzycki, Z. A study of the mechanism of microsomal hydroxylation. In Oxidases and Related Redox Systems, edited by T. E. King, H. S. Mason, and M. Morrison, John Wiley and Sons Inc., New York, 1964, Volume 2, pgs. 815-832.

32. Kampffmeyer, H. and Kiese, M. The hydroxylation of aniline and N-ethylaniline by microsomal enzymes at low oxygen pressures. Biochem. Z. 339: 454-459 (1964).

33. Nash, T., The colorometric estimation of formaldehyde by means of the Hantzch reaction. Biochem. J. 55: 416-421, 1953.

34. Werringloer, J. and Estabrook, R. W., The formation of hydrogen peroxide during microsomal electron transport reactions, Z. physiol. chem. 357: 1063, 1976.

35. Estabrook, R. W. and Werringloer, J., Active oxygen – fact or
     fancy. In the Proceedings of the Third International Symposium
     on Microsomes and Drug Oxidations, edited by V. Ullrich, A.
     Hildebrandt, R. Estabrook, and A. Conney, Pergamon Press,
     Oxford, 1976, in press.

36. Alcohol and Aldehyde Metabolizing Systems, edited by R. G.
     Thurman, T. Yonetani, J. R. Williamson, and B. Chance. Academic
     Press, Inc., New York, New York, 1974.

37. Lieber, C. S. and DeCarli, L. M., Hepatic microsomal ethanol-
     oxidizing system. In vitro characteristics and adaptive
     properties in vivo. J. Biol. Chem. 245: 2505-2512, 1970.

38. Thurman, R. G., Ley, H. G., and Scholz, R., Hepatic microsomal
     ethanol oxidation. Hydrogen peroxide formation and the role
     of catalase. Eur. J. Biochem. 25: 420-430, 1972.

39. Teschke, R., Hasumura, Y., and Lieber, C. S., Hepatic micro-
     somal alcohol-oxidizing system. Affinity for methanol, ethanol,
     propanol and butanol. J. Biol. Chem. 250: 7397-7404, 1975.

40. Hildebrandt, A. G. and Roots, I., Reduced nicotinamide adenine
     dinucleotide phosphate (NADPH)-dependent formation and break-
     down of hydrogen peroxide during mixed function oxidation
     reactions in liver microsomes. Archives Biochem. Biophys.
     171: 385-397, 1975.

41. Estabrook, R. W., Cooper, D. Y., and Rosenthal, O., The
     light reversible carbon monoxide inhibition of the steroid
     C21-hydroxylase system of the adrenal cortex. Biochem. Z. 338:
     741-755, 1963.

42. Werringloer, J., Hildebrandt, A., and Estabrook, R. W.,
     Hydrogen peroxide formation and breakdown by the liver micro-
     somal electron transport system. Abstracts of the Tenth
     International Congress of Biochemistry, Hamburg, Germany,
     July, 1976., pg. 292.

43. Kadlubar, F. F., Morton, K. C., and Ziegler, D. M., Microsomal-
     catalyzed hydroperoxide-dependent C-oxidation of amines.
     Biochem. Biophys. Res. Comm. 54: 1255-1261, 1973.

44. Hrycay, E. G. and O'Brien, P. J., Cytochrome P-450 as a
     microsomal peroxidase in steroid hydroperoxide reduction.
     Arch. Biochem. Biophys. 153: 480-494, 1972.

45. Hrycay, E. G. and O'Brien, P. J., Microsomal electron transport
     I. Reduced nicotinamide adenine dinucleotide phosphate-cyto-
     chrome c reductase and cytochrome P-450 as electron carriers
     in microsomal NADPH-peroxidase activity. Arch. Biochem.
     Biophys. 157: 7-22, 1973.

46. Hrycay, E. G. and O'Brien, P. J., Microsomal electron transport
     II. Reduced nicotinamide adenine dinucleotide-cytochrome b5
     reductase and cytochrome P-450 as electron carriers in micro-
     somal NADH-peroxidase activity. Arch. Biochem. Biophys. 160:
     230-245, 1974.

47. Rahimtula, A. D., O'Brien, P. J., Hrycay, E. G., Peterson,
     J. A., and Estabrook, R. W., Possible higher valence states
     of cytochrome P-450 during oxidative reactions. Biochem.
     Biophys. Res. Comm. 60: 695-702, 1974.

48. Yonetani, T. and Schleyer, H., Studies on cytochrome c peroxi-
     dase. IV: The reaction of ferrimyoglobin with hydroxyperoxide
     and a comparison of the peroxide-induced compounds of ferri-
     myoglobin and cytochrome c - peroxidase. J. Biol. Chem. 242:
     1974-1979, 1967.

OXYGEN SENSING HEME PROTEINS: MONOXYGENASES, MYOGLOBIN AND HEMOGLOBIN[†]

I. C. Gunsalus, S. G. Sligar, T. Nordlund and
H. Frauenfelder

Departments of Biochemistry and Physics
University of Illinois, Urbana, IL 61801

Heme iron in the ferrous state is one of nature's best dioxygen sensors.[1] A wide variety of protein structural environments incorporate heme and permit either oxygen binding, single electron redox processes, or both. The oxygen transport proteins myoglobin (Mb) and hemoglobin (Hb), for example, alternately bind and release oxygen. The P450 oxygenase[2,3] heme proteins and cytochrome c oxidase, also bind oxygen in their biological role and, in addition, shuttle heme in a ferric-ferrous reduction and reoxidation cycle. The cytochromes, in contrast, do not accept small molecules as a heme axial ligand as both available positions are occupied by amino acid residues from the primary protein structure. The sole function of these proteins is electron transfer by univalent ferric-ferrous redox processes, which are often coupled with energy storage for cellular work. A unique additional property of monooxygenase proteins (as well as the deoxygenases which will not be discussed in this paper) is the sensing of carbon substrates in addition to oxygen. The P450 heme proteins, which comprise one of the largest classes of oxygenases[2], undergo sequentially; (a) substrate binding, (b) single electron (ferric-ferrous) reduction, (c) oxygen binding, and (d) a second single electron reduction to liberate products and regenerate the ferric resting state.[4] Monooxygenase stoichiometry is thus: $2e^- + 2H^+ + O_2 +$ Substrate (S) $\rightarrow$ $H_2O +$ Hydroxylated Substrate (S-O).[5] These heme proteins vary in their degree of substrate selectivity, redox couples, and mode of regulation.

Heme dioxygen sensors and redox cytochromes are common to all aerobic cells and many anaerobic ones. Only the oxygen carrying heme proteins, Mb and Hb, act in relatively simple complexes.

Mb contains a single polypeptide chain and one protoporphyrin IX molecule.[8] Hemoglobin is a tetramer containing two molecules each of two structurally similar heme containing polypeptides.

As we turn to the monoxygenase systems, two large classes are recognizable: (a) the mitochondrial and microbial type where the heme-coupled redox processes are performed by an iron sulfide protein[9,10], which in turn is reduced by a flavoprotein reductase driven with pyridine nucleotide energy, and (b) the microsomal systems which lack an iron sulfide protein, the oxygen active center apparently being reduced directly by a flavoprotein reductase. Examples of (a) include the oxygenases of the microorganisms which serve to introduce "inert" hydrocarbon substrates into the metabolic mainstream[4] and the adrenal mitochondrial systems active in the selective synthesis of steroid hormones.[7] Group (b) are represented by the inducible hepatic microsomal oxygenases which play a crucial role in detoxification processes.[6]

We have prepared this presentation in two sections. _First_, the monoxygenases; their components, the two electron process and composition of intermediates. _Second_, analysis of the dynamics and energetics of the primary reactions of dioxygen and carbon monoxide binding in a time, temperature, and resolution range wide enough to reveal fundamental processes. In this second investigation, we have used the relatively simple protein myoglobin, whose three-dimensional or tertiary structure is well documented, hemoglobin's α and β subunits, and finally the purified P450 monoxygenase protein.

P450 MONOXYGENASES: THE TWO ELECTRON REDOX CYCLE

A typical P450 methylene hydroxylase reaction process is shown in Figure 1.[3] This example is taken from the monoterpene monoxygenase isolated in quantity and crystallizable form from Pseudomonous putida[13], a system regarded as analogous to the adrenal cortex 11 β steroid hydroxylases.[10] This P450 heme protein of roughly 50,000 molecular weight receives the first and second single electron reducing equivalents from a specific redoxin protein (termed putidaredoxin) with a sulfide iron active center of the $Fe_2S_2^*Cys_4$ variety.[14] Much is known of the structure[15,16], function[17,18], and physical properties of these iron sulfide proteins and the effect of modification on selective multiprotein binding[17] and "catalytic" activity. Figure 1 indicates the two sequential electron transfer steps, e_1 and e_2, the first following substrate binding, the second following dioxygen addition, leading to the serial of reactions of O_2 cleavage, oxygenation and product release. Later, we shall address in more detail the processes indicated by the question mark, in a discussion of single oxygen

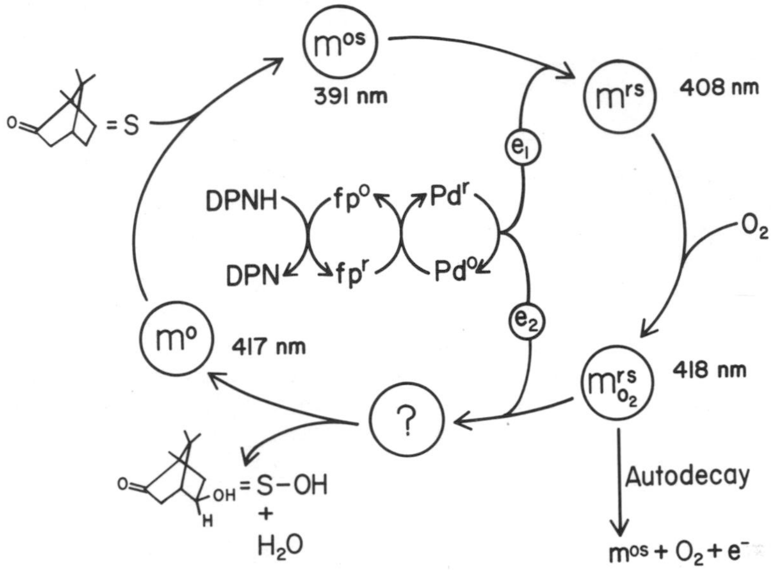

Figure 1.   A P450 monoxygenase reaction cycle and stable intermediates.   m = heme P450$_{cam}$, o = ferric, r = ferrous (e$_1^-$ added),
s = substrate, camphor, O_2 = dioxygen, Pd = putidaredoxin (Fe$_2$S$_2^*$Cys$_4$),
o = oxidized (2Fe^{3+}), r = reduced le, fp = flavoprotein, Pd reductase.

atom intermediate states.   As can be seen in Figure 1, we have been
able to stabilize four physical states of heme in this system.
The wealth of spectral and resonance[20,21,22] information accumulated
has permitted not only an understanding of the iron states but also
the kinetics and thermodynamics of interconversion as well.   Much
of this physical and chemical data has been reviewed elsewhere[4]
where appropriate references to original publications can be found.
For our purposes, it is sufficient to know that regulation in the
flow of the first electron to the heme center is substrate dependent[9], the second electron dioxygen dependent, with the redoxin
donating both redox equivalents.   The binding constants for substrate, oxygen, and for the redoxin-P450 dienzyme complex are in
the micromolar range and the latter complex has been shown to
participate in the catalytic events.[17,37]

a.   Dioxygen Heme Protein Intermediates

A central intermediate in O_2 metabolism is the dioxygen-heme
complex which is common to the transport proteins myoglobin and
hemoglobin and the monoxygenase.   As determined by Mössbauer

spectroscopy[20], all of these ferrous heme-dioxygen complexes, MbO_2, HbO_2 and P450 ($m_{O_2}^r$, or with substrate $m_{O_2}^{rs}$) exhibit a very high degree of ferric iron character indicative of a charge separation with the O_2 or porphyrin carrying a partial negative charge.

The chemical properties of O_2 and the intermediates in reduction were summarized in a particularly attractive manner by George Boyd[23] in setting the tone and level of an oxygenase symposium of the British Biochemical Society in 1972. Dioxygen, a stable paramagnetic compound with two unpaired electrons, has an oxygen-oxygen bond distance of about 1.2Å. The introduction of a single electron requires a considerable quantity of energy. Even after modulation by substrates in the biological system, the potential is near -170 mV.[9] The product, at the reduction level of superoxide, O_2^r, exhibits an oxygen-oxygen bond distance of about 1.3Å. The input of a second reducing equivalent brings the molecule to the redox level of peroxy anion, $O_2^=$, with a bond distance extended to approximately 1.5Å.

The one-electron reduced O_2 molecule may be found as a metabolite in the monoxygenase systems as either an autooxidation product[24], or, as mentioned, as a spin paired adduct with ferric heme. The second electron reduction to the peroxy-anion redox level is exemplified in the P450 reaction cycle as the $Fe^{+2}O_2^r$ or $Fe^{3+}O_2^{2-}$ compound. Release of water from the $Fe^{3+}O_2^{2-}$ adduct could yield a new intermediate containing a single oxygen atom. Present evidence[25-28] implicates this species as the "active oxygen" that transfers [0] to substrate in a process analogous to the carbene reactions familiar to chemists.

b.   Heme [0] Intermediates

Attempts to define further intermediate states have been encouraged by the recognition of an additional spectral species in both the microsomal and microbial proteins, when organic peroxides or peracids are reacted with the ferric heme protein to generate hydroxylated substrate.[25-28] This oxygen intermediate bears such striking similarity to the Compound I species seen as a peroxidase enzyme intermediate that many investigators have suggested an oxene structure.[30] An energetically favorable mechanism for generation of this compound has been proposed by Sligar et al.[28] and is represented by the triangular three-event reaction sequence in the upper left portion of Figure 2b. It should be noted that this "second oxygen intermediate" apparently brings together at one point the peroxidase and catalase heme protein mechanisms. These latter enzymes utilize H_2O_2 as substrate, i.e. dioxygen reduced to the redox level of $O_2^=$, with subsequent oxidation/reduction yielding water and O_2.

REACTIONS OF OXYGENATED HEME PROTEINS

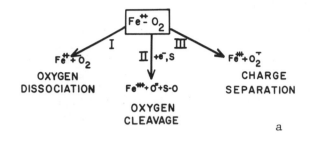

STATES DURING HYDROXYLATION

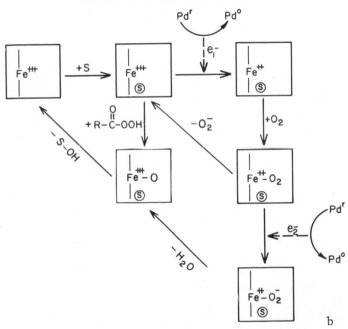

Figure 2.   Heme protein oxygenated states: Hydroxylation.

We wish to reemphasize two points before turning to the second main topic of this paper. First, the selective but multiple reactions of dioxy ferrous heme proteins, illustrated in Figure 2a, can all occur in each of the proteins considered but at vastly different rates. The branching ratio is made extremely unfavorable by certain proteins and the thermodynamic partition similarly is influenced. The dissociation rate, reaction I, is similar among the proteins discussed. In contrast, the autooxidation rate III is at least 500 times faster in P450 than Hb. The rates of II are even more dissimilar. With Hb this reduction is slight, while with P450 it is much more rapid than even reaction III. In spite of these rather large differences, hemoglobin has recently been shown to catalyze hydroxylation of analine, an aromatic substrate in the presence of pyridine nucleotide and rat liver flavoprotein reductase.[36] Thus, the differences are relative and the protein structures selected by nature exhibit excellent partitions for their designated purposes.

In the following section the photodissociable nature of the dioxygen and CO adducts of heme are utilized to explore the in-depth fine structure of ligand reactions which play fundamental roles in the biological processes.

HEME PROTEIN KINETICS

The discussion given so far has centered on components, states, and overall reactions. It would also be desirable to understand the monoxygenase reactions on a molecular level. However, the monoxygenase systems are rather complex and their structure is not yet fully known. They are thus not the easiest starting point for elucidating the connection between structure and function. Fortunately, protoheme can be studied without the protein surrounding and honorary enzymes such as myoglobin (Mb) and hemoglobin (Hb) are simpler, their structures have been determined with X-rays and neutrons, and their reactions with small ligands such as CO and O_2 can be observed easily. We are, therefore, undertaking a systematic investigation of the dynamics of ligand binding to protoheme and heme proteins over a wide range in temperature and reaction time. Results have been unexpectedly rich, and we believe that they will lead to a deeper understanding of the monoxygenases. Here we will briefly describe our approach and sketch some results.

We use flash photolysis to study the binding of small ligands to protoheme and heme proteins.[31,32,33] The idea underlying such experiments is simple. Consider, for example, Mb with bound ligand L, denoted by MbL. Irradiation with light absorbed by MbL breaks the bond; L dissociates from Mb and later rebinds. Photodissociation and rebinding can be followed optically since the absorption spectra

of ligand-bound and -free hemes differ.   The sample is placed in a
cryostat with optical windows and temperature control from 2 to
340 K.   The monitoring light is detected with a photomultiplier,
whose output is digitized and recorded in a system with a loga-
rithmic time base.[34]   Ligand binding is observed over nine decades
in time after each flash.   Wide temperature and time ranges are
crucial to data acquisition and interpretation as is illustrated
by the binding of CO to microbial P450 in Figure 3.   Here, $N(t)$
is the fraction of P450 molecules that have not rebound CO at time
t after photodissociation.   The curves indicate at least three
different processes in the reaction $P450 + CO \rightarrow P450 \cdot CO$.   (Note that
a log-log plot is needed to accommodate nine orders of magnitude
in time and three in dynamic range.   A straight line describes a
power law, $N(t) \propto t^{-n}$, not an exponential.   An exponential is given
by a rapidly falling curve as, for instance, the one at $T = 280$ K
in Figure 3.)   All heme proteins that we have studied so far show
a richness comparable to or greater than that in Figure 3.   The
processes differ from protein to protein and also depend on the
ligand molecule.   Some features, however, are general and occur
with modifications in all cases: (a) At the lowest temperatures,
typically below about 150 K and for times longer than 10 μs, a
single process dominates.   We denote this process by I; it is
independent of ligand concentration in the solvent and not exponential, but often approximates a power law, $N(t) \approx (1 + t/t_o)^{-n}$.
Process I is nearly independent of the nature of the solvent.
(b) At the highest temperatures, typically above 300 K, only one
process can be observed which we denote with IV.   It is proportional
to the ligand concentration in the solvent, exponential, and depends
markedly on the solvent properties.   (c) The naked protoheme only
shows processes I and IV.[33]   When embedded in a protein, additional
processes can be observed at temperatures between about 150 and
300 K.   The number and temperature dependencies of the additional
processes depend on solvent, protein, and ligand; they are independent of ligand concentration for gaseous ligand pressures below
about 10 atmospheres.

To evaluate flash photolysis data of the type shown in Figure
3, we assume that the protein molecule can be pictured as consisting
of the active center (heme), the globin that surrounds the active
center and forms a pronounced pocket on one side, and a hydration
shell (Figure 4a).   A ligand moving from the solvent to the binding
site at the heme iron then must overcome a series of barriers.   The
outermost barrier may be formed by the hydration shell, the next by
the entrance to the pocket, and the last by the heme.   The number
and properties of the barriers can be determined from the experimental data in Figure 3.   Details of the procedure are given in
references 31 and 33 and are elaborate.   The basic idea, however,
is straightforward: we assume that the ligand molecule moves in a
series of wells separated by potential barriers; the differential
equations describing the motion are solved by computer and the

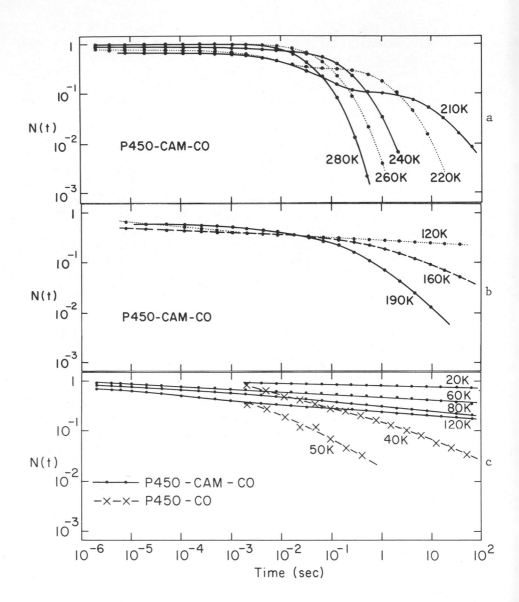

Figure 3.   Rebinding of photodissociated CO to P450. N(t) = fraction
of Mb molecules CO free at time t.   -CAM = camphor bound to P450.

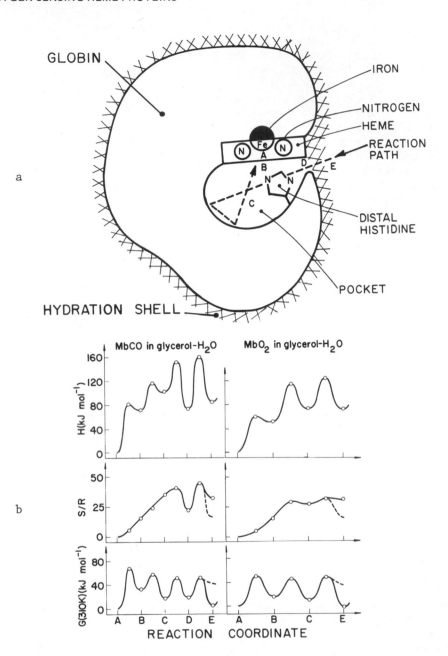

Figure 4. a. Mb reaction path schematic. b. Barriers encountered by ligands binding to Mb. G = Gibbs free energy, S = entropy, H = enthalpy.

solution is fitted to the experimental data at each temperature.
These fits yield values of the rate parameters over all barriers.
The temperature dependence of the rate parameters gives activation
enthalpies and entropies.

The data show that free protoheme in solution possesses two
barriers, I and IV. Myoglobin provides evidence for four barriers
for CO binding; one of these barriers becomes small if the ligand
is O_2. Enthalpies, entropies, and Gibbs energies for the binding
of CO and O_2 to Mb in a glycerol-water solvent are given in Figure
4b. Comparison of the barriers for free protoheme and Mb implies
that barrier I must be at the heme, IV at the solvent interface,
and the intermediate ones must be formed by the protein.[33]

The nonexponential rebinding observed for process I, which
leads from well B to the binding site A, implies that the innermost barrier is not of equal height in all Mb molecules but must
be described by a distribution, $g(H_{ba})$.[31,35] Here, $g(H_{ba}) dH_{ba}$
denotes the probability of finding a Mb molecule with activation
enthalpy between H_{ba} and $H_{ba} + dH_{ba}$. The spectral function $g(H_{ba})$
can be obtained from N(t); a few examples are shown in Figure 5.
Each protein exhibits its unique fingerprint in enthalpy distribution. We believe that this distribution reflects the existence
of many protein conformational states with different activation
enthalpies.

Examination of a variety of proteins demonstrates the protein
dependence of the barriers. Experiments with CO binding to the
separated chains of Hb, for example, show that protein structure
can affect all barriers, though barriers I and IV retain their
respective identification with the heme group and the protein-
solvent interface. Additional experiments with proteins altered
chemically or mutationally at specific points in the amino acid
sequence permit detailed studies of various parts of the protein
and may lead to a clear picture of how access to the active site is
controlled. Physiological and chemical effects of these modifications have been cataloged for years (see, for example, Dayhoff[38]),
but the mechanisms for the effects are not generally understood.
We have begun study of this problem using chemical modification
of the Hb β chain. The modification involves binding paramercuro-
benzoate (PMB) to two cysteines, one of which is attached directly
to the heme's proximal histidine. The effect of the bound PMB upon
the innermost barrier is large: the activation enthalpy for process
I almost doubles (Figure 5). The other barriers change much less,
showing that a local modification can have a local kinetic effect.

The ligand dependence of the barriers in Mb illustrates the
design of Mb as an O_2 storage protein. The Gibbs energy barriers,
Figure 4b, for O_2 are of about equal heights, allowing O_2 to move
in and out with nearly equal ease. Passage over the barriers is

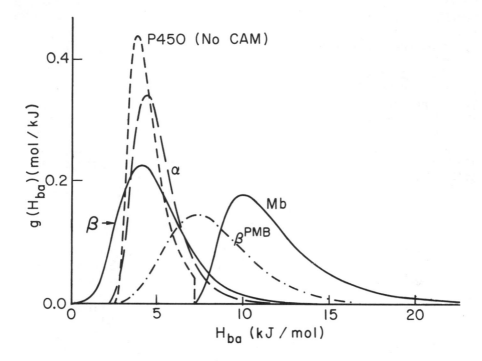

Figure 5. Activation enthalpy distributions at innermost barrier in representative heme proteins. Mb = myoglobin, α and β = hemoglobin subunits, β^{PMB} = cysteinyl p - mercury benzoate derivative.

smooth, as is evidenced by the entropy plot. CO coming from the solvent, on the other hand, encounters Gibbs energy barriers of ever increasing heights and thus is rejected at each barrier. Moreover, the entropy plot demonstrates that passage over the two outer barriers is violent.

We have confined the discussion of the kinetics to the binding of one small ligand to proteins containing one heme group. Even for such simple processes, the parameters controlling binding vary greatly, as is demonstrated by the results in Figures 4 and 5. These variations indicate how strongly the protein structure in a simple heme protein can affect the function of the active center. Equally important for an understanding of oxygen sensing proteins, however, are interactions involving more complex systems. In particular two related aspects must be explored: (a) The first is the influence of other proteins on the binding process. A typical example of this influence occurs in Hb, where the tetramer possesses the well-known cooperativity. A similar regulatory function is exerted by one protein on another in the hydroxylation sequence in which P450 is involved. (b) A second and related aspect is modulation of reactivity by the binding of smaller molecules to specific sites on the protein. Examples are diphosphoglycerate binding to Hb and camphor binding to P450, the latter a case in which the modulator is simultaneously a substrate. We see the strong dependence of P450 reactivity on substrate reflected in CO binding to the protein, Figure 3c: binding at low temperatures is much faster if camphor is absent. The influence of both types of molecules, proteins and small effector molecules can be investigated with the techniques we have described here and such studies promise to lead to a much deeper understanding of oxygen sensing proteins.

FOOTNOTES AND REFERENCES

†   Supported in part by Grants from the National Institutes of Health AM 00562, GM 21161, GM 18051, and the National Science Foundation BMS 74-01366.

1.   Szent-Gyogyi, A. (1937) "Studies on Biological Oxidation and Some of its Catalysts" Eggenbergersome, Buchhandlung, Budapest.

2.   Gunsalus, I. C., Pederson, T. C. and Sligar, S. G. (1975) Ann. Review Biochem. 44, 377.

3.   Hayaishi, O. (ed.) (1974), "Molecular Mechanisms of Oxygen Activation", Academic Press, New York.

4.   Gunsalus, I. C., Meeks, J. R., Lipscomb, J. D., Debrunner, P. G. and Münck, E. (1974) in "Molecular Mechanisms of Oxygen Activation" (O. Hayaishi, ed.), Academic Press, New York, pp. 559-613.

5.   Mason, H. S. (1957) Adv. Enzymology 19, 79.

6.   Gillett, J. R. et al. (eds.) (1969) "Microsomes and Drug Oxidations", Academic Press, New York.

7.   Hamberg, M., Samuelsson, B., Bjorkhen, I., and Danielsson, H. (1974) in "Molecular Mechanisms of Oxygen Activation" (O. Hayaishi, ed.), Academic Press, New York.

8.   Dickerson, R. E. and Geis, I. "The Structure and Action of Proteins" (1969) Harper-Row, New York.

9.   Sligar, S. G. and Gunsalus, I. C. (1976) Proc. Nat. Acad. Sci. USA 73, 1078.

10. Takemori, S., Sato, M., Gomi, T., Suhara, K. and Katagiri, M.
     (1975) Biochem. Biophys. Res. Comm. 67, 1151.

11. Guengerich, F. P., Ballou, D. P. and Coon, M. J., J. Biol.
     Chem. 250, 7405.

12. Fridovich, J. (1974) in "Molecular Mechanisms of Oxygen Activa-
     tion" (O. Hayaishi, ed.) Academic Press, New York.

13. Yu, G. A., Gunsalus, I. C., Katagiri, M., Suhara, K. and
     Takemori, S. (1974) J. Biol. Chem. 249, 94.

14. Lovenberg, W., (ed.) (1973) "Iron-Sulfur Proteins", Vol. I,
     Academic Press, New York.

15. Tanaka, M., Haniu, M. and Yasunobu, K. (1973) J. Biol. Chem.
     248, 1141.

16. Tanaka, M., Haniu, M., Yasunobu, K. T., Dus, K. and Gunsalus,
     I. C. (1974) J. Biol. Chem. 249, 3689.

17. Sligar, S. G., Debrunner, P. G., Lipscomb, J. D., Namtvedt,
     M. J. and Gunsalus, I. C. (1974) Proc. Nat. Acad. Sci. USA
     71, 3906.

18. Lipscomb, J. D., Sligar, S. G., Namtvedt, M. J. and Gunsalus,
     I. C. (1976) J. Biol. Chem. 251, 1116.

19. Sligar, S. (1975) Ph.D. Thesis, University of Illinois, Urbana.

20. Sharrock, M., Münck, E., Debrunner, P. G., Marshall, V. P.,
     Lipscomb, J. D., and Gunsalus, I. C. (1973) Biochemistry 12, 258.

21. Sharrock, M., Debrunner, P. G., Schulz, C., Lipscomb, J. D.,
     Marshall, V. and Gunsalus, I. C. (1976) Biochem. Biophys. Acta
     420, 8.

22. Champion, P. M., Lipscomb, J. D., Münck, E., Debrunner, P. G.
     and Gunsalus, I. C. (1975) Biochemistry 14, 4151.

23. Boyd, G. S. and Smellie, R. M. S. (eds.) "Biological Hydroxy-
     lation Mechanisms", Biochem. Soc. Symp. 34, Academic Press,
     New York.

24. Sligar, S. G., Lipscomb, J. D., Debrunner, P. G. and Gunsalus,
     I. C. (1974) Biochem. Biophys. Res. Commun. 61, 290.

25. Rahimtula, A., O'Brien, P., Hrycay, E., Peterson, J. and
     Estabrook, R. (1974) Biochem. Biophys. Res. Comm. 60, 695.

26. Coon, M. J. _et al_. (1976) Adv. Exp. Medicine and Biology,
     74, 270.

27. Hrycay, E., Gustafsson, J., Ingelman-Sundberg, M. and Ernster,
     L. (1975) Biochem. Biophys. Res. Comm. 66, 209.

28. Sligar, S. G., Shastry, B. S. and Gunsalus, I. C. (1976) in
     "Microsomes and Drug Oxidations"(V. Ullrich, ed.) Plenum Press,
     New York.

29. Hollenberg, P., and Hager, L. (1973) J. Biol. Chem. 248, 2630.

30. Dolphin, D., Forman, D., Borg, J., Fajer, J. and Felton, R.
     (1971) Proc. Nat. Acad. Sci. USA 68, 614.

31. Austin, R. H., Beeson, K. W., Eisenstein, L., Frauenfelder, H.
     and Gunsalus, I. C. (1975) Biochemistry 14, 5355.

32. Austin, R. H. Beeson, K., Eisenstein, L., Frauenfelder, H.,
     Gunsalus, I. C. and Marshall, V. P. (1973) Science 181, 541.

33. Alberding, N., Austin, R. H., Chan, Shirley S., Eisenstein, L.,
     Frauenfelder, H., Gunsalus, I. C. and Nordlund, T. M. (1976)
     J. Chem. Phys. 65, 000.

34. Austin, R. H., Beeson, K. W., Chan, S. S., Debrunner, P. G.,
     Downing, R., Eisenstein, L., Frauenfelder, H. and Nordlund,
     T. M. (1976) Rev. Sci. Instrum. 47, 445.

35. Austin, R. H., Beeson, K. W., Eisenstein, L., Frauenfelder, H.,
     Gunsalus, I. C. and Marshall, V. P. (1974) Phys. Rev. Letters
     32, 403.

36. Mieyal, J. J., Ackerman, R. S., Blumen, J. L. and Freeman, L. S.
     (1976) J. Biol. Chem. 251, 3436.

37. Pederson, T. C., Austin, R. H. and Gunsalus, I. C. (1976) in
     "Microsomes and Drug Oxidations" (V. Ullrich, ed.) Plenum
     Press, New York.

38. Dayhoff, M. O. (ed.) (1972) "Atlas of Protein Sequence and
     Structure" Vol. V, The National Biochemical Research Foundation.

PEROXISOMAL ENZYMES AND OXYGEN METABOLISM IN LIVER

Helmut Sies

Institut für Physiologische Chemie und Physikalische

Biochemie der Universität München, Munich, Germany

SUMMARY

1) Catalase and three oxidases(urate, L-α-hydroxyacid and D-aminoacid oxidases), enzymes decomposing and producing H_2O_2, respectively, in the peroxisomes of rat liver, are discussed with emphasis on properties relevant for physiological conditions.

2) The method of determination of H_2O_2 production rates in intact tissues by measurement of steady state levels of catalase Compound I is presented. H_2O_2 production is 0.05-0.1 μmol/min per g of perfused liver and may be stimulated severalfold by infusion of oxidase substrates; in the intact anaesthetized rat, the rate is about 0.3-0.4 μmol/min per g liver. H_2O_2 production amounts to 5-20 % of O_2 uptake under different metabolic conditions.

3) During steady states of hypoxia, H_2O_2 formation becomes O_2-limited. The comparison of catalase Compound I levels or the rate of urate oxidation(indicator of peroxisomal O_2 concentration) with the degree of reduction of cytochrome oxidase or cytochrome $\underline{c}$(indicators of mitochondrial O_2 concentration) reveals quite similar O_2 dependence in the organ, in contrast to largely different O_2 affinities of the isolated enzymes. This is explained by intercellular O_2 gradients. Experiments with isolated hepatocytes show that intracellular O_2 gradients may also exist but contribute to a lesser extent.
The determination of urate oxidation in rat liver is a simple biochemical measure of tissue oxygenation.

4) H_2O_2 or other oxygen metabolites(e.g. lipid-OOH) could play a role in oxygen sensing mechanisms. A possible pathway involving

GSH peroxidase and subsequent changes in ion permeabilities due to perturbation of the thiol redox state is briefly stated.

INTRODUCTION

The concept of the physiological occurrence of hydrogen peroxide in mammalian tissues has received experimental support in a number of systems in recent years. Thus, it is now apparent that a small but significant part of the reduction of oxygen to water proceeds via H_2O_2 in intact biological systems under physiological conditions.

In 1947, Chance(1) discovered the active intermediate of catalase, catalase Compound I, and more recently the detection of a steady state level of catalase Compound I by organ-photometric methods in the perfused liver(2) evidenced the occurrence of H_2O_2 in an intact mammalian system. In a series of cell-biological studies, deDuve and coworkers(see (3)) concluded that catalase as well as some H_2O_2-producing oxidases were associated in the microbodies, subcellular organelles which accordingly were renamed 'peroxisomes'. Peroxisomes are viewed as functional units in cellular H_2O_2 metabolism(3), but it is clear that there are other important extraperoxisomal enzyme activities dealing with H_2O_2, and there are peroxisomal enzymes not directly related to O_2 metabolism. Some features related to the role of the peroxisomes in O_2 metabolism are shown in Scheme 1. The biochemistry of the peroxisome in the liver cell has recently been reviewed(4).

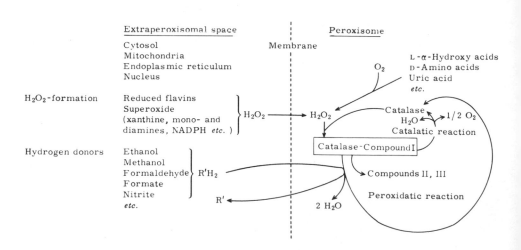

Scheme 1. The role of oxidases and catalase in peroxisomal H_2O_2 metabolism(from (4)).

PEROXISOMAL ENZYMES

Catalase

Catalase is a tetrameric enzyme with four probably identical subunits and four heme groups; the iron in the heme is trivalent. In contrast to hemoglobin, there are no indications of cooperativity between the heme groups. Its molecular weight is about 240,000. The methods of its isolation as well as its physical and chemical properties have most recently been reviewed by Deisseroth and Dounce (5) and Chance and Schonbaum(6).

The catalytic action of catalase(1a and 1b) was one of the first enzymatic functions discovered; H_2O_2 reacts both as a reductant and as an oxidant with the formation of O_2 and water in a dismutation process. The peroxidatic action of catalase(1a and 1c)utilizes other reductants, e.g. lower alcohols, as discovered by Keilin and Hartree(7).

$$\text{Catalase-Fe}^{3+} + H_2O_2 \xrightarrow{k_1} \text{Compound I} \tag{1a}$$

$$\text{Compound I} + H_2O_2 \xrightarrow{k_4'} \text{Catalase-Fe}^{3+} + 2\,H_2O + O_2 \tag{1b}$$

$$\text{Compound I} + \underset{\text{(donor)}}{AH_2} \xrightarrow{k_4} \text{Catalase-Fe}^{3+} + 2\,H_2O + A \tag{1c}$$

For the application to physiological systems, the kinetic properties of catalase resulting from the values of the reaction constants are of special interest. Thus, the steady state fraction of total catalase heme e existing as Compound I, p, is:

$$p_m/e = \left(1 + \frac{k_4'}{k_1} + \frac{k_4 a_o}{k_1 x_m} \right)^{-1}, \tag{2}$$

with a = donor concentration and x = H_2O_2 concentration, assuming that the back reaction of Compound I is negligible(8). The maximal steady state concentration of Compound I is obtained at high H_2O_2 concentration:

$$p_M/e = \left(1 + \frac{k_4'}{k_1} \right)^{-1}, \tag{2a}$$

indicating a simple relationship between maximal steady state concentration of Compound I and the second-order rate constants for formation and decomposition of Compound I.

It is clear from reactions (1a-1c) that the peroxidatic and the catalytic pathways will compete. Addition of hydrogen donor may increase the concentration of Compound I during constant H_2O_2 generation rates, and <u>vice versa</u>. It has been particularly useful to identify the concentration of hydrogen donor, a, required to decrease Compound I to half-maximal:

$$a \left.\right]_{\text{at } p_M/2} = \text{constant} \times \frac{1}{e} \frac{dx}{dt} n \qquad , \qquad (3)$$

with $\frac{1}{e} \frac{dx}{dt} n$ = steady state turnover number , being the ratio of the steady state rate of H_2O_2 formation and total catalase heme concentration. From this equation, the rate of H_2O_2 production in the intact organ can be estimated(see below). It may be mentioned here that the turnover number of the isolated enzyme with excess substrate is $>10^8 \text{ min}^{-1}$, whereas in the steady state in the organ it is of the order of $10 - 10^2 \text{ min}^{-1}$.

Peroxisomal Oxidases

There are three oxidases described to be contained in the peroxisomes, urate oxidase, L-α-hydroxyacid oxidase and D-aminoacid oxidase. They roughly account for 15 % of the peroxisomal protein, similar to the fraction accounted for by catalase(10). The enzyme activities in rat liver and some relevant kinetic data are collected in Table 1. The literature on chemical and biological properties of these oxidases can be found in a monograph(17). While urate oxidase is a copper enzyme, the other two oxidases are flavoproteins.

Urate oxidase occurs in the peroxisomal core of non-primates and catalyzes the reaction:

$$\text{Urate} + O_2 + 2 H_2O \longrightarrow \text{Allantoin} + CO_2 + H_2O_2 \quad .$$

Table 1

PROPERTIES OF PEROXISOMAL OXIDASES IN RAT LIVER. References in Parentheses.

Enzyme	Activity(9) μmol/min per g liver at 37°	Fraction of Peroxisomal Protein(%)(10)	K_m	Rate in O_2 / Rate in Air
Urate Oxidase	3.1	10 (core)	Urate: 0.02 mM(11)	1.8(11)
L-α-Hydroxyacid Oxidase	1.1	3	Glycolate: 0.25 - 0.5 mM(12,13) L-α-OH-Isocaproate: 3.4 mM(13)	$K_m(O_2)$: 0.4mM(15)
D-Aminoacid Oxidase	1.4	2	D-Norvaline:0.06 mM; D-Alanine:1.8 mM(14) (kidney enzyme)	2.4(16)

H_2O_2 FORMATION IN RAT LIVER

The organ-spectrophotometric identification of catalase Compound I in perfused rat liver by its absorbance band at 660 nm(2,18) has permitted an estimation of H_2O_2 production rates in the intact organ(19) on the basis of equation(3). The trace shown in Fig.1 demonstrates the following features: first, the level of Compound I in the endogenous steady state is close to the maximal level; second, it can be depleted rapidly by added hydrogen donor and then be replenished by endogenous H_2O_2 generation; third, in a state of increased H_2O_2 production rates, e.g. with added glycolate, higher concentrations of hydrogen donor are needed for depletion of Compound I.

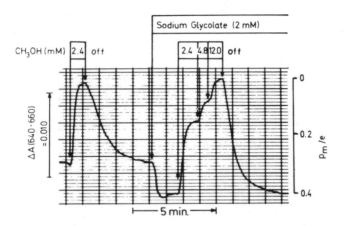

Fig. 1. Dependence of level of catalase Compound I in hemoglobin-free perfused rat liver on hydrogen donor(methanol) and on H_2O_2 generation(glycolate). Absorbance difference ΔA(640-660 nm) is recorded through a lobe of perfused liver. The horizontal bars on top indicate the respective time intervals and concentrations for infusion of methanol and glycolate. Total catalase heme e was estimated from the HCN-complex(not shown). Heme occupancy p_m/e is plotted as the ordinate at right. From ref.(18).

The rate of H_2O_2 production is about 50-80 nmol/min per g of perfused liver(19,15) and is increased by the addition of substrates for peroxisomal oxidases up to 15-fold(Table 2). Similar values were obtained by Portwich and Aebi with isotope methods(20).

Oshino et al(21) have extended this approach to the liver of anaesthetized rats to measure the H_2O_2 production in situ; it is 0.38 μmol/min per g liver(or 1.45 μmol/min per 100 g body wt) when the rat breathes air or O_2 even at 6 x 10^5Pa. However, the infusion of glycolate was accompanied by a doubling of the H_2O_2 production rate. Thus, the formation of H_2O_2 in liver is substrate-limited not

Table 2

RATES OF H_2O_2 PRODUCTION IN ISOLATED HEMOGLOBIN-FREE PERFUSED RAT LIVER AS OBTAINED FROM MEASUREMENT OF CATALASE HEME OCCUPANCY

Substrates or Inhibitors	$a_{1/2}$ for methanol (mM)	$(dx_n/dt)(1/e)$ (turnover number) [per min]	dx_n/dt (nmol H_2O_2/min/ g liver wet wt)
Lactate 2mM, pyruvate 0.3mM	0.12 (0.09-0.16)	3.8	49
+Antimycin A 8μM	0.18	5.8	75
+Octanoate 0.3mM	0.40	13.0	170
+Octanoate 0.3mM and Antimycin A 8μM	0.24	7.4	96
+Oleate 0.1mM	0.16	5.1	66
+Xylitol 5.2mM	0.15	4.8	62
+Urate 1mM	----	54*	750
+Glycolate 3mM	----	34*	490

From Oshino et al. (19). *Titration performed with 0.6 mM methanol initially present.

only in the perfused organ(19) where blood supply of substrates is excluded, but also in the intact animal(21).

It may be mentioned that the rate of H_2O_2 production sets the limit for hydrogen donor metabolism. A decrease in H_2O_2 formation rates results in a decrease of the upper limit of hydrogen donor (e.g. alcohol) oxidation rates.

H_2O_2 Production Under Hypoxic Conditions

In view of the relatively high $K_m(O_2)$ of the peroxisomal oxidases in the range of 0.1-0.4 mM O_2 it might be expected that the formation of H_2O_2 by these oxidases would be severely restricted upon instalment of hypoxic conditions. However, as will be seen below, this appears not to be the case to a large degree in the perfused organ.

There are no suitable extracellular indicators of tissue oxygenation for the present purposes, but organ photometry of components of the mitochondrial respiratory chain provides the relevant information. Cytochromes aa_3(22) and c(23) have been employed for such purpose. As shown in Fig.2, during a hypoxic steady state corresponding to 30 % reduction of cytochrome oxidase(band at 607 nm) a

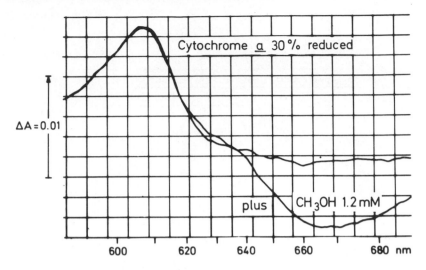

Fig. 2. Demonstration of the presence of catalase Compound I under hypoxic conditions in perfused rat liver. An absorbance difference spectrum was first recorded under a stationary condition of hypoxia to give 30 % reduced cytochrome oxidase. Then another spectrum was obtained during infusion of methanol; band at 665 nm corresponds to 70 % of maximal Compound I. From ref.(24).

considerable fraction of catalase is present as Compound I. This is evidenced by the decrease of the 665 nm band upon infusion of methanol as hydrogen donor. The stationary concentration of Compound I under the hypoxic condition is about 70 % of that obtainable under full oxygenation.

The question arises, of course, whether the H_2O_2 production under hypoxic conditions could not be due to extraperoxisomal oxidases with lower $K_m(O_2)$.

Quantitation of H_2O_2 production under hypoxic conditions revealed that it was half-maximal when cytochrome c was 40 % reduced, whereas with urate or glycolate as H_2O_2 generating substrate the half-maximal rate was observed at 25 % and 10 % reduction of cytochrome c, respectively(15).

Correlation of Urate Removal and Cytochrome Oxidase Reduction During Hypoxic Steady States

The stoichiometry between urate removal rates and extra H_2O_2 formation as detected by catalase Compound I in perfused liver(15) indicates that little, if any, H_2O_2 escapes from the peroxisome. Furthermore, it underlines that the measurement of urate removal pro-

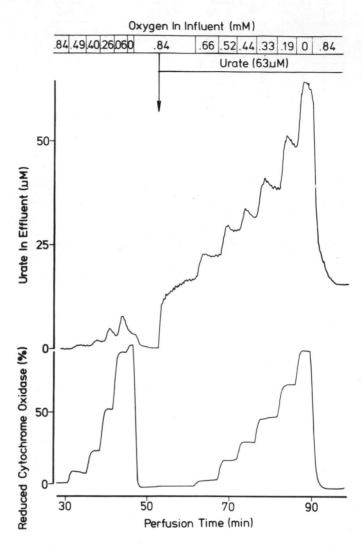

Fig. 3. Simultaneous measurement of urate concentration in effluent and of reduced cytochrome oxidase in a lobe of perfused rat liver during steady states of hypoxia. Oxygen concentration in influent and the infusion of urate(63 μM) as indicated on top. Note that initial steady state is reestablished after the anoxic interval. Urate was measured in a flow-through cuvette at 293 nm, cytochrome oxidase was measured by dual-wavelength photometry at 607-622 nm.

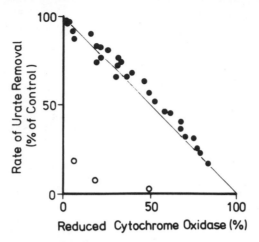

Fig. 4. Relationship between the rate of urate removal and the degree of reduction of cytochrome oxidase during hypoxic steady states in hemoglobin-free perfused rat liver. Data from several experiments such as in Fig.3 are given as closed circles. Similar data obtained from isolated hepatocytes such as the experiment in Fig.6 are given as open circles.

vides another useful parameter for the study of O_2 metabolism in peroxisomes. In fact, urate oxidase activity is well-suited for this purpose since it is unilocular(peroxisomal core) and the reaction is not complicated by side-reactions and is irreversible. The simultaneous recording of urate concentration in the effluent perfusate and of the degree of reduction of cytochrome oxidase during steady states of hypoxia(Fig.3) indicates that, surprisingly, the sensitivity of urate oxidase and of cytochrome oxidase to hypoxia is similar: The stepwise increase in the effluent concentration of urate towards the influent level is approximately matched by the increments in the degree of reduction of cytochrome oxidase towards the fully reduced value. The slight overshoot in the effluent urate concentration during the transitions is probably due to the release of urate from endogenous sources; in the absence of added urate, there also is a small release of urate, as shown by the hypoxic interval from 30-50 min in the experiment of Fig.3.

Data from a number of experiments similar to that of Fig.3 are plotted in Fig.4. Clearly, the rate of urate removal is halved only when cytochrome oxidase is half-reduced. Similar results were obtained by measurement of cytochrome $\underline{c}$ at 550-540 nm(not shown). The half-maximal concentrations for O_2 for isolated urate oxidase and cytochrome oxidase, however, are about three orders of magnitude apart: about 0.2 mM(11) or 0.1 mM(for the enzyme from hog liver; H.Sies, unpubl.)for urate oxidase, and about 0.1-1 µM for cytochrome oxidase according to the recent discussion by Nicholls & Chance(25).

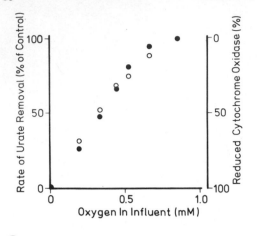

Fig. 5A. Data of Fig.3 plotted against O_2 concentration
in influent perfusate.
Open circles: rate of urate
removal; closed circles: reduced cytochrome oxidase. .
Hemoglobin-free perfusion as
described previously(34) except that L-lactate/pyruvate
was 2.1mM/0.3mM. Flow rate:
4 ml/min per g liver; temperature: 37°C.

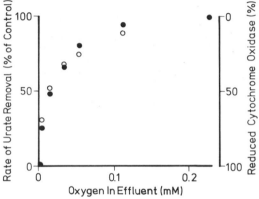

Fig.5B. Data of Fig.3 plotted against O_2 concentration
in effluent perfusate.

Oxygen Gradients

The existence of stationary O_2 gradients may provide an explanation for these observations. There are two alternative possibilities: (a) intracellular O_2 gradients between the peroxisomal core
site of urate oxidase and the mitochondrial inner membrane site of
cytochrome oxidase, and (b) intercellular O_2 gradients along the sinusoids of the hepatic lobule, possibly in combination with a non-
homogeneous distribution of the peroxisomes and the mitochondria
within the liver lobule. Another explanation would be, of course,
differences of the $K_m(O_2)$ values for the two copper enzymes in situ
as compared to the isolated enzymes; at present, this is difficult
to assess.

Although it is clear that intracellular O_2 gradients must exist,
it appears unlikely that the O_2 concentrations in the hepatocyte differ by about three orders of magnitude between two relatively closely
localized sites within the hepatocyte. Thus, the major part of the
difference of the O_2 sensitivity is expected to result from the se-

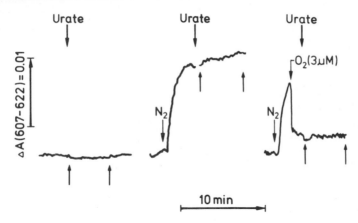

Fig. 6. Protocol of the experiments with hepatocytes isolated from fed rats for measurement of rate of urate removal under defined conditions of hypoxia. Arrows at bottom indicate time of sampling for measurement of urate concentration. Data from such experiments are shown as open circles in Fig.4.

cond possibility, namely intercellular O_2 gradients along the sinusoids of the lobule.This is supported by observations with isolated rat hepatocytes. As shown in Fig.6, isolated hepatocytes prepared with our modification(26) of the collagenase method(27) were incubated and the redox state of cytochrome oxidase was measured. O_2 concentration was manipulated by adjustment of the gas mixture(O_2/N_2, both containing 5 % CO_2) to result in the desired steady state reduction of cytochrome oxidase; the three conditions in Fig.6 represent, from left to right, full oxidation, full reduction, and 22 % reduction, respectively. Urate removal rates were calculated from samples taken at 5 min intervals after the addition of urate. Data from such experiments are shown as open circles in Fig.4. Clearly, the rate of urate removal is much more decreased during slight hypoxia as indicated by the redox state of cytochrome oxidase. These observations still leave the possibility of small intracellular O_2 gradients between peroxisomes and mitochondria, but certainly they place the emphasis on intercellular O_2 gradients.

Intercellular O_2 gradients along the liver sinusoid from the periportal to the pericentral region have frequently been discussed (28). The O_2 gradient during stationary hypoxia should be quite steep at a certain distance away from the periportal region in order to explain the results of Fig.4. It should be less steep in case of an inhomogeneous distribution of the two enzymes along the sinusoid: urate oxidase would have to be relatively more concentrated in the periportal area and cytochrome oxidase in the pericentral area. However, morphometrically there appears to be a gradient of mitochondrial and peroxisomal volumes, if any, in the opposite direction(29).

CONCLUSIONS

Liver Peroxisomes and Oxygen Metabolism. The presence of catalase together with some peroxisomal and also extraperoxisomal(e.g.
xanthine oxidase) oxidases provides the capacity for sustaining a
steady state of H_2O_2 concentration, ranging from 10^{-7}-10^{-9} M under
quasi-physiological conditions(19). In the liver of an anaesthetized rat, the H_2O_2 production rate is similar when the rat is breathing air or O_2(21), indicating that H_2O_2 formation is substrate-limited rather than O_2-limited; glycolate infusion stimulated H_2O_2 formation under these conditions. Since the sources of H_2O_2 in the
cell are heterogeneous, it may well be, however, that some specific
reactions providing H_2O_2 may be O_2-limited. H_2O_2 formation accounts
for about 5-20 % of total O_2 uptake by the liver in different metabolic conditions.

The relevance of O_2^- formation and subsequent H_2O_2 production
by superoxide dismutase(30) will be discussed elsewhere(Boveris,
this volume).

Intracellular and intercellular O_2 gradients. The monitoring
of the O_2 dependence of enzymes in different subcellular locations
may provide information on localized O_2 concentrations. The observation in isolated hepatocytes that the rate of urate oxidation is
still about 15 % at a steady state of O_2 supply causing 10 % reduction of cytochrome oxidase(Fig.4) suggests that the steady state
concentration of O_2 in the peroxisomal core may be higher than that
in the mitochondrial inner membrane, unless the $K_m(O_2)$ for urate
oxidase is lower or that of cytochrome oxidase is higher in situ
than in vitro.

The similar apparent O_2 dependence of urate oxidase and of cytochrome oxidase in the perfused liver(Fig.4) suggests steep intercellular O_2 gradients, most probably along the sinusoids. The O_2
gradient along the sinusoid should be broadened in presence of an
O_2 carrier, allowing the more central cells to receive a better O_2
supply. In a few preliminary experiments of liver perfusion(at 33°)
with 2.5 g % human hemoglobin from washed erythrocytes, we have indeed observed only about 30 % of the initial rate of urate oxidation
at 50 % reduction of cytochrome oxidase. Thus, it is worthwhile to
mention that in the experimental model of the hemoglobin-free perfused rat liver the O_2 gradients may be particularly steep. This
may cause problems under hypoxic conditions but, of course, not under well-oxygenated conditions.

Hypoxic transitions. The properties of H_2O_2 formation under
hypoxic conditions may become of interest for the general problem
of oxidative metabolism at low oxygen pressure(see review by Jöbsis
(31)). Peroxisome-like structures have been observed in numerous

cell types, and the cytochemical demonstration of a peroxidatic activity of catalase(diaminobenzidine as hydrogen donor) has been performed with many tissues(see (4) for references).

Regarding biochemical reactions intervening in O_2 sensing mechanisms during hypoxic transitions, it is well possible that H_2O_2 may play a role in some yet unspecified peroxidatic reaction. Catalase as a regulator of H_2O_2 concentration would have a role in such mechanism. One suitable peroxidatic reaction could be that of GSH peroxidase. This non-peroxisomal enzyme catalyzes the reduction of H_2O_2 and other hydroperoxides by glutathione(32). The formation of glutathione disulfide in a steady state of hydroperoxide reduction leads to a transition of the thiol redox state in the cell, e.g. in the liver cells(33,34). The transition in the thiol redox state, in turn, has profound effects on active and passive cation permeability as well as on the chemical stimulation of excitable cells(35,36). In fact, the GSH/GSSG system was implicated by Kosower and Werman(37) in the mechanism of transmitter release at the motoneural junction.

Thus, the hypoxic state will be associated with a decreased rate of GSSG formation due to a decreased rate of formation of H_2O_2 or other hydroperoxides(e.g. lipid-OOH), and theoretically this could constitute a biochemical pathway for oxygen sensing mechanisms. It will be of interest to test this hypothesis in an appropriate O_2 sensing experimental system.

Acknowledgements

Substantial parts of the experiments on H_2O_2 formation reported here result from a fruitful collaboration with B. Chance, N. Oshino and Th. Bücher, which is gratefully acknowledged. Thanks are also extended to J. Duhm for discussions on O_2 gradients.

Own work reported here was supported by Deutsche Forschungsgemeinschaft, Sonderforschungsbereich 51 "Medizinische Molekularbiologie und Biochemie", Grant No. D/8.

REFERENCES

1. Chance B: An intermediate compound in the catalase-hydrogen peroxide reaction. Acta Chem. Scand. 1:236-267, 1947

2. Sies H, Chance B: The steady state level of catalase compound I in isolated hemoglobin-free perfused rat liver. FEBS Lett. 11:172-176, 1970

3. deDuve C, Baudhuin P: Peroxisomes(microbodies and related par-

ticles. Physiol.Rev. 46:323-357, 1966

4. Sies H: Biochemistry of the Peroxisome in the Liver Cell. Angew.
Chem.Int.Ed. 13:706-718, 1974; Angew.Chem.86:789-801, 1974

5. Deisseroth A, Dounce AL: Catalase: Physical and Chemical Properties, Mechanism of Catalysis, and Physiological Role. Physiol. Rev.
50:319-375, 1970

6. Chance B, Schonbaum G: Catalase. In Boyer PD(Editor): The Enzymes, 3rd edition. New York and London, Academic Press,1976, vol XIII
pp

7. Keilin D, Hartree EF: Coupled Oxidation of Alcohol.Proc.Roy.
Soc.B 119:141-   ,1936

8. Chance B, Oshino N: Analysis of the catalase-hydrogen peroxide
intermediate in coupled oxidations. Biochem.J.131:564-567, 1973

9. Leighton F, Poole B, Beaufay H, Baudhuin P, Coffey JW, Fowler S,
deDuve C: The large-scale separation of peroxisomes, mitochondria,
and lysosomes from the livers of rats injected with triton WR-1339.
J.Cell Biol.37:482-513,1968

10. Leighton F, Poole B, Lazarow PB, deDuve C: The Synthesis and
Turnover of Rat Liver Peroxisomes.I. Fractionation of Peroxisome
Proteins. J.Cell Biol. 41:521-535, 1969

11. Mahler H: Uricase. In Boyer PD, Lardy HA, Myrbäck K(Editors):
The Enzymes, 2nd edition, New York and London, Academic Press, 1963,
vol 8, pp 285-296

12. Kun E, Dechary JM, Pitot HC: The Oxidation of Glycolic Acid by
a Liver Enzyme. J.Biol.Chem. 210:269-280, 1954

13. McGroarty E, Hsieh B, Wied DM, Gee R, Tolbert NE: Alpha Hydroxy
Acid Oxidation by Peroxisomes. Arch.Biochem.Biophys.161:194-210,1974

14. Dixon M, Kleppe K:D-Amino Acid Oxidase.II.Specificity, Competitive Inhibition and Reaction Sequence. Biochem.Biophys.Acta 96:368-
382, 1965

15. Oshino N, Jamieson D, Chance B: The Properties of Hydrogen Peroxide Production under Hyperoxic and Hypoxic Conditions of Perfused
Rat Liver. Biochem.J. 146:53-65, 1975

16. Meister A, Wellner D: Flavoprotein Amino Acid Oxidases. In Boyer
PD, Lardy HA, Myrbäck K(Editors): The Enzymes, 2nd edition, New York
and London, Academic Press, 1963, vol 7, pp 609-648

17. Hruban H, Rechcigl M: Microbodies and related particles. Int. Rev. Cytol. Suppl.I:1-296, 1969

18. Sies H, Bücher Th, Oshino N, Chance B: Heme Occupancy of Catalase in Hemoglobin-free Perfused Rat Liver and of Isolated Rat Liver Catalase. Arch.Biochem.Biophys. 154:106-116, 1973

19. Oshino N, Chance B, Sies H, Bücher Th: The Role of H_2O_2 Generation in Perfused Rat Liver and the Reaction of Catalase Compound I and Hydrogen Donors.Arch.Biochem.Biophys. 154:117-131, 1973

20.Portwich F, Aebi H: Erfassung der Peroxydbildung tierischer Gewebe mittels peroxydatischer Umsetzungen. Helv.Physiol.Pharmakol. Acta 18:1-16, 1960

21. Oshino N, Jamieson D, Sugano T, Chance B: Optical Measurement of the Catalase-Hydrogen Peroxide Intermediate(Compound I) in the Liver of Anaesthetized Rats and its Implication to Hydrogen Peroxide Production in situ. Biochem.J. 146:67-77, 1975

22. Chance B, Schoener B, Schindler F: The intracellular oxidation-reduction state. In: Oxygen in the Animal Organism, Dickens F, Neil E(Editors), Pergamon Press, Oxford, 1964, pp 367-388

23. Sugano T, Oshino N, Chance B: Mitochondrial functions under hypoxic conditions.The steady states of cytochrome c reduction and of energy metabolism. Biochim.Biophys.Acta 347:340-358, 1974

24. Sies H: Das Peroxisom im Hepatocyten. Katalase-Komplex I in der hämoglobinfrei durchströmten Rattenleber. Habilitationsschrift, Universität München, 1971

25. Nicholls P, Chance B: Cytochrome c oxidase. In: Hayaishi O(Editor)Molecular Mechanisms of Oxygen Activation. New York and London, Academic Press, 1974, pp 479-534

26. Sies H, Grosskopf M: Oxidation of cytochrome b_5 by hydroperoxides in rat liver. Eur.J.Biochem.57:513-520, 1975

27. Berry MN, Friend DS: High-yield preparation of isolated rat liver parenchymal cells. A biochemical and fine structural study. J.Cell Biol.43:506-520, 1969

28. Miller JA, Kessler M: Tissue pO_2 levels in the liver of warm and cold rats artificially respired with different mixtures of O_2 and CO_2. In: Bicher HI, Bruley DF(Editors): Oxygen Transport to Tissue. New York, Plenum Publ. Co. 1973, pp 361-370

29. Loud AV: A quantitative stereological description of the ultra-

structure of normal rat liver parenchymal cells. J.Cell Biol. 37: 27-46, 1968

30. McCord JM, Fridovich I: Superoxide dismutase. An enzymic function for erythrocuprein(hemocuprein). J.Biol.Chem.244:6049-6055,1969

31. Jöbsis FF: Oxidative metabolism at low pO_2. Fed.Proc.31:1404-1413, 1972

32. Mills GC: Glutathione peroxidase and the destruction of hydrogen peroxide in animal tissues. Arch.Biochem.Biophys. 86:1-5, 1969

33. Sies H, Gerstenecker C, Menzel H, Flohé L: Oxidation in the NADP system and release of GSSG from hemoglobin-free perfused rat liver during peroxidatic oxidation of glutathione by hydroperoxides. FEBS Lett. 27:171-175, 1972

34. Sies H, Summer KH: Hydroperoxide-metabolizing systems in rat liver. Eur.J.Biochem. 57:503-512, 1975

35. Dikstein S: Stimulability, adenosine triphosphatases and their control by cellular redox processes. Naturwissenschaften 58:439-443, 1971

36. Flohé L, Benöhr HC, Sies H, Waller HD, Wendel A(Editors): Glutathione. G.Thieme Verlag, Stuttgart, 1974

37. Kosower EM, Werman R: A new step in transmitter release at the myoneural junction. Nature New Biology 233:121-122, 1971

MITOCHONDRIAL PRODUCTION OF SUPEROXIDE RADICAL AND HYDROGEN PEROXIDE

Alberto Boveris

Institute of Biochemistry, School of Medicine
University of Buenos Aires, Paraguay 2155
1121 CF Buenos Aires, Argentina

The development and application of sensitive methods for the determination of hydrogen peroxide led, a few years ago in the laboratories of the Johnson Research Foundation, to the recognition of intact mitochondria as an effective source of H_2O_2 (Fig. 1; refs. 1-4). Previous observations by Jensen (5) and by Hinkle et al. (6) had indicated that the mitochondrial respiratory chain was capable of producing H_2O_2. However, these results were taken with caution, in the sense that they might reflect an artificial activity induced by the ultrasonic or alkaline treatment used in the preparation of the submitochondrial particles. In 1971, Chance and Oshino (1) demonstrated variations in the level of the catalase intermediate of the peroxisomal-mitochondrial fraction of rat liver following the addition of mitochondrial substrates and uncouplers. In the same year, Loschen et al. (2) showed H_2O_2 formation in pigeon heart mitochondria and its relationship to the mitochondrial metabolic state by using the peroxidase-scopoletin method. It was realized that this assay could be easily interfered by endogenous hydrogen donor of the horseradish peroxidase and by exogenous hydrogen donors in the mitochondrial preparations, and consequently, an alternative method was developed. Boveris et al. (3) applied the cytochrome c peroxidase assay to the subcellular fractions of rat liver and established that mitochondria, microsomes, peroxisomes and soluble enzymes are all cellular sources of H_2O_2. The same assay system was utilized to determine the general properties of the mitochondrial generation of H_2O_2 in pigeon heart mitochondria (4). The initial observations have been now extended to mitochondria isolated from other vertebrate tissues, such as rat kidney and pigeon lung, and

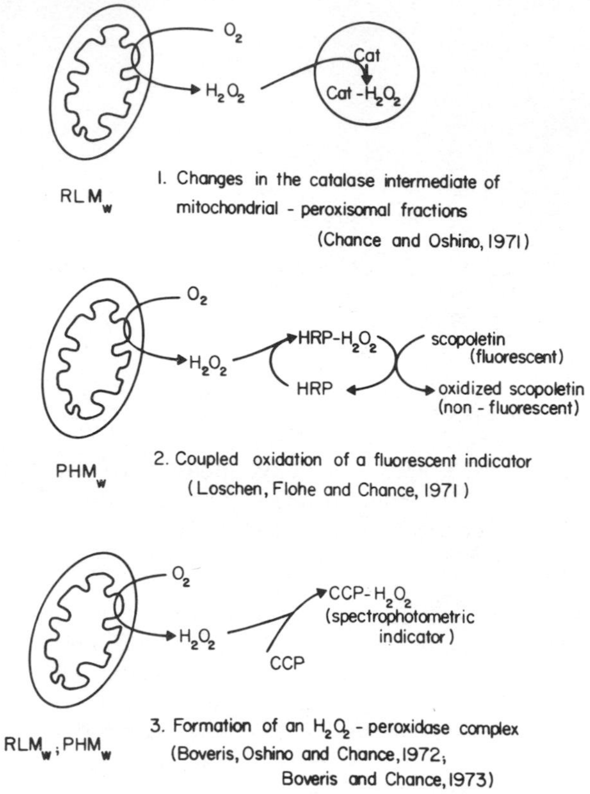

Fig. 1. Scheme of the different methods utilized in the determination of the mitochondrial production of H_2O_2.

from rather miscellaneous sources, such as <u>Ascaris</u> muscle, the protozoan <u>C</u>. <u>fasciculata</u> (7), baker's yeast and various plant tissues as potato tuber, mung bean hypocotyl (8) and skunk cabbage spadix.

MITOCHONDRIAL PRODUCTION OF HYDROGEN PEROXIDE
Effect of Substrates, Uncouplers and Inhibitors

Isolated mitochondria produce H_2O_2 at rates that depend on the metabolic state. This activity is higher in State 4 (9), which is defined by the absence of phosphate acceptor (ADP_ and characterized by a high reduction of the components of the respiratory chain, and lower in State 3 (9), where the respiratory carriers are largely oxidized (2-4). Fig. 2 illustrates the H_2O_2 production by rat liver and pigeon lung mitochondria. The cytochrome <u>c</u> peroxidase assay detects H_2O_2 generation as a spectrophotometric change due to the

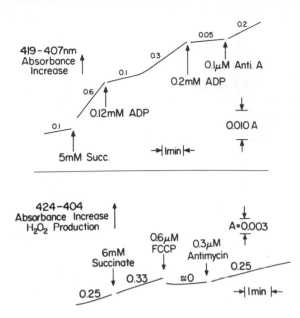

Fig. 2. Production of H$_2$O$_2$ by rat liver (upper trace) and pigeon
lung (bottom trace) mitochondria. Pigeon lung mitochondria were
prepared according to ref. (10) and suspended (0.1 mg protein/ml)
in 0.23 M mannitol, 0.07 M sucrose, 30 mM Tris-Mops buffer pH 7.4,
and supplemented with 0.2 μM cytochrome c peroxidase. Rat liver
mitochondria trace was taken from ref. ($\overline{3}$). The numbers near the
traces indicate nmol H$_2$O$_2$/min per mg of protein.

formation of the peroxidase-H$_2$O$_2$ enzyme-substrate complex, which is
indicated as an upward deflection of the trace. The low rate of H$_2$O$_2$
formation supported by endogenous substrates is increased upon
addition of succinate; subsequent supplementation with ADP or un-
coupler decreases H$_2$O$_2$ formation. The transient effect of ADP
observed in the trace corresponding to rat liver mitochondria is
due to ADP exhaustion after its phosphorylation to ATP. Addition
of antimycin A exerts a moderate stimulatory effect on both rat
liver and pigeon lung mitochondria.

Production of H2O2 in isolated rat liver and pigeon heart
mitochondria accounts for about 1-2 % and 2-4 % respectively, of
the corresponding oxygen uptake in State 4 (3-4,11).

Succinate and NADH-dependent substrates are equally effective
in supporting maximal H$_2$O$_2$ production (3-4). This is shown by the
similar rate of H$_2$O$_2$ generation of pigeon heart mitochondria in
State 4 with either malate-glutamate or succinate-glutamate as

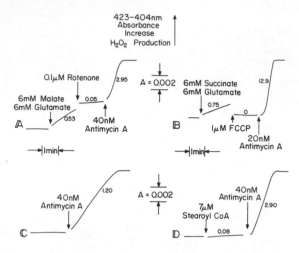

Fig. 3. Production of H_2O_2 by pigeon heart mitochondria (0.056 mg protein/ml) suspended in mannitol-sucrose-Tris-Mops buffer pH 7.4. 0.21 μM cytochrome $\underline{c}$ peroxidase. B: 0.028 mg protein/ml mitochondrial protein.

substrate (Fig. 3). It is noteworthy that when malate-glutamate is used as the source of reducing equivalents, H_2O_2 production is inhibited by rotenone (Fig. 3, trace A). When electron flow is blocked by antimycin A, pigeon heart mitochondria exhibit high rates of H_2O_2 production (4). Fatty acids, fatty acid derivatives as stearoyl-Co A or palmitoyl-carnitine, and endogenous substrate support a low H_2O_2 production (3-4), but in the presence of antimycin A they are able to sustain a considerable peroxide formation.

It is then apparent that the mitochondrial generator of H_2O_2 is a member of the respiratory chain or at equilibrium with it, since H_2O_2 production is maximal in the highly reduced states, such as in State 4 or in the presence of antimycin A, and minimal in the oxidized states, as in States 3 and 3u.

From the effect of the respiratory inhibitors, it can be concluded that at least one of the members of the isopotential group acting between the rotenone- and the antimycin A-sensitive sites, reacts in its reduced form with molecular oxygen to produce H_2O_2. Interestingly enough, the flavoprotein succinate dehydrogenase (2), the energy-linked cytochrome $\underline{b}_{566}$ (12-13), an unidentified iron-sulfur center (14) and the reduced forms of ubiquinone (15) have been pointed or postulated as the autoxidizable component responsible for mitochondrial H_2O_2 generation.

SUPEROXIDE RADICAL AS PRECURSOR OF MITOCHONDRIAL HYDROGEN PEROXIDE

Since in the succinate dehydrogenase-cytochromes $\underline{b}$ segment of the respiratory chain, the transition from 2 to 1 electron transfer takes place, it was considered likely that O_2^- would be the primary product of H_2O_2 generation. Superoxide dismutase seems to be present in the intracellular sites in which O_2^- formation occurs. Mitochondria contain two types of superoxide dismutase, a mangano-enzyme in the matrix space and a cupro-zinc enzyme in the intermembrane space (16-17). Loschen et al.(12,18) and Boveris and Cadenas (19) detected O_2^- production in submitochondrial particles by adrenochrome formation and cytochrome $\underline{c}$ reduction, respectively. Fig. 4 illustrates the O_2^- generation by beef heart submitochondrial particles that were extensively washed to remove endogenous superoxide dismutase. The addition of substrate and antimycin A starts O_2^- formation, which is detected as an increase in absorbance due to the formation of adrenochrome. The inhibition of this process by the addition of superoxide dismutase provides the specificity of the assay. The inset in Fig. 4 shows a titration of the superoxide dismutase effect.

The production of O_2^- and H_2O_2 by submitochondrial particles was measured in parallel determinations; values of 1.1 (15), 1.6-2.1 (19), and 2.0 (20) have been reported for the ratio of the rates of O_2^- and H_2O_2 generation, varying somewhat with the different experimental conditions. Nevertheless, these values are close enough

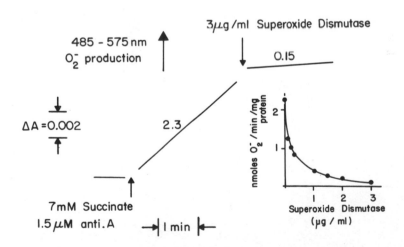

Fig. 4. Production of O_2^- by beef heart submitochondrial particles (0.45 mg protein/ml) suspended in mannitol-sucrose-Tris-Mops buffer, pH 7.6, and supplemented with 1 mM epinephrine.

to the theoretical value of 2 (reaction [1]; ref. 21) to consider O_2^-, if not a stoichiometric precursor, at least the main intermediate in mitochondrial H_2O_2 production.

$$O_2^- + O_2^- + 2 H^+ \longrightarrow H_2O_2 + O_2 \qquad [1]$$

UBIQUINOL AND UBISEMIQUINONE AS SOURCES OF SUPEROXIDE RADICAL AND HYDROGEN PEROXIDE

Early experiments with mitochondrial membranes depleted of endogenous ubiquinone and reconstituted with variable amounts of ubiquinones had shown a linear relationship between quinone content and H_2O_2 formation (4). However, that evidence does not allow an unique interpretation. The ubiquinone effect could be attributed to: a) regulation of succinate dehydrogenase activity by ubiquinone; b) necessity of ubiquinone for electron transport from succinate dehydrogenase to cytochromes b; and c) non-enzymatic autoxidation of ubiquinol. Parallel measurements of succinate dehydrogenase and succinate-cytochrome c reductase activities and H_2O_2 production in ubiquinone-depleted and ubiquinone-reconstituted membranes show that the two former activities reach a plateau at a low level of reducible ubiquinone (1-2 nmol/mg of protein), whereas H_2O_2 generation is linearly related to the quinone content over a wide range of

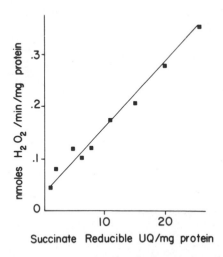

Fig. 5. Relationship between reducible ubiquinone and production of H_2O_2 in ubiquinone-depleted and ubiquinone-reconstituted mitochondrial membranes from beef heart. Data from ref. (15).

Table 1. HYDROGEN PEROXIDE PRODUCTION BY ISOLATED COMPLEXES OF THE MITOCHONDRIAL RESPIRATORY CHAIN (Data from refs. (15) and (22)).

	H_2O_2 Production (nmol/min/mg protein)
NADH–ubiquinone reductase (Complex I)	4.62
idem + rotenone	1.10
Ubiquinol–cytochrome c reductase (Complex III)	4.24
Succinate dehydrogenase (Complex II)	0.03

ubiquinone levels (up to 26 nmol/mg of protein)(Fig. 5; ref. 15). Such evidence rules out an important contribution of succinate dehydrogenase or cytochromes b and points to the reduced forms of ubiquinone as the main source of mitochondrial O_2^- and H_2O_2.

Further evidence for the same conclusion was obtained after fractionation of the mitochondrial respiratory chain. Cadenas et al. (22) have found that NADH–ubiquinone reductase (Complex I) and ubiquinol–cytochrome c reductase (Complex III), that contain ubiquinone as the sole common component, are effective generators of O_2^- and H_2O_2. Furthermore, rotenone, which decreases electron flow to endogenous ubiquinone, inhibits H_2O_2 production by NADH–ubiquinone reductase (Table 1; ref. 22).

Succinate dehydrogenase is much less effective in producing H_2O_2 (Table 1; ref. 15). In agreement with this low activity of the solubilized flavoprotein, it has been reported that submitochondrial particles depleted of succinate dehydrogenase are still able to produce H_2O_2 (13,15).

Cyanide inhibits O_2^- production in submitochondrial particles paralleling the steady-state level of oxidized cytochrome c. The finding that the production of O_2^-, the main intermediate of mitochondrial H_2O_2, is inhibited by cyanide should be taken into account when evaluating oxygen uptake in the tissues in the presence of cyanide as being somewhat equivalent to H_2O_2 formation. The relationship between cytochrome c oxidation and formation of O_2^-, is interpreted assigning a role to the cytochrome in the generation of ubisemiquinone, that would constitute the autoxidizable component.

$$UQH_2 + Cyt\ c^{3+} \longrightarrow UQH^{\bullet} + Cyt\ c^{2+} + H^{+} \quad\quad [2]$$

$$UQH^{\bullet} + O_2 \xrightarrow{\ k\ } UQ + O_2^- + H^{+} \quad\quad [3]$$

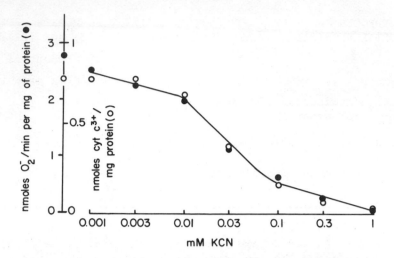

Fig. 6. Effect of cyanide on O_2^- production and on the steady state oxidation level of cytochrome c. Beef heart submitochondrial particles (1.8 mg protein/ml) suspended in mannitol-sucrose-Tris-Mops buffer, pH 7.6. 3.3 μM antimycin A and 7 mM succinate. The adrenochrome assay was utilized to determine O_2^- formation.

Apparently, ubisemiquinone which is rather stable in the mitochondrial membranes linked to a protein iron-sulfur center (23-25), reacts non-enzymatically with molecular oxygen yielding O_2^-. Disregarding for the moment the rate of the back reaction (quinones can act as oxidants for O_2^-; ref. (26)), chemical equation [3] gives the following differential equation for the rate of O_2^- generation:

$$dO_2^-/dt = (O_2) (UQH^\bullet) k \qquad [4]$$

The data discussed here seem to indicate that ubisemiquinone is chiefly responsible for mitochondrial peroxide production, but the function of other O_2^- and H_2O_2 generators is not excluded. For instance, Forman and Kennedy have reported formation of about 0.1 nmol O_2^-/min per mg of protein as due to dihydroorotate dehydrogenase, which is an auxiliary dehydrogenase in rat liver mitochondria (27). However, under comparable conditions, H_2O_2 production that could be attributed mainly to the reduced forms of ubiquinone is more active (0.3-0.6 nmol H_2O_2/min per mg of protein; ref. (3)).

OXYGEN DEPENDENCE OF O_2^- AND H_2O_2 PRODUCTION

According to equation [4], at a constant level of ubisemiquinone, O_2^- (and H_2O_2) formation should be linearly related to oxygen concentration. Fig. 8 shows rates of O_2^- formation as a function of

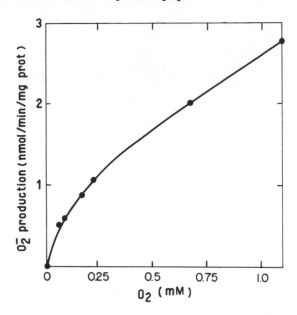

Fig. 7. Oxygen dependence of O_2^- production in beef heart submitochondrial particles. The mannitol-sucrose-50 mM Tris-Mops buffer,
pH 7.4, containing the particles and 1 mM epinephrine was equilibrated with oxygen-nitrogen gas mixtures of known composition.

oxygen concentration. Although not linearly, O_2^- formation is proportional to oxygen tension. A similar oxygen dependence of the mitochondrial production of H_2O_2 in the hyperbaric region has been already reported (4,28-29).

PHYSIOLOGICAL RELEVANCE OF O_2^- AND H_2O_2 AT THE CELLULAR LEVEL

There is an important question related to the extent to which
the mitochondrial generation of H_2O_2 occurs under physiological
conditions. From the data obtained with isolated mitochondria (3),
and the observation that in the perfused liver, mitochondria are in
a metabolic state close to State 4 (30), it is possible to estimate
that mitochondrial production of H_2O_2 might be close to 2 % of the
total organ oxygen uptake. However, direct measurements in support
of that possibility are still lacking.

The rates of H_2O_2 production measured in the perfused liver by
monitoring the catalase intermediate, largely reflect peroxisomal
H_2O_2 metabolism. Nevertheless, the increases in H_2O_2 production
measured after antimycin A addition with lactate-pyruvate as

substrate (31) and after hyperbaric oxygenation in the tocopherol-deficient rats (32), can be interpreted as due to an increased mitochondrial generation of H_2O_2. Moreover, it has been reported that oxidized glutathione release in perfused liver, that seems to largely reflect the turnover of mitochondrial and cytosolic gluta-thione peroxidases, is increased under hyperbaric oxygenation (32). This latter change could also be attributed to an enhanced O_2^- and H_2O_2 production in the mitochondria. However, alternative explana-tions such as an increased oxygen availability, after antimycin A administration or hyperbaric oxygenation, for other H_2O_2-forming systems, and a direct effect of molecular oxygen in lipoperoxide formation (32) can equally explain the experimental observations.

Although present in minute concentrations, O_2^- and H_2O_2 are normal intracellular metabolites. Fig. 8 provides a scheme repre-senting a rat liver cell, since most of the available data refers to that tissue, in which the enzymes and organelles that generate and utilize oxygen intermediates and hydroperoxides are indicated.

Cytosolic enzymes such as xanthine oxidase, aldehyde oxidase, etc., produce O_2^- (21). Mitochondria seem to constitute the main intracellular locus of origin of O_2^-; they would produce as much as 24 nmol O_2^-/min per g of rat liver, a rate that could account for about 75 % of the total cellular production of O_2^-. Mitochondrial superoxide dismutase keeps a low steady-state concentration of O_2^-, that has been calculated as 8×10^{-12} M in the matrix space (16). Similar considerations have estimated the cytosolic steady-state concentration of O_2^- at 66×10^{-12} M (16). Recent reports (33-35; see also Estabrook, this volume) indicate that endoplasmic reticu-lum may produce considerable amounts of O_2^- under physiological conditions.

Concerning H_2O_2, it is well understood that a series of organ-elles and enzymes are sources of this oxygen intermediate, and that the effective rate of H_2O_2 formation by these systems depends on the substrate and oxygen supply. The data obtained with the isolated fractions of rat liver indicate that mitochondria, microsomes, per-oxisomes and soluble enzymes provide 14 %, 47 %, 34 % and 5 %, res-pectively, of the cytosolic H_2O_2 when fully supplemented with their substrates (3). Considering the rate of H_2O_2 production in the perfused rat liver (31,36) and in the same organ in situ (37), and the catalase content of rat liver (36), the intracellular steady state concentration of H_2O_2 can be estimated at about 10^{-8} M (31).

The possible rate of the non-enzymatic Haber-Weiss reaction (equation [5]; ref. (38)) in the cytosol of rat liver can also be estimated from the steady-state concentrations of O_2^- and H_2O_2, and assuming a second order reaction constant of 10^{10} $M^{-1}s^{-1}$, it results to be about 0.1 nmol $HO^{\cdot}$/min per g of liver. The Haber-Weiss

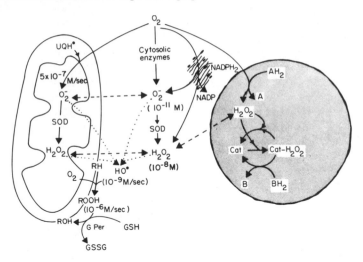

Fig. 8. Metabolism of oxygen intermediates and hydroperoxides in rat liver. Mitochondria, peroxisomes and endoplasmic reticulum are represented, respectively, by the oval body at the left, the round body at the right, and the reticulum close to the round body. SOD: superoxide dismutase; Cat: catalase; G Per: glutathione peroxidase; AH_2: peroxisomal H_2O_2-forming substrate (urate, D-aminoacids, etc.); BH_2: hydrogen donor for the catalase reaction (ethanol, methanol, etc.).

reaction has been claimed also as a source of singlet oxygen ($^1O_2$) (39). Although the mechanism is far from being clear, different

$$H_2O_2 + O_2^- \longrightarrow HO^{\cdot} + HO^- + O_2 \qquad [5]$$

lines of evidence seem to indicate that both $^1O_2$ and $HO^{\cdot}$ can act as initiators of the process of lipoperoxidation (39-40). For instance, considering $HO^{\cdot}$ as initiator of the chain reaction, it can be formulated:

$$RH + HO^{\cdot} \longrightarrow H_2O + R^{\cdot} \qquad [6]$$

$$R^{\cdot} + O_2 \longrightarrow RO_2^{\cdot} \qquad [7]$$

$$RO_2^{\cdot} + RH \longrightarrow RO_2H + R^{\cdot} \qquad [8]$$

In the first reaction, $HO^{\cdot}$ abstracts a hydrogen atom from a methylene carbon group. The formed organic radical incorporates oxygen and regenerates a radical (reactions [7] and [8]) that keeps the chain reaction leading to extensive lipid and organic peroxide generation.

Although clear evidence for the formation of significant amounts of lipid or organic peroxide under physiological conditions is still lacking, some recent data on oxidized glutathione release from the perfused liver, constitutes an important contribution and a promising approach for the matter. Perfused rat liver releases 2-4 nmol GSSG/min per g of tissue (41-42). This value would correspond, considering that GSSG release reflects usually about 3 % of the turnover of glutathione peroxidase (41-42), to about 100 nmol ROOH/min per g of liver. Apparently, the radical chain reaction acts as an amplification factor that leads to the formation of about 1000 ROOH per HO$\cdot$ (and/or $^{1}O_{2}$) generated.

The determination of the product of a reaction whose velocity depends on oxygen concentration may provide an additional parameter to estimate oxygen tension in the tissues. Mitochondrial formation of O_{2}^{-} and $H_{2}O_{2}$ is proportional to oxygen tension; however determination of peroxide generation rates and steady state concentrations as indirect measurement of oxygen tension is basically complicated by the existence of various intracellular sources of O_{2}^{-} and $H_{2}O_{2}$ and by the existence of intercellular or intracellular oxygen gradients (43; see also Sies, this volume).

Oxygen intermediates and hydroperoxides may constitute part of a chemical system able to sense oxygen tension in the tissue.

ACKNOWLEDGEMENTS

Most of this work has been carried out as collaborative research with Prof. B. Chance, to whom the author wishes to express his gratitude for ideas and encouragement. This investigation was supported by grants from U.S. Public Health Service (HL-SCOR-15061) and from Consejo Nacional de Investigaciones Cientificas y Tecnicas, Argentina. The author is a career investigator of the latter institution.

REFERENCES

1.   Chance B, Oshino N: Kinetics and mechanism of catalase in peroxisomes of the mitochondrial fraction. Biochem.J.122:225-233, 1971

2.   Loschen G, Flohe L, Chance B: Respiratory chain linked $H_{2}O_{2}$ production in pigeon heart mitochondria. FEBS Lett. 18:261-264, 1971

3.   Boveris A, Oshino N, Chance B: The cellular production of hydrogen peroxide. Biochem.J. 128:617-630, 1972

4.   Boveris A, Chance B: The mitochondrial generation of hydrogen peroxide. Biochem.J. 134:707-716, 1973

5. Jensen PK: Antimycin-insensitive oxidation of succinate and reduced nicotinamide adenine dinucleotide in electron transport particles.I. pH dependency and hydrogen peroxide formation. Biochim. Biophys. Acta 122:157-166, 1966

6. Hinkle PC, Butow RA, Racker E, Chance B: Partial resolution of the enzymes catalyzing oxidative phosphorylation. XV. Reverse electron transfer in the flavin-cytochrome b region of the respiratory chain of beef heart submitochondrial particles. J.Biol.Chem. 242: 5169-5173, 1967

7. Kusel JP, Boveris A, Storey BT: H_2O_2 production and cytochrome c peroxidase activity in mitochondria isolated from the trypanosomatid hemoflagellate Crithidia fasciculata. Arch.Biochem.Biophys. 158:799-805, 1973

8. Rich PR, Boveris A, Bonner WDJr, Moore AL: Hydrogen peroxide generation by the alternate oxidase of higher plants. Biochem. Biophys.Res.Commun. 71:695-703, 1976

9. Chance B, Williams GR: The respiratory chain and oxidative phosphorylation. In Nord FF(Editor): Advances in Enzymology. New York, Interscience, 1956, vol 17, pp 65-134

10. Fisher AB, Scarpa A, LaNoue KF, Bassett D, Williamson JR: Respiration of rat lung mitochondria and the influence of Ca^{2+} on substrate utilization. Biochemistry 12:1438-1445, 1973

11. Chance B, Boveris A, Oshino N, Loschen G: The nature of the catalase intermediate in its biological function. In King TE, Mason HS, Morrison M(Editors): Oxidases and related redox systems. Baltimore, University Park Press, 1973, vol 1, pp 350-353

12. Loschen G, Azzi A, Flohe L: Mitochondrial H_2O_2 formation: relationship with energy conservation. FEBS Lett. 33:84-88, 1973

13. Loschen G, Azzi A, Flohe L: Mitochondrial hydrogen peroxide formation. In Thurman RG, Yonetani T, Williamson JR, Chance B(Editors): Alcohol and aldehyde metabolizing systems. New York and London, Academic Press, 1974, pp 215-229

14. Erecinska M, Wilson DF: The effect of antimycin A on cytochromes b_{561}, b_{566} and their relationship to ubiquinone and the iron-sulfur centers S-1(+N-2) and S-3. Arch.Biochem.Biophys. 174:143-157, 1976

15. Boveris A, Cadenas E, Stoppani AOM: Role of ubiquinone in the mitochondrial generation of hydrogen peroxide. Biochem.J. 156:435-444, 1976

16. Tyler DD: Polarographic assay and intracellular distribution of superoxide dismutase in rat liver. Biochem.J. 147:493-504, 1975

17. Peeters-Joris C, Vandevoorde AM, Baudhuin P: Subcellular localization of superoxide dismutase in rat liver. Biochem.J. 150:31-39, 1975

18. Loschen G, Azzi A, Richter C, Flohe L: Superoxide radicals as precursors of mitochondrial hydrogen peroxide. FEBS Lett. 42: 68-72, 1974

19. Boveris A, Cadenas E: Mitochondrial production of superoxide anions and its relationship to the antimycin-insensitive respiration. FEBS Lett. 54:311-315, 1975

20. Dionisi O, Galeotti T, Terranova T, Azzi A: Superoxide radicals and hydrogen peroxide formation in mitochondria from normal and neoplastic tissues. Biochim.Biophys.Acta 403:292-301, 1975

21. Fridovich I: Superoxide dismutase. In Meister A(Editor): Advances in Enzymology. New York, Interscience, 1974, vol 41, pp 35-97

22. Cadenas E, Boveris A, Ragan CI, Stoppani AOM: Production of superoxide radicals and hydrogen peroxide by isolated Complexes I and III of the respiratory chain. Arch.Biochem.Biophys. in press

23. Ruzicka FJ, Beinert H, Schepler KL, Dunham WR, Sands RH: Interaction of ubisemiquinone with a paramagnetic component in heart tissue. Proc.Natl.Acad.Sci.U.S.A. 72:2886-2890, 1975

24. Ingledew WJ, Ohnishi T: Properties of the S-3 iron sulfur centre of succinate dehydrogenase in the intact respiratory chain of beef heart mitochondria. FEBS Lett. 54:167-171, 1975

25. Ingledew WJ, Salerno JC, Ohnishi T: Studies on electron paramagnetic resonance spectra manifested by a respiratory chain hydrogen carrier. Arch.Biochem.Biophys. 176: in press, 1976

26. Sawada Y, Iyanaghi T, Yamazaki I: Relation between redox potentials and rate constants in reactions coupled with the system oxygen-superoxide. Biochemistry 14:3761-3764, 1975

27. Forman HJ, Kennedy J: Role of superoxide radical in mitochondrial dehydrogenase reactions.Biochem.Biophys.Res.Commun. 60: 1044-1050, 1974

28. Boveris A, Chance B: Optimal rates of hydrogen peroxide production in hyperbaric oxygen. In Thurman RG, Yonetani T, Williamson JR, Chance B(Editors): Alcohol and aldehyde metabolizing systems. New York and London, Academic Press, 1974, pp 207-214

29. Chance B, Boveris A, Oshino N: Hydrogen peroxide in mitochondria. Proc. IV Inter. Congress Biophysics. Pushchino.1973. Symposial papers, vol 4(2), pp 903-909

30. Scholtz R, Thurman RG, Williamson JR, Chance B, Bucher T: Flavin and pyridine nucleotide oxidation-reduction changes in rat liver.I. Anoxia and subcellular localization of fluorescent flavoproteins. J.Biol.Chem. 244:2317-2324, 1969

31. Oshino N, Chance B, Sies H, Bucher T: The rate of H_2O_2 generation in perfused rat liver and the reaction of catalase Compound I and hydrogen donors. Arch.Biochem.Biophys. 154:106-116, 1973

32. Nishiki K, Jamieson D, Oshino N, Chance B: Oxygen toxicity in the perfused rat liver and lung under hyperbaric conditions. Biochem.J. 158: in press, 1976

33. Mishin V, Pokrovsky A, Lyakhovich VV: Interactions of some acceptors with superoxide anion radicals formed by the NADPH-specific flavoprotein in rat liver microsomal fractions. Biochem.J. 154: 307-310, 1976

34. Sligar SG, Lipscomb JD, Debrunner PG, Gunsalus IC: Superoxide anion production by the autoxidation of cytochrome P450$_{cam}$. Biochem.Biophys.Res.Commun. 61:290-296, 1974

35. Bartoli GM, Galeotti T, Palombini G, Parisi G: The relation between O_2^- radicals production and mixed function oxidation in rat liver microsomes. Abstr.X Inter.Congress Biochem.Hamburg.1976. Abs. 06-7-096, p 348

36. Oshino N, Jamieson D, Chance B: The properties of hydrogen peroxide production under hyperbaric and hypoxic conditions of perfused rat liver. Biochem.J. 146:53-65, 1975

37. Oshino N, Jamieson D, Sugano T, Chance B: Optical measurement of the catalase-hydrogen peroxide intermediate (Compound I) in the liver of anesthetized rats and its implication to hydrogen peroxide production in situ. Biochem.J. 146:67-77, 1975

38. Haber F, Weiss J: The catalytic decomposition of hydrogen peroxide by iron salts. Proc.Roy.Society.London. A147:332-351, 1934

39. Kellogg EW, Fridovich I: Superoxide, hydrogen peroxide and singlet oxygen in lipid peroxidation by a xanthine oxidase system. J. Biol.Chem. 250:8812-8817, 1975

40. Fong KL, Mc Cay PB, Poyer JL, Keele BB, Misra H: Evidence that peroxidation of lysosomal membrane is initiated by hydroxyl free

radicals produced during flavin enzyme activity. J.Biol.Chem. 248:
7792-7797, 1973

41. Oshino N. Chance B: Properties of glutathione release observed
during reduction of organic hydroperoxide, demethylation of aminopyrine and oxidation of some substances in perfused rat liver and
their implications for the physiological function of catalase.
Biochem.J. in press

42. Sies H, Summer KH: Hydroperoxide metabolizing systems in rat
liver. Eur.J.Biochem. 57:503-512, 1975

43. Chance B: Pyridine nucleotide as an indicator of the oxygen requirements for energy-linked functions of mitochondria. Circulat.
Res.Suppl. 38-39: 31-38, 1976

Mechanism of Oxygen Sensing

in Tissues

Chairman: R.F. Coburn

CHEMORECEPTION AND TRANSDUCTION
ON NEURONAL MODELS

N. CHALAZONITIS

Institut de Neurophysiologie et Psychophysiologie
C.N.R.S.   31, Chemin Joseph-Aiguier,
13274 Marseille 2   FRANCE

Experiments on Aplysia neuronal models during pO_2, CO_2 and pH transients lead to results useful in understanding some functional mechanisms which may, in some instances, be transposed on chemo-receptor nerve terminals of the arterial chemo-receptor ganglia of mammals.

In past work, by means of intracellular recording we reported data concerning the sensitivity of identifiable neurons of Aplysia to changes in pO_2, pCO_2 and pH : changes in membrane potential and membrane resistance, the frequency of rhythmicities, direct excitability, and post-synaptic activation have been investigated (1, 2, 3, 4, 5). Furthermore, pO_2 and pCO_2 in the extracellular and intracellular space have been quantitatively determined and their changes have been recorded simultaneously with electrical activity in single cells (6, 7, 8, 9, 10, 11, 12, 13, 14, 15, 16).

As methods and techniques have been already described in the above references, only the terms hypoxia and hypercapnia will be defined here. Whereas normoxia in Aplysia blood in vivo is about 25 mm Hg pO_2, determination of the normoxic intraneuronal pO_2 gives 5 to 7 mm Hg when the ganglion is in situ (non-isolated). In order to establish a comparable intracellular pO_2 in the neuron when the ganglion is isolated (the usual Aplysia preparation), the extracellular pO_2 must reach about 100 mm Hg. Therefore, hypoxia for the Aplysia preparation will be any extracellular pO_2 lower than 100 mm Hg. Furthermore, we will define as hypercapnia, extracellular pCO_2's higher than 3mm Hg in sea water (i. e. when the CO_2 composition of the atmosphere is greater than 5%). Similarly, any pH lower than 7. 8 (the normal pH of sea water) may be considered as an H^+ ion stimulus. Whatever, hypoxia, hypercapnia or low pH, as above delimited, will be named respiratory stimuli. The Aplysia data will be compared with what is known about single mammalian chemoreceptor responsiveness. In addition, the model neuronal chemosensitivity will also be examined during synaptic activation. Neuronal chemosensitivity to respiratory gases after acetylcholine treatment will be reported. Finally, some membrane mechanisms will be considered at a molecular scale, which will in turn complete some views of recent work (12, 13, 14).

I - COMPARATIVE EFFECTS OF RESPIRATORY STIMULI ON SENSITIVE NEURONAL MODELS

The preparation of the isolated Aplysia ganglion is in its main aspects comparable to the glomus chemoreceptive ganglion of mammals, particularly in studies of hypoxic and/or ischaemic effects. Moreover, the Aplysia chemosensitive neurons, when intracellularly explored, yield a description of some bioelectric changes during chemoreception, whereas the glomus chemosensitive terminals offer only information through their centripetal (toward respiratory centers) discharge (electroneurogram).

Comparable diagrams relating the hypoxic discharge to pO_2, pCO_2 and pH have been already published for both the Aplysia neuron (12, 13, 14) and for chemoreceptor centripetal nerve fibres (17). In both cases a hypoxic transient increases the frequency of any initially autorhythmic cell. The maximum slope of the curves (impulses/sec expressed as a function of $-\Delta pO_2$) is observable from normoxia to hypoxia (Fig. 1). Similarly, in ischemia, when the environmental pCO_2 increases transitorily along with hypoxia (18), the chemoreceptor discharge increases in frequency in mammals (17). Analogously, in Aplysia the neuronal discharge also increases during hypoxic and hypercapnic transients (4, 14). In ischemia a synergism is therefore conspicuously established by simultaneous hypoxia and hypercapnia.

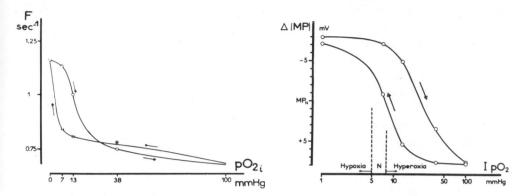

FIGURE 1 -   Left diagram -   The frequency of a spontaneous
firing cell as a function of the logarithm of the intracellular pO_2.
Ascending arrow deoxygenation (from O_2 to N_2), descending
arrow : reoxygenation. In both cases (for either deoxygenation
or reoxygenation) the maximum slopes are observed around
normoxia. Note a hysteresis in frequency recovery during the
cycle normoxia (7 mm Hg) $\longrightarrow$ hypoxia $\longrightarrow$ normoxia.
Right diagram - Change in membrane potential as a function of
the logarithm of the intracellular pO_2. Maximum slope observed,
around normoxia (7 mm Hg). Note the hysteresis in membrane
potential recovery after the cycle normoxia $\longrightarrow$ hypoxia $\longrightarrow$
normoxia.

It is obvious that the CO_2 output from mitochondria
occurring during oxydative decarboxylation cannot outlast the
nicotinamide deshydrogenase reduction which is displayed
after the complete abolition of the oxygen supply.

Whatever the stimulus (hypoxia, hypercapnia or both)
the intracellular exploration of Aplysia chemosensitive neurons
offers supplementary information about the relationship between
discharge increase and membrane depolarization.

1 - Membrane Potential Changes During Transients
in pO_2, pCO_2 and pH

On many neurons, but not on all, small measurable
changes in the intracellular pO_2 significantly affect the resting
potential of the somatic neuromembrane. Hypoxia (pO_2 displa-

cement inside the cell from 7 to 1 mm Hg) occurs when the
extracellular pO_2 decreases below 100 mm Hg (Fig. 2). Hypercapnia (pCO_2 higher than 6 mm Hg) and acidosis (pH lower than
7) similarly elicit depolarization. Conversely, when pO_2, pCO_2
and pH values return to normal, the somatic membrane tends
to repolarize and the normal membrane potential is recovered.
Estimations of neuronal sensitivity to respiratory gas transients
may be considered with respect to two aspects. The first is a
biophysical aspect : evaluation of the ratio $\Delta(MP) / \Delta pO_2$.
During various experimental conditions the ratio oscillates
between 1mV/1mm Hg intracellular pO_2, and zero depending
upon the type of neurons studied. The hypercapnic sensitivity

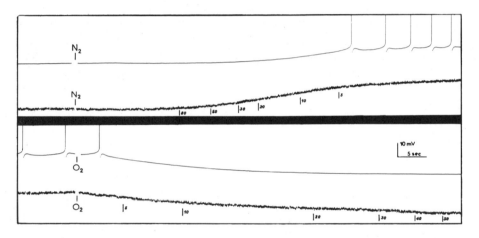

FIGURE 2 - Simultaneous recording during a hypoxic transient
of the photometric trace indicating the instantaneous saturation
of the intraneuronal hemoglobin and of the electrical activity in
a neuron which is silent in normoxia. Numbers of the photometric trace indicate the instantaneous intracellular pO_2 value
inside the neuron, as calculated from the photometric trace.
Arrows indicate admission of nitrogen or oxygen. Note that
during hypoxia (from 7 mm Hg to zero) a generator potential
(depolarization) leads to a discharge. Returning to normoxia
(7 mm Hg) the repolarization abolishes the discharge. During
hyperoxia the hyperpolarization is continued slowly.

was evaluated analogously from the ratio $\Delta(MP)/\Delta(pCO_2)$.
According to neuronal type, the maximum value obtained was
0.2 mV/mm Hg. The second aspect concerns the functional
significance of the respiratory stimulus which is measurable
by the spike discharge obtained if the chemoreceptive neuron
is initially at rest, or by the increased spike production if the
chemoreceptive neuron is rhythmically active. Therefore, the
functional value of given respiratory transients depends not
only on the ratio $\Delta(MP)/\Delta pO_2$, etc.., but also on the initial
value of the resting potential. For a given depolarization the
closer the membrane potential is to the firing level, the greater
will be the response (i.e. the length and frequency of the discharge).

Although a tautology, it is to be stressed that if a given
depolarization (say 10 mV) is obtained from a neuron by a given
respiratory transient, and if this neuron displays a threshold
potential higher than 10 mV, it will never give a discharge
during the transient. It turns out that the highest sensitivity to
a respiratory transient occurs when the neuronal membrane
potential is closest to the firing level. For that reason the best
examples of chemosensitive neurons in mammals are the ones
concerning neuronal units initially in autorhythmic activity (17),
and in that case pure hypoxia is a stimulus for a given chemoreceptive unit. In hypoxia the relationship between impulse/sec
and pO_2 is hyperbolic-like for both Aplysia neurons or arterial
chemoreceptor endings. However, from normoxia to hyperoxia
the relationship between membrane potential of Aplysia neurons
and pO_2 would in many cases be described by the relationship

$$MP_R = (MP_n + K \cdot \log (pO_2)$$

where MP_R and MP_n are respectively the "hyperoxic" and the
"normoxic" membrane potential values. It was also found that
the constant, K, is higher when the transition is from normoxia
to hyperoxia rather than the reverse.

Membrane potential measurements have not yet been
possible in aortic ganglia of mammals. From what is known
about firing frequency of chemoreceptor endings as a function
of pO_2, the MP of such units might also be a function of pO_2

in a manner analogous to that in Aplysia neurons (Fig. 1, 2).
Similarly, the results obtained by Biscoe et al. (17, 19)
concerning increase in single unit frequency of discharge during
hypercapnia are comparable to the ones obtained in Aplysia
neurons (14).

2 - Neuronal Chemosensitivity under Synaptic Action.

Aplysia neurons offer again precise information about
chemosensitivity recorded in neurons submitted simultaneously
to respiratory stimuli and synaptic activation. As a matter of
fact, a depression of arterial chemoreceptor discharge during
stimulation of the sinus nerve efferents has been already investigated by Neil and O'Regan (20, 21). Comparatively, with
neuronal models it has been established that when a respiratory
stimulus is able to produce a discharge or an extra-discharge,
a given inhibitory synaptic afferent would attenuate the respiratory response and/or even abolish it. During a first stage the
discharge of the explored neuron increases. Consecutively, the
respiratory stimulus activates an inhibitory interneuron which
fires and attenuates or even stops the activity of the explored
neuron. Such an action of the respiratory stimulus on both of
the coupled neurons leads to a temporary attenuation. Such a
model might be considered in the case of depression in arterial
chemoreceptors, whatever the nature of the inhibitory transmitter.

Conversely, possible synaptic facilitatory (or synergistic actions) may also be considered in synaptically coupled
neurons. Suppose that a given respiratory stimulus exerts a
depolarization insufficient to bring the membrane to its firing
level. In this case, this stimulus will elicit no functional effect.
But if, during this respiratory stimulus, an afferent synaptic
activation eliciting EPSP's (excitatory post-synaptic potentials)
would add its depolarizing action, a discharge of spikes will be
possible. The overall chemoreceptive discharge cannot outlast
the synaptic bombardment; therefore this kind of chemosensitivity will be temporary as opposed to a permanent chemosensitivity of firing neurons.

Whatever the case (facilitation or attenuation), if a given
chemosensitive cell is synaptically controlled, it will be endowed

with a composite, or "network-derived" chemosensitivity which
is both direct (its own) and indirect (i.e. of multisynaptic origin).

3 - Respiratory Stimuli During Acetylcholine Effects.

The release of acetylcholine during respiratory stimulation in mammals, demonstrated by Eyzaguirre and Zapata (22),
raises interesting questions which might be answered from experiments on neuronal models, i.e. on neurons which are sensitive
to both acetylcholine and respiratory stimuli.

The sensitivity of molluscan neurons to acetylcholine
treatment has been demonstrated long ago by Kerkut and
coworkers, and also by Tauc and Gerschenfeld (see Gerschenfeld, (23) for review), and by Kandel et al (24). These authors
reported that the response to acetylcholine may be either depolarization or hyperpolarization and depends on the type of neuron.
These results (de- or hyper-polarization) for different identifiable Aplysia neurons are summarized by Boisson (25). Recently, Gola and Chalazonitis (unpublished) demonstrated that if
identifiable and chemosensitive neurons are initially depolarized
in hypercapnia, they can still display a further depolarization
with acetylcholine (0.5 to 5 x 10^{-4} M) (Fig. 3). Not only is the
initial depolarization with CO_2 reversible, but also the further
depolarization with acetylcholine. In preliminary experiments
Gola and Chalazonitis found an independence between hypoxia
and acetylcholine effects (26); on the so-called "petites cellules
rouges" of Aplysia, or R_3, acetylcholine treatment elicits a
hyperpolarization under normoxia. If initially the cell is depolarized in hypoxia, the acetylcholine treatment again elicits a
hyperpolarization. In summary, it seems that some chemosensitive neurons display an independence to alternate treatment ;
i.e. hypoxia or hypercapnia followed by acetylcholine application.
Whatever the kind of molecular receptors, specific or not,
these data suggest a dual behaviour according to the type of the
chemosensitive cell. If a given cell depolarizes during a respiratory stimulus, any released acetylcholine acting on its membrane may increase the depolarization (facilitation or synergism
between both stimuli). Such a depolarization may be abolished
if acetylcholine exerts a nyperpolarizing action (antagonism).
In the same line of thinking, the data reported by Douglas (27)
(namely that acetylcholine receptor blockers do not affect
chemoreflex responses provoked by hypoxia) point out in the

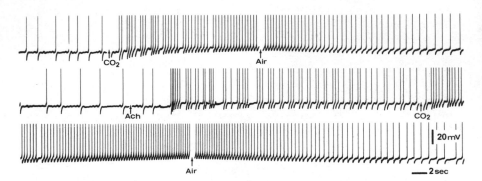

FIGURE 3 - Alternate sensitivity to acetylcholine and CO_2 of a rhythmic neuron.
Upper recording : first arrow : from air to 20% CO_2 (in 20% O_2 + 60% N_2). Depolarization and increase in frequency.
Second arrow : from CO_2 to air : repolarization and recovery.
Middle recording : Same cell. First arrow : application of $0.5 \ 10^{-4}$ acetylcholine in sea water. The membrane depolarizes and the frequency increases. Second arrow : from air to 20% CO_2 . Further depolarization and increase in frequency.
Lower recording : Continuation of the previous recording.
Arrow : from 20% CO_2 to air. The cell repolarizes and the frequency recovers.

case of mammalian chemoreceptors the concept of independence of the effects of acetylcholine and respiratory stimuli.

In conclusion, in both cases, a possible release and action of acetylcholine during a respiratory transient does not preclude a simultaneous direct effect of the respiratory stimulus on the same neuromembrane.

II - DISCUSSION OF MEMBRANE MECHANISMS

The demonstration of changes of the membrane electrical resistance (MR) as a function of changes in pO_2, pCO_2, pH (increase in hypoxia, decrease in hyperoxia, etc..) have yielded some insight into the behavior of membranes at the cellular scale (13). As a matter of fact, it has been concluded that MR is logarithmically related with pO_2 :

$$(MR) \text{ hyperoxic} = (MR) \text{ normoxic} - K \cdot \log (pO_2).$$

Taking into account that the oxygen requirements of the neuronal respiratory chain are satisfied in normoxia, leads to the conclusion that oxygen would be adsorbed on some membrane sites of rather specific affinity. As a consequence of this adsorption, some change in the molecular "conformational state", would explain MR changes (13).

In addition, if "oxygenophilic" molecules exist in the membrane, we might define them as "oxyphores", i.e. "bearers of oxygen". Therefore, the hemoglobin molecule should be considered as a useful analogue in predicting possible affinities of oxyphores; for instance, possible competition of O_2 and CO_2 for the same site, and control of these affinities by ionic factors (H^+, Ca^{++}, etc..) could be predicted.

The presence of oxyphores in membranes which are sensitive to O_2 and CO_2 might explain the direct actions of these molecules in leading to permeability changes. Such changes may occur independently and/or in addition to other membrane alterations originating from the deceleration of the respiratory chain, which leads to ionic pump attenuation.

It is obvious that the concept of oxyphore presence could hardly be extended to non-chemosensitive membranes. Particularly for Aplysia neuromembranes, it seems highly probable that oxyphores could correspond to a real hemoprotein which is hemoglobin- or myoglobin-like (28, 29). The presence of Aplysia hemoglobin (Hb) in the neuromembrane is very probable for two reasons. First, it has been demonstrated (27) that Hb is present in the neurosomes of the neuronal cytoplasm. If Hb is synthesized outside of the neuron, it must cross the membrane during its accumulation in the neurosomes. It is then likely that Hb can bind firmly with other molecules in the

membrane. The other reason arises from the demonstration
of a possible displacement of the membrane potential and
decrease in resistance by specific photoactivation of the Hb
in situ (30, 31) .

Irrespective of the type of oxyphore or of permeability
changes which occur during their unloading of oxygen (hypoxia)
and/or overloading with CO_2 (hypercapnia), it will be recalled
that the respiratory chain, and consequently, the ionic pump,
both decelerate. Torrance (32) and Biscoe (19), considering
arterial chemoreceptors, and Kerkut and York (33), and Chalazonitis and Arvanitaki (13) working with molluscan neurons,
investigated how changes in respiratory molecules would be
related to the function of the ionic pump.

Whatever the case, the generator potential, sustaining
a discharge, is the apparent response during any respiratory
stimulus. This potential may be the consequence of an outflow
of generator current mainly across the axon hillock area of the
cell body. Details of such a transduction (stimulus $\longrightarrow$ generator
current) have been already discussed (13). The generator current
might arise through vectorial permeability changes, which would
be triggered by the unloading (hypoxia) and/or overloading (hypercapnia) of the oxyphore site. The time course of such changes
in the oxyphore site should depend on diffusion processes of
O_2, CO_2 through the ganglionic tissue. The half-desaturation
of the intracellular hemoglobin in the isolated ganglion preparation (from 25% -normal saturation in air- to 12%) takes
about 20 sec. Then, if one assumes that half number of oxyphores in the membrane are unloaded in 20 seconds, the direct
action of O_2 in the membrane may be considered as a rather
fast process. The reverse "loading" of the intracellular Hb
from 0 to 12 mm Hg is even faster; it occurs in about 10 sec
in vivo. On the other hand, the overall duration of one cycle
of unloading and loading from air (25% saturation) to zero
saturation and back to 25% saturation, is about 120 sec. During
that cycle, there is a hysteresis of the membrane potential
hypoxic decrease as follows : For a given depolarization obtained
during the cycle normoxia $\longrightarrow$ anoxia, the subsequent repolarization occuring during anoxia $\longrightarrow$ normoxia varies between 15 and
60% of the amount of the initial depolarization. Such a hysteresis
in repolarization may denote (as Chance has suggested) the
occurrence of another hypoxic process of endogenous, i.e. of

mitochondrial origin. Metabolic molecules (ADP, Ca^{++}, etc..) elaborated in hypoxia may diffuse from the mitochondria to the membrane. Then, the changes elicited by such molecules in the membrane structure may concern not only ionic pumps but also permeabilities. The time course of this process might be slower than the previous one, i.e. the saturation and/or desaturation of membrane oxyphores.

A third molecular influence on the membrane is the exogenous action of released neuroamines (acetylcholine, catecholamines, etc..), which may be triggered by the respiratory stimuli. One could imagine that the closer the cell containing these amines, lies to the chemosensitive cell, the faster will be the time course of their action on the chemosensitive cell. This is not the case for the examined Aplysia neuronal somata, for they are not directly surrounded by neuroamine containing cells. Therefore, released neuroamines might come from remote places, and their action then would correspond to a slow process. In any case, as already determined, any action of these neuroamines on the membrane potential, either on the post-synaptic areas, or on other areas (via arrival from the intercellular space), would be either facilitatory or inhibitory during the direct action of the respiratory stimuli.

Suggestions on a mechanism of transduction during the time courses of direct, indirect and neurochemical influences may concern the possible creation of a transitory transcellular ionic current. Such a current can be created by the entrance of a given ionic species through an area and its continuous exit through another area (Fig. 4a) (i.e. spatial separation of cationic charge flow in opposite directions) . Such a trans-cellular ionic flux is thus equivalent to a transcellular electric current.

Another picture of current flow is the one concerning only transmembrane current production, i.e. outflow of positive charge of one or more cationic species (Fig. 4b, 4c). In such a case an outflow of positive ionic charge across the whole membrane will first give rise to a discharge. A subsequent decrease and annihilation of such an outflow will abolish the generator potential. Furthermore the first cationic outflow may alternate with a second cationic inflow of a different species. Thus cationic fluxes of opposite direction cross the somatic membrane in succession, accelerating the abolition of the generator potential.

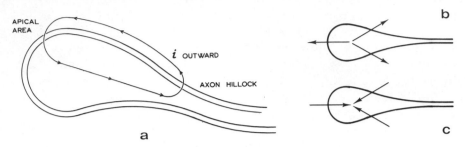

FIGURE 4 - Left : (a) Continuous transcellular current.
Simultaneous outflux of charge through the axon hillock area
and influx of charge through the apical area.
Right : (b) First stage : arrows indicate charge outflow which
elicits a generator potential. (c) Second stage : compensatory
inflow of charge (repolarization).

Whatever the spatial separation of the ionic fluxes
(transcellular current), or their possible time-separation
(transmembrane current), the overall property of the membrane
transduction during respiratory stimuli will be defined as
"rheogeny", that is "generator current" production.

Rheogeny is a general property recognized in many
sensors. The Aplysia chemosensitive neurons behave as
sensors therefore, and many of them are multiceptors, that is
sensitive to different kinds of environmental stimuli. It turns
out that for a given identifiable neuron, production of generator
current (rheogeny) may be possible by different stimuli (chemical, thermal, mechanical, electrical and even photostimuli).
If rheogeny is a common property of Aplysia neurons which
respond to respiratory and mechanical stimuli, it should also
be so in the case of arterial chemoreceptors which are submitted
to mechanical influences during respiratory transients. Therefore it is worthwhile to consider that arterial chemoreceptors
as well as Aplysia neuromembranes may have multiceptor
properties.

CONCLUSIONS

Some data and mechanisms established on Aplysia neuronal models, possibly valid for arterial chemoreceptors of mammals, will be summarized as follows :- Any type of respiratory stimulus triggers a discharge of certain Aplysia chemosensitive neurons and of arterial chemoreceptor terminals. In both cases, the maximum chemosensitivity then depends on a maximum depolarization of the membrane per unit of stimulus which is sufficient to attain the firing level. The elicitation of a discharge-chemoresponse denotes that any chemosensitive membrane is comparable to a pace-maker membrane (i.e. displaying some oscillatory behavior), but that it differs fundamentally from a stable axonal membrane.

- Any mechanical deformation of the chemosensitive membrane triggered by the respiratory stimulus, directly or indirectly, may facilitate the direct depolarizing effect exerted by the respiratory stimulus itself.

- Synaptic influences, and/or exogenous neurochemical influences triggered by the respiratory stimulus may be facilitatory or inhibitory on the final discharge elicited by the chemosensitive neuromembrane during the direct action of the stimulus.

- The direct action of the respiratory stimulus affects both permeabilities and ionic pumps. Any pump function may be decreased during the respiratory chain deceleration.

- Suggestions have been made in order to explain the mechanism of transduction. Such a transduction implies the elicitation of a discharge, whatever the chemical action in the membrane. One suggestion involves transcellular current formation. An alternative explanation implies transmembrane current formation in two stages :

During a first stage an outflow of cationic charge depolarizes the membrane (generator potential).

During a second stage an opposite cationic inflow compensates for the initial depolarization.

REFERENCES

(1) Chalazonitis N : Chemopotentiels des neurones géants fonc-
tionnellement différenciés. Arch. Sci. physiol. 13 : 41-78, 1959.

(2) Chalazonitis N : Chemopotentials on giant nerve cells (Aplysia
fasciata). In Florey E (Editor) : Nervous Inhibition. New-York,
Pergamon Press, 1961. pp 178-193.

(3) Chalazonitis N : Effects of changes in pCO_2 and pO_2 on rhythmic potentials from giant neurons. Ann. N. Y. Acad. Sci. 109:
451-479, 1963.

(4) Chalazonitis N, Sugaya E : Stimulation-inhibition de neurones
géants identifiables d'Aplysia par l'anhydride carbonique.
C. R. Acad. Sci. 247 : 1657-1659, 1958.

(5) Chalazonitis N, Romey G : Excitabilité directe et conductance
de la membrane somatique en fonction de la pression partielle
de l'anhydride carbonique (neurone d'Aplysia). C. R. Soc. Biol.
158 : 2367-2372, 1964.

(6) Chalazonitis N, Gola M : Enregistrements simultanés de la
pO_2 intracellulaire et de l'autoactivité électrique du neurone
géant (Aplysia depilans). C. R. Soc. Biol. 159 : 1770-1776, 1965 a.

(7) Chalazonitis N, Gola M, Arvanitaki A : Microspectrophoto-
métrie différentielle sur des neurones géants in vivo, d'Aplysia
depilans. Mesure de la diffusibilité de l'oxygène. C. R. Soc. Biol.
159 : 2440-2445, 1965 b.

(8) Chalazonitis N, Nahas GG : Small pCO_2 change and neuronal
synaptic activation. Nature (London) 205 : 1016-1017, 1965 c.

(9) Chalazonitis N, Gola M, Arvanitaki A : Régulation de l'acti-
vabilité synaptique des neurones par de faibles variations de la
pO_2 intracellulaire (Aplysia depilans). C. R. Soc. Biol. 160 :
1020-1023, 1966 a.

(10)Gola M : Mesures spectrophotométriques de la saturation
en oxygène de l'hémoprotéine d'Aplysia depilans. C. R. Soc.
Biol. 159 : 1777-1782, 1965

(11) Chalazonitis N, Takeuchi H : Application microélectropho-
rétique locale d'ions H^+ et variations des paramètres bioélec-
triques de la membrane neuronique. C. R. Soc. Biol. 160 :610-
615, 1966.

(12) Chalazonitis N : Intracellular pO_2 control on excitability and synaptic activability in Aplysia and Helix identifiable giant neurons. Ann. N-Y. Acad. Sci. 147 : 419-459, 1968.

(13) Chalazonitis N, Arvanitaki A : Neuromembrane electrogenesis during changes in pO_2, pCO_2 and pH. In Costa E, Giacobini E (Editors) : Biochemistry of simple neuronal models. Advances in Biochem. Psychopharmacology . New-York, Raven Press, 1970, vol 2, pp 245-284.

(14) Chalazonitis N : Simultaneous recordings of pH, pCO_2 and neuronal activity during hypercapnic transients (identifiable neurons of Aplysia).In Nahas GG, Schaefer KE (Editors) :Carbon dioxide and metabolic regulations. New-York, Springer Verlag, 1974, pp 63-80.

(15) Brown AM : Carbon dioxide action on neuronal membranes. In Nahas GG, Schaefer KE (Editors) : Carbon dioxide and metabolic regulations. New-York, Springer Verlag, 1974, pp 81-86.

(16) Carpenter DO, Hubbard JH, Humphrey DR, Thompson HK, Marschall WH : Carbon dioxide effects on nerve cell function. In Nahas GG, Schaefer KE (Editors) : Carbon dioxide and metabolic regulations. New-York, Springer Verlag, 1974, pp. 49-62.

(17) Biscoe TJ, Purves MJ, Sampson SR : The frequency of nerve impulses in single carotid body chemoreceptor afferent fibres recorded in vivo with intact circulation. J. Physiol. (Lond.) 208 : 121-131, 1970.

(18) Siesjö BK : Biochemical aspects of cerebral hypoxia. In Penzholz H, Brock M, Hamer J, Klinger M, Spoerri O (Editors): Brain Hypoxia, Pain. Advances in Neurosurgery. New-York, Springer Verlag, 1975, vol 3, pp 54-58.

(19) Biscoe TJ : Carotid body : structure and function. Physiol. Rev. 51 : 437-495, 1971.

(20) Neil E, O'Regan RG : Effects of sinus and aortic nerve efferents, on arterial chemoreceptor function. J. Physiol (Lond.) 200 : 69-71.

(21) Neil E, O'Regan RG : The effects of efferent electrical stimulation of the cut sinus and aortic nerves on peripheral arterial chemoreceptor activity in the cat. J. Physiol. (Lond.) 215 : 15-32, 1971.

(22) Eyzaguirre C, Zapata P: The release of acetylcholine from carotid body tissues. Further study of the effects of acetylcholine and cholinergic blocking agents on the chemosensory discharge. J. Physiol. (Lond.) 195 : 589-607, 1968.

(23) Gerschenfeld HM : Chemical transmitters in invertebrate nervous systems. Soc. exper. Biol. Symp. 20 : 299-326, 1966.

(24) Kandel ER, Frazier WT, Coggeshall RE : Opposite synaptic actions mediated by different branches of an identifiable inter-neuron in Aplysia. Science 155 : 346-349, 1967.

(25) Boisson M : Variations distinctes de l'oscillabilité consécu-tives à l'hyperpolarisation de quelques neurones géants sécré-toires par la noradrénaline (Aplysia depilans, Linné, 1767, fascia-ta, Poiret, 1790, rosea, Rathké, 1799). Thèse IIIe cycle. Océanographie Biologique. Université Paris. 1973.

(26) Gola M, Chalazonitis N : unpublished.

(27) Douglas WW : The effect of a ganglion blocking drug hexa-methonium on the response of the cat's carotid body to various stimuli. J. Physiol. (Lond.) 118 : 373-383, 1952.

(28) Chalazonitis N, Arvanitaki A : Chromoprotéides et succi-noxydases dans divers grains isolables du protoplasme neuro-nique. Arch. Sci. Physiol. 10 : 291-319, 1956.

(29) Wittenberg BA, Briehl RW, Wittenberg TB : Hemoglobins of invertebrate tissues. Biochem. J. 96 : 363, 1965.

(30) Arvanitaki A, Chalazonitis N : Photopotentiels d'excitation et d'inhibition de différents somata identifiables (Aplysia). Bull. Inst. océanogr. Monaco 57 (1164) : 1-83, 1960.

(31) Chalazonitis N : Light energy conversion in neuronal mem-branes. Photochem. Photobiol. 3 : 539-549, 1964.

(32) Torrance RW : Prolegomena to arterial chemoreceptors. Torrance (Editor). Oxford, Blackwell, 1968.

(33) Kerkut GA, York B : The oxygen sensitivity of the electro-genic sodium pump in snail neurones. Compar. Biochem. Physiol. 28 : 1125 , 1969.

OXYGEN TENSION SENSORS IN VASCULAR SMOOTH MUSCLE*

R.F. Coburn

Department of Physiology, School of Medicine, University

of Pennsylvania, Philadelphia, PA   19174

It is well documented in the literature that mechanical tension in at least some vascular smooth muscle preparations is sensitive to organ bath oxygen tension (1-4). Figure 1 illustrates
the O_2 sensitivity of in vitro strips of rabbit aorta as studied
by Detar and Bohr (2), who have contributed to the characterization of this phenomenon. PO_2 dependent mechanical tension cannot
be demonstrated in vascular smooth muscle which does not have spontaneous tension without adding an agonist to produce active tension.
Most investigators have studied this phenomenon in arterial strips
contracted with catecholamines. Identical PO_2 dependent mechanical
tension, however, can be demonstrated in rabbit aorta with norepinephrine and with angiotensin contractions (5), suggesting that
oxygen sensitivity is not due to effects of oxygen on release, uptake or metabolism of catecholamines.

PO_2 dependent mechanical tension is usually studied with strips
of arterial wall, 0.15 to 0.3 mm thick, and it has been shown that
the critical organ bath PO_2 below which mechanical tension falls
with falls in organ bath PO_2 is dependent on thickness of the preparation (6), as expected if there is an oxygen tension sensor in
the tissue which is sensitive to falls in PO_2 below a critical value.
Strips of vascular tissue contain cells other than smooth muscle,
i.e. neural, endothelial, and we cannot be certain if PO_2 dependent
mechanical tension is due to oxygen sensors in smooth muscles cells,
but this is most likely. Effects of pharmacological blocking agents

*Supported by HL 10331 and HL 10561 from the National Institutes
of Health, Bethesda, Maryland

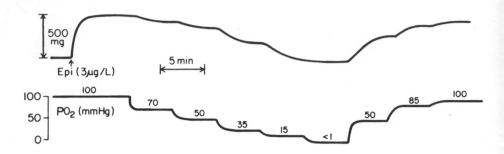

Figure 1. PO_2 dependent mechanical tension in rabbit aorta.   Fig-
            ure taken from Detar and Bohr (2).   Published with per-
            mission of the author.

such as tetrodotoxin, atropine, or scopolamine suggest that release
of acetylcholine and other humoral agents from nerves may not be
the mechanism of PO_2 dependent mechanical tension.

It has been suggested by several investigators (2,3) that the
mechanism of O_2 dependent mechanical tension involves oxygen limitation of aerobic energy production, as depicted in Figure 2.   This
postulates that PO_2 in the tissue core drops to levels which limit
respiratory chain function.   Information is transduced from oxygen
sensor to contractile proteins by a fall in ATP concentration, according to this theory.   A variation of this model is that fall in
high energy phosphates has an "effect" on the cell surface membrane
with consequent effects on contractile protein mediated by change
in membrane potential or membrane calcium permeability.   For oxygen
to limit respiratory chain function requires, according to current
concepts (7), a mitochondrial PO_2 fall to levels as low as 0.05 mm
Hg.   In order to have an effect on the redox state of the cell requires mitochondrial PO_2 falls to even lower values, due to cushion-
ing.   The concept that decreases in [ATP] can influence tension is
feasible since biochemical studies show that [ATP] effects on myosir
ATPase, and disaggregation of actomyosin are qualitatively altered
by changes in ATP concentration, at least in skeletal muscle (8,9).
But, to my knowledge, there is no direct evidence in smooth muscle
preparations that small changes in [ATP] below control levels, whicl
have been found with anoxia in vascular smooth muscle, have an effec
on tension.

a_3-ATP Model

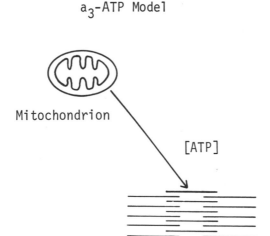

Mitochondrion

[ATP]

Contractile Proteins

Figure 2. The cytochrome a_3-ATP model to explain PO_2 dependent mechanical tension.

There already are some problems with the a_3-ATP or aerobic energy model described above. Biochemical studies of energetics in vascular strips indicate the importance of glycolysis, even under aerobic conditions (9-14). For the A_3-ATP model to work requires that the pasteur effect is not sufficient to compensate under conditions of oxygen limitation of aerobic energy production. Some published biochemical studies suggest that glycolysis can completely or nearly compensate during complete anoxia. Needleman (13) found no change in ATP concentration in rabbit aorta during anoxia, although creatine phosphate levels decreased significantly. Peterson and Paul (14) found there was no difference during anoxia in energy production computed from oxygen uptake plus lactate efflux in bovine mesentery artery. Other workers have measured rather small decreases in [ATP] in various vascular tissues during anoxia (11, 15). It is clear in rabbit aorta that there are sufficient energy stores during complete anoxia for contraction (10, 11, 13). After detectable oxygen uptake is inhibited by CN^-, isoproterenol relaxations are seen which are not very different from isoproterenol re-

laxations during control conditions, indicating the energy state
of the cell is sufficient for pumping of Ca out of the cell, or
into intracellular Ca depots (5).

Calculation of tissue PO_2 gradients in vascular strips to determine if the PO_2 in tissue core is low enough to limit respiratory
chain function has been performed as an approach to give insight
whether cytochrome a_3 could be the oxygen tension sensor involved
in PO_2 dependent mechanical tension. Figure 3 illustrates diffusion
of oxygen into tissue and the principal factors which influence
tissue PO_2 gradients. Pittman and Duling (6) calculated tissue PO_2
gradients in vascular strips and obtained evidence which suggested
that core tissue PO_2 may be low enough to limit respiratory chain
function; but it was necessary to use rather high oxygen uptake
values and a low diffusion coefficient to obtain low core PO_2 values.
Due to the many assumptions and uncertainties, this approach cannot
answer the question whether core PO_2 is low enough to limit cytochrome a_3 reactions with oxygen, but these interesting calculations

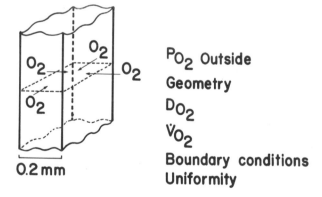

Figure 3.   Schematic representation of oxygen diffusion into
            strips of vascular smooth muscle. This figure illus-
            trates major factors which influence PO_2 gradients and
            core PO_2.

at least suggest the possibility that there is a PO_2 gradient as great as 200 mm Hg across 80 to 100 microns diffusion distances in vascular strips mounted in an organ bath. Fay (16) has measured polarographically, very steep PO_2 gradients in the guinea pig ductus arteriosis.

Consideration of factors which influence tissue PO_2 gradients in tissues points out the difficulty inherent in studying the mechanism of PO_2 dependent mechanical tension, using either biochemical or spectrophotometric techniques. Smooth muscle cells are electrically connected, and may be humorally connected, and at an organ bath PO_2 just below the critical PO_2 for a loss in mechanical tension, only a few muscle cells in the core may have a low enough PO_2 to cause a metabolic change. But it is possible that a biochemical event in these few cells could result in changes in mechanical tension in cells in the periphery of the strip. Therefore biochemical or spectrophotometric measurements at an organ bath PO_2 near the critical PO_2 might fail to demonstrate changes or be influenced by cells that have changes in tension but no oxygen limitation of respiratory chain function. Whereas, if studies are performed at very low organ bath PO_2, biochemical or spectrophotometric changes could be seen which are not related to the mechanism of PO_2 dependent mechanical tension. For this reason the biochemical data reviewed above in vascular tissue during complete anoxia are not completely pertinent to the mechanism of PO_2 dependent mechanical tension.

Figure 4 shows data obtained in our laboratory on strips of rabbit aorta, which are similar to data obtained by Kroeger and Stephens (17) on trachealis muscle, and Fay (3) on guinea pig ductus arteriosis. This type of data has been used to support the a_3-ATP or aerobic energy hypothesis. This figure shows the relationship of oxygen uptake ($\dot{V}O_2$) and mechanical tension in experiments where organ bath PO_2 was altered. Falls in mechanical tension with falls in organ bath PO_2, coincide with falls in $\dot{V}O_2$. But it seems to me that this is not very strong evidence that decreases in mechanical tension are a result of decreases in aerobic energy production since the $\dot{V}O_2$ fall could be a result of smaller metabolic demand. This presupposes the possibility that PO_2 dependent mechanical tension could involve a mechanism independent of respiratory chain function.

I now want to discuss data obtained in our laboratory from experiments aimed at identifying the oxygen tension sensor involved in PO_2 dependent mechanical tension (5, 18). It seemed to us that at this stage of knowledge about the mechanisms of PO_2 dependent

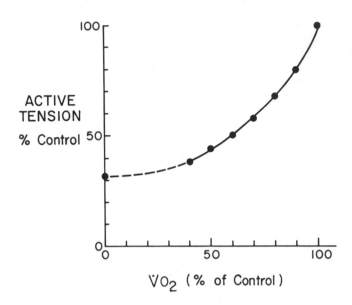

Figure 4. Relationships of oxygen uptake and mechanical tension
            in experiments where organ bath PO_2 is lowered in a
            graded manner. Experiments were performed on rabbit
            aorta strips. Bars indicate mean values with ±1 SEM.

mechanical tension, it is important to determine if the oxygen sensor is cytochrome a_3 or another oxygenase or receptor. We have
asked this question and our general approach has been to determine
if inhibition of oxygen uptake with respiratory chain inhibitors
causes the same effects on mechanical tension as occurs with decreasing organ bath PO_2. We used carbon monoxide (CO) and cyanide
(CN^-) because gases diffuse and equilibrate rapidly in tissue (CN^-
probably diffuses into tissue primarily as HCN at pH used in our
experiments). It was possible also to remove the inhibitors rapidly
and the preparation recovered and was stable with these inhibitors.
We attempted to use antimycin A, but the preparation never survived
and we could perform only one run with this inhibitor. The apparatu
used in these studies consists of an organ bath in which strips of
rabbit aorta can be mounted so that isometric tension can be determined. A PO_2 electrode in the apparatus allows measurement of ox-

ygen uptake when the top of the apparatus is closed. The bath is stirred with a small magnet to minimize stagnant layers. All studies were performed at 40°C. Rabbit aortic strips are dissected free of adventitia, but endothelium remains. Thickness of the strips varied from 0.17 to 0.23 mm. Resting oxygen uptake was $121 \pm$ (SD) 70 μl/g (wet weight) x hr. With addition of norepinephrine (4 x 10^{-6} g/ml), $\dot{V}O_2$ increased three fold to 325 ± 75 μl/g x hr. Mechanical tension-oxygen uptake relationships have already been shown in Figure 4.

In 1960 Lantz (19) noted that PO_2 dependent mechanical tension in rabbit aorta is blunted or absent during K contractions, as compared to norepinephrine contractions. We have taken advantage of this finding and have used K contractions as controls in our studies of effects of metabolic inhibitors on strips contracted with norepinephrine. In studying the reason for blunting of PO_2 dependent mechanical tension during K contractions, we determined that it is not due to a lesser oxygen uptake or to different organ bath PO_2-oxygen uptake relationships. So it is suggested that tissue PO_2 gradients and core PO_2 at a given organ bath PO_2 are similar with K and norepinephrine contractions. The reason for blunting of PO_2 dependent mechanical tension remains to be determined.

CN^- caused a dose dependent inhibition of oxygen uptake with the following characteristics. Threshold [CN^-] for an effect on oxygen uptake was $\cong$ 0.02 mM; 50% inhibition occurred at 0.1 mM and detectable $\dot{V}O_2$ was completely inhibited at [CN^-] in excess of 1 mM. There was no difference in [CN^-]-$\dot{V}O_2$ relationships with norepinephrine and K contractions.

Figure 5 compares effects of graded [CN^-] at a constant organ bath PO_2 of 200 mm Hg, and graded lowering of organ bath PO_2, on mechanical tension and oxygen uptake, during norepinephrine and 59 mM K contractions. During norepinephrine contractions, smaller relaxations were seen with CN^- for a given inhibition of aerobic metabolism than resulted from fall in organ bath PO_2. During K contractions there was no difference in effects of CN^- and lowered organ bath PO_2 on mechanical tensions at a given oxygen uptake. The findings during K contractions suggest that the mechanical effects of CN^- are due to inhibition of respiratory chain function since mechanical effects are the same as occur with an equivalent inhibition of $\dot{V}O_2$ due to lowering organ bath PO_2. Effects of CN^- and lowering organ bath PO_2 during K contractions are not different from effects of CN^- during norepinephrine contractions. Therefore, it seems likely that CN^- effects on norepinephrine mechanical tension are also related to decreasing respiratory chain function, and that much

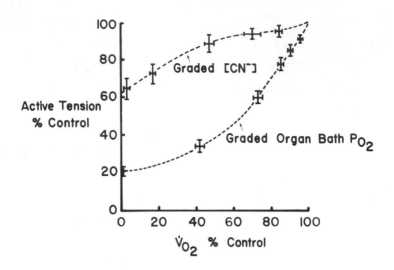

Figure 5A. Comparison of $\dot{V}O_2$-mechanical tension relationships
            resulting from graded CN^- or graded changes in organ
            bath PO_2 in rabbit aortic strips contracted with nor-
            epinephrine (1×10^{-6} g/ml).

larger relaxations seen with lowered organ bath PO_2 are due primarily
to an effect on an oxygenase or receptor, other than cytochrome a_3.
This conclusion was supported in experiments where we administered
CN^- after lowering organ bath PO_2 to nearly zero which had no effect
or caused a small relaxation.

If PO_2 dependent mechanical tension is related to an oxygen tension sensor other than cytochrome oxidase, mechanical tension should
be sensitive to changes in oxygen tension even under conditions where
the respiratory chain has been completely blocked. Figure 6 illustrates that this is indeed true. After administration of CN^-, during
norepinephrine contractions, at concentrations which completely blocked detectable oxygen uptake changes in organ bath PO_2 always resulted

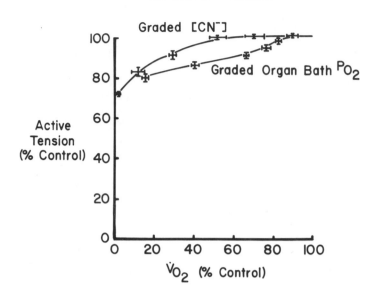

Figure 5B. Same comparison as in Figure 5A, but experiments were performed on rabbit strips contracted with 59 mM K. Maximal tension and oxygen uptake were not significantly different with maximal norepinephrine and with 59 mM K.

in changes in mechanical tension. Under control condition with K contractions, a similar experimental sequence failed to show PO_2 dependent mechanical tension. The persistence of PO_2 dependent mechanical tension with blocking of the respiratory chain during norepinephrine cannot be explained by competition of CN^- and O_2 for binding to cytochrome a_3 (20). Under conditions of zero $\dot{V}O_2$, tissue PO_2 should equal organ bath PO_2 so it is possible to determine the oxygen affinity of the oxygenase or receptor which is involved in PO_2 dependent mechanical tension. Experiments are now in process and

preliminary findings show PO_2 dependent mechanical tension at organ
bath PO_2 over the range of 5 to 30 mm Hg.

The usefulness of CO as an inhibitor was limited somewhat by
the small inhibition of oxygen uptake that occurred even at organ
bath P_{CO} as high as 540 mm Hg and PO_2 considerably less than 100 mm
Hg. On administering very high partial pressures of CO at constant
PO_2, mechanical tension fell 20-30% as shown in Figure 7. $\dot{V}O_2$-
mechanical relationships seen on administering CO indicate that for
a given fall in $\dot{V}O_2$ mechanical tension fell more than it did with
CN^-, but slightly less than occurred with falls in organ bath PO_2.
A major finding with CO was that administration of CO after CN^- had
completely inhibited detectable $\dot{V}O_2$, resulted in a large relaxation,
similar to the finding on reducing organ bath PO_2 during CN^- inhibition of respiration. These findings suggest that the effect of CO
on mechanical tension is not due to reaction with cytochrome a_3. We

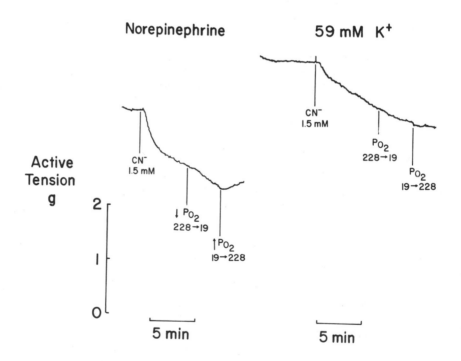

Figure 6.   Effects of altering organ bath PO_2 after administration
of CN^- at a concentration which completely inhibited detectable oxygen uptake.

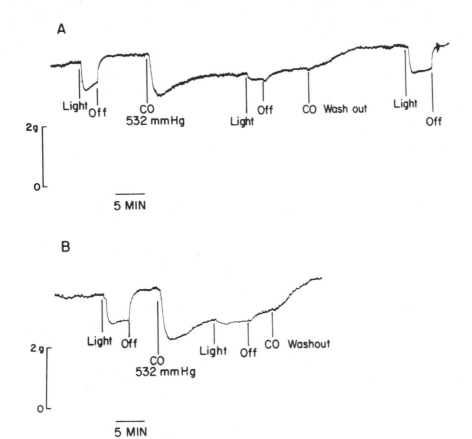

Figure 7. Effects of "light" on mechanical tension, before and
after administration of carbon monoxide. Data from two
different experiments.

attempted to strengthen this interpretation by photodissociating CO
and cytochrome a_3 using "light" (21). Focusing tungsten "light" on
the preparation reversed the fall in oxygen uptake due to CO, but
did not reverse the tension, as shown in Figure 7. The data were
complicated by the well known finding (22) that smooth muscle relaxes
with "light" under control conditions. After CO the "light" relaxation was always smaller, but there was never a slow contraction as
seen by Fay (3) in his studies of effects of CO on mechanical tension

in the guinea pig ductus arteriosis. The CO data are consistent with
data seen with CN$^-$ and seem to be best explained by reaction of CO
with a oxygenase or receptor other than cytochrome oxidases, which
is involved in CO relaxations.

Our experiments to date have produced three findings which seem
not to be consistent with the cytochrome a_3 - ATP model, and which
suggest that another oxygen sensor is involved in PO_2 dependent mechanical tension. These findings are: the inability of CN$^-$ to cause
relaxations as large as those seen with lowering of organ bath PO_2
and evidence that effects of CN$^-$ on mechanical tension are due to
inhibition of the respiratory chain; the finding that mechanical tension is still affected by alteration in organ bath PO_2 after inhibition of detectable oxygen uptake by CN$^-$ treatment; the finding that
CO has an effect on mechanical tension under conditions where the
respiratory chain is blocked with cyanide. Our inability to reverse
CO relaxations by photodissociation of CO from cytochrome a_3 is weaker
evidence. The reader is referred to previous publications (5) for
a more complete discussion of the strengths and limitations of our
approaches.

Our interpretations of the CN$^-$ data lean heavily on the use of
K contractions as "controls". There is evidence that energy production during K contractions is more aerobic and less glycolytic than
during norepinephrine contractions (10, 11, 13), and there may be
other metabolic differences. However if PO_2 dependent mechanical
tension is due solely to falls in energy production, it would seem
that K contractions should be more susceptible. But PO_2 dependent
mechanical tension was blunted during K contractions in our experiments. With CN$^-$ inhibition of respiration, tension was always greater
at a given $\dot{V}O_2$ than was seen with falls in organ bath PO_2. This indicates either that energy is used more efficiently (perhaps a slower
rate of cross bridge cycling) or that more glycolytic energy was
utilized to maintain tension during CN$^-$. It seems most likely that
if glycolytic energy production was higher during CN$^-$ inhibition of
the respiratory chain, than with lowered PO_2 inhibition, that this
reflected increased metabolic demand.

Fay has published very interesting experiments (3, 16) using
the guinea pig ductus arteriosus which show evidence for oxygen tension limitation of energy production as the cause for relaxations
which occur in this tissue during falls in organ bath PO_2. These
data are really not in conflict with ours, assuming that mechanisms
are the same in the different tissues. Our data suggest (on the
basis of CN$^-$ experiments) that a portion of PO_2 dependent mechanical
tension is due to inhibition of respiratory chain function. However,
our data show that the organ bath PO_2 threshold for an effect mediated by inhibition of the respiratory chain is lower and effects are

relatively small compared to relaxations not explained by inhibition of aerobic energy production.

Most of my comments have been about possible oxygen tension sensors in vascular smooth muscle. There is very little hard data about transduction of information from oxygen sensor to contractile protein. B. Johannson (personal communication) and Yamaguchi and Stephens (23) have described membrane depolarization, in rat mesenteric vein and trachealis muscle respectively, due to falls in bathing solution PO_2, suggesting that the surface membrane may be involved in the transduction process. Our finding that K abolishes portion of PO_2 dependent mechanical tension which cannot be explained by inhibition of aerobic energy production also could be explained if a membrane potential dependent process is involved.

In conclusion; we add another hypothesis to those already published to explain PO_2 dependent mechanical tension in vascular strips. Our interest in this phenomenon in vascular smooth muscle is that this tissue may be considerably simpler for study of physiological effects of altered PO_2, in that in all likelihood only one cell type is involved, compared to the complexity of determining oxygen sensors and transduction processes in such systems as carotid body or the pulmonary circulation. Evidence that a "physiological" effect of hypoxia may be mediated by a mechanism other than inhibition of aerobic energy production appears to be the first found in any mammalian tissue.

1. Carrier, O., Jr., Walker, J.R., and Guyton, A.C. Role of oxygen in autoregulation of blood flow in isolated vessels. Am. J. Physiol. 206: 951-954, 1964.

2. Detar, R., and Bohr, D.F. Oxygen and vascular smooth muscle contraction, Am. J. Physiol. 214: 241-244, 1968.

3. Fay, F.S. Guinea pig ductus arteriosus. I. Cellular and metabolic basis for oxygen sensitivity. Am. J. Physiol. 221: 470-479, 1971.

4. Smith, D.J., and Vane, J.R. Effects of oxygen tension on vascular and other smooth muscle. J. Physiol. 186: 284-294, 1966.

5. Coburn, R.F., Grubb, B., and Aronson, R. Oxygen tension sensing in rabbit aorta. Submitted for publication.

6. Pittman, R.N., and Duling, B.R. Oxygen sensitivity of vascular smooth muscle. I. In Vitro studies. Microvascular Res. 6: 202-211, 1973.

7. Chance, B., Oshino, N., Sugano, T., and Mayevsky, A. Basic
    principles of tissue oxygen determination from mitochondrial
    signals. In: Oxygen Transport to Tissue, Plenum Press, New
    York, 1973, p. 277-291.

8. Finlayson, B., Lymn, R.W., and Taylor, E.W. Studies on the
    kinetics of formation and dissociation of the actomyosin com-
    plex. Biochem. 8: 811-819, 1969.

9. Lymn, R.W., and Taylor, E.W. Transient state phosphate produc-
    tion in the hydrolysis of nucleoside triphosphates by myosin.
    Biochem. 9: 2975-2983, 1970.

10. Shibata, S., and Briggs, A.H. Mechanical activity of vascular
    smooth muscle under anoxia. Am. J. Physiol. 212: 981-984, 1967.

11. Lundholm, L., and Mohme-Lundholm, E. Energetics of isometric
    and isotonic contraction in isolated vascular smooth muscle un-
    der anaerobic conditions. Acta Physiol. Scand. 65: 275-282, 1965.

12. Lundholm, L. and Mohme-Lundholm, E. Dissociation of contraction
    and stimulation of lactic acid production in experiments on
    smooth muscle under anaerobic conditions. Acta Physiol. Scand.
    57: 111-124, 1963.

13. Needleman, P., and Blehm, D.J. Effect of epinephrine and potas-
    sium chloride on contraction and energy intermediates in rabbit
    thoracic aorta strips. Life Sciences 9: 1181-1189, 1970.

14. Peterson, J.W., and Paul, R.J. Aerobic glycolysis in vascular
    smooth muscle: relation to isometric tension, Biochem. et Bio-
    phys. Acta 357: 167-176, 1974.

15. Van Harn, G.L., Rubio, R., and Berne, R.M. Adenine nucleotide
    formation in vascular smooth muscle during hypoxia. The Physi-
    ologist 19: 398, 1976.

16. Fay, F. Oxygen tension sensors in ductus arteriosis. This Sym-
    posium. 1976.

17. Kroeger, E., and Stephens, N.L. Effect of hypoxia on energy
    and calcium metabolism in airway smooth muscle. Am. J. Physiol.
    220: 1199-1204, 1971.

18. Grubb, B. and Coburn, R.F. O_2 dependent mechanical tension.
    The Physiologist 19: 212, 1976.

19. Laszt, L. Effect of potassium on muscle tension especially on
    that of vascular muscle. Nature 185: 696, 1960.

20. Yonetani, T. and Ray, G.S.   Studies of cytochrome oxidase VI.
     Kinetics of the aerobic oxidation of ferrocytochrome c by cyto-
     chrome oxidase. J. Biol. Chem. 240: 3392-3398, 1965.

21. Keilin, D., and Hartree, E.F. Cytochrome and cytochrome oxi-
     dase. Proc. Roy. Soc. London, Ser. B., 127: 167-191, 1939.

22. Furchgott, R.F., Ehrreich, S.J., and Greenblatt, E. The photo-
     activated relaxation of smooth muscle of rabbit aorta. J. Gen.
     Physiol. 44: 499-519, 1961.

23. Yamaguchi, H., Stephens, N.L., and Dhalla, N.S. Electrophsiolog-
     ical effects of hypoxia in tracheal smooth muscle. Fed. Proc.
     35: 776, 1976.

COMMENTS ON: OXYGEN TENSION SENSORS IN VASCULAR SMOOTH MUSCLE

Richard J. Paul

Department of Physiology, University College

London

In assessing the effects of hypoxia in vascular smooth muscle (VSM), one often uses isometric force as an index of the energy available to the muscle and oxygen uptake as a measure of the cellular ATP production. Such interpretation, as with all biological models, is subject to shortcoming. I think it would be useful as a first step in the discussion to examine the relation between isometric force and ATP utilization under normoxic conditions where aerobic metabolism is not oxygen-diffusion limited.

To be brief, the simple text-book picture originally developed for skeletal muscle can be applied in a straightforward manner to vascular smooth muscle. That is, increased isometric force is a reflection of an increase in the actomyosin cycling, which through its ATPase activity causes the ADP levels to rise which in turn is the signal to intermediary metabolism for the observed increased thru put. There are several aspects peculiar to VSM however, that are relevant to the discussion.

The amount of phosphagen (predominantly ATP & PCr, about 2 μMole/g) in VSM is small in comparison to skeletal muscle. The preformed phosphagen pool is less than required by the muscle to develop the peak of an isometric contraction, while in the absence of ATP synthesis, even basal levels of ATP utilization would exhaust all available phosphagen in several minutes. This implies that contractile ATP utilization and its metabolic resynthesis must be tightly coupled, particularly in a temporal sense. This aspect will be important when interpreting the results from metabolically inhibited tissues. An example of the coupling between isometric force and the rate of oxygen uptake (J_{O_2}) is shown in the Figure 1

117

for graded isometric contractions in bovine mesenteric vein.

Now although oxygen uptake is a monitor of metabolic thru put, it does not give a complete picture of the total ATP production. A rather unusual aspect of VSM energy metabolism is the relatively large contribution of aerobic glycolysis. In fact most (on the order of 80% to 90%) of the glucose carbon ends up as lactate, though in terms of ATP synthesis, only 15% to 30% is accounted for by

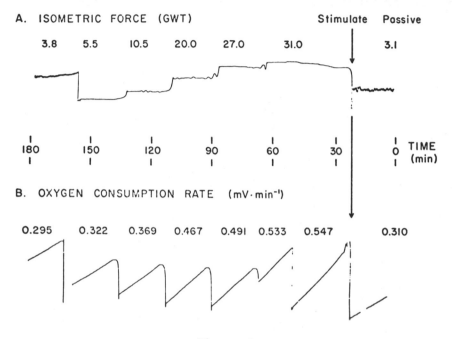

Figure 1

A. A record of the graded isometric forces maintained at fixed length (resting length L_o, at which passive tension = 1 gram weight) during a sequence of decreasing epinephrine concentrations following maximal stimulation. Time runs from right to left, and the values of isometric force are given. The change in force scale from passive to stimulated is 5 : 1.

B. Simultaneous record of oxygen electrode output during the sequence in (A). The rate of decline of the oxygen concentration in the muscle chamber is given, and may be converted to units of oxygen consumption using 0.05 µmole O_2 per mV. Fast vertical rises in the O_2 trace are due to either partial flushes of the chamber with aerated physiological saline, which both dilutes the stimulant and returns the O_2 tension to near that of air, or simply changes in electrical bias to keep the O_2 trace on recorder scale. (J. Mechanochemistry and Cell Motility 3:19-32, 1974.)

aerobic glycolysis. Under certain conditions, for example under
epinephrine, norepinephrine or histamine stimulation, the rate of
lactate production is proportional to J_{O_2}, thus the contribution of
aerobic glycolysis to the total ATP production is constant. An example of this is shown in Figure 2. However, under k^+-depolariza-
tion, aerobic glycolysis does not increase with force as does J_{O_2},
but remains at or below the unstimulated levels. In this case the
rate of O_2 uptake per unit force is greater than its value under
pharmacological stimulation; though importantly, the rate of ATP
utilization per unit actomyosin interaction is not apparently a
function of the means of stimulation. I want to stress that one
must keep in mind the whole of aerobic metabolism (oxidative phosphorylation and glycolysis) when interpreting tissue sensitivity to
oxygen; oxygen uptake alone may give one an erroneous impression.
For a detailed review of the energy metabolism in VSM, one is referred to the work of Paul & Rüegg[1].

One should also keep in mind that there is a great variability
among the various types of vascular muscle in their sensitivity to
oxygen. For example, bovine mesenteric artery and vein can maintain
isometric tension equally well in the presence or absence of oxygen
as well as showing a nearly text-book Pasteur effect. Rabbit aorta
and porcine carotid artery cannot maintain full isometric tension in
the absence of oxygen, while the residual tension in anoxia appears
to be a function of the stimulation. Others, notably the ductus
arteriosis can under certain conditions have an absolute oxygen
requirement for tension. It will be of interest to see if a coherent
pattern to explain this variability in oxygen sensitivity can emerge
in the course of these workshop discussions.

Dr. Coburn has argued that a limitation of ATP available to the
contractile apparatus mediated by the O_2 sensitivity of cytochrome a_3
is not the mechanism of the oxygen-sensitive tension. These experiments provide evidence against oxidative phosphorylation as the
oxygen sensor, though not against the total ATP supply being a limiting factor in view of what was said about aerobic glycolysis.
However, a limitation of energy supply as a mechanism for tension
regulation is unlikely on other grounds. If the tissue ATP synthesis lagged the actomyosin ATPase, the low phosphagen stores would
rapidly be reduced to zero. This would lead to competition amongst
the various ATP requiring cellular processes, formation of rigor-
links and teleologically, a not too happy picture for the cell.
Fortunately there is data available on the phosphagen content of
rabbit aorta during hypoxia which show that even under anoxic conditions, the ATP content is reduced by less than 50% compared to
aerobic conditions[2,3]. In fact, the data indicate that the fall in
tension with oxygen partial pressure occurs well before any reduction in cellular ATP is observed. Though not absolutely conclusive,
the available data indicates that a reduction of the actomyosin
ATPase itself is a direct end product of hypoxia in some tissues.

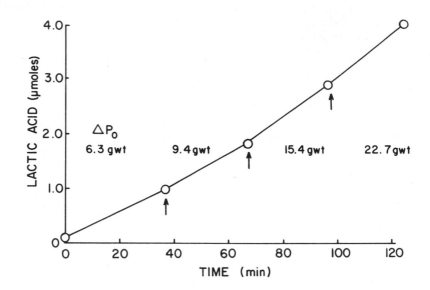

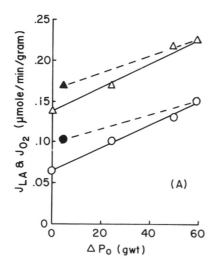
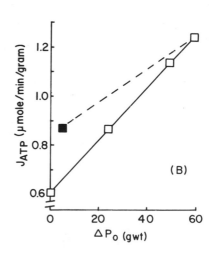

Figure 2

Upper: The total lactic acid content of the muscle chamber (20 ml volume) is plotted against time for a sequence of graded isometric tensions, similar to that shown in Fig. 1(A), for another tissue. In this case, isometric tension was increased stepwise by the addition of submaximal doses of epinephrine (arrows) immediately following the withdrawal of a small sample of the bathing solution for chemical analysis of lactic acid. The slope between points is therefore the average lactic acid production rate over the time interval, which is seen to increase in parallel with the stable graded isometric tension.

Lower: (A) Plot of oxygen consumption rate J_{O_2} (o) and lactic acid production rate J_{LA} (Δ) measured in a single vein segment by the procedures illustrated above and in Fig. 1. Both J_{O_2} and J_{LA} depend linearly on the graded active isometric forces maintained at rest length for varying degrees of activation. At the minimum contracted tissue length (L_{min}), at which maximal pharmacological stimulation yields no active isometric force (about ½ the resting length), the values of J_{O_2} and J_{LA} (closed symbols) are each found to be about 20% greater than their respective basal values.

(B) J_{O_2} and J_{LA} data from (A) are each converted, using standard biochemical ratios, to equivalent rates of ATP synthesis and summed. The linear dependence of J_{ATP} on active isometric force, and an elevation of J_{ATP} above the basal level at L_{min} are evident. While the data here is for epinephrine stimulation, similar results are obtained for norepinephrine and histamine stimulation. The reduction in data scatter around the linear plots of J_{O_2} and J_{LA} upon summing to J_{ATP} is statistically significant. (Biochimica et Biophysica Acta 357:167-176, 1974.)

The most obvious control point for the actomyosin ATPase is at the level of intracellular Ca^{++}. To be sure, more subtle control points exist, such as the pH dependence of the troponin-tropomyosin regulatory proteins as well as a possible phosphorylation dependence of the myosin light chains in a myosin-linked regulatory scheme. In the first instance, however, a dependence of intracellular Ca^{++} on the external oxygen concentration would be the first place to look for a mechanism of oxygen-sensitive tension.

On a purely speculative level, a Ca^{++} compartment whose ability to accumulate Ca^{++} was a function of cellular ADP levels could provide the necessary link between oxygen concentration and tension. This could explain a fall in tension with hypoxia as well as the oxygen-sensitivity of tension in ductus arteriosis accompanying increased ATP synthesis as proposed by Fay (c.f. This symposium). In view of the ADP requirement for Ca^{++} accumulation[4], one is quite tempted to identify the mitochondria as providing such a compartment. (One might expect increased ADP levels in hypoxia which could cause an increase in mitochondrial Ca^{++} uptake and thus lower levels of actomyosin interaction; similarly, increased ATP production with oxygen concentration in the ductus would lower the ADP levels and have the opposite effect on tension.) However, such a simple model could not be readily reconciled with the data on the effects of cyanide poisoning as just presented by Dr. Coburn. In any case, it appears that the dependence of tension on O_2 concentration cannot be explained in terms of a limitation on energy supply in some tissues. This suggests the existence of a rather novel class of oxygen sensors in VSM.

REFERENCES

1. Paul, R.J. & Rüegg, J.C. (1976). Biochemistry of vascular smooth muscle: proteins of the contractile apparatus and their relationship to energy metabolism. In, Altura, B.M. & Kaley, G. (eds.) Microcirculation. University Park Press, Baltimore.

2. Namm, D.H. & Zucker, J.L. (1973). Biochemical alterations caused by hypoxia in the isolated rabbit aorta. Correlation with changes in arterial contractility. Circ. Res. 32:464-470.

3. Needleman, P. & Blehm, D.J. (1970). Effect of epinephrine and potassium chloride on contraction and energy intermediates in rabbit thoracic aorta strips. Life Sci. 9:1181-1189.

4. Leblanc, P. & Clauser, H. (1974). ADP and Mg^{2+} requirement for Ca^{2+} accumulation by hog heart mitochondria. Correlation with energy coupling. Biochim. Biophys. Acta 347:87-101.

MECHANISM OF OXYGEN INDUCED CONTRACTION OF DUCTUS ARTERIOSUS

Fredric S. Fay, Pankajam Nair*, and William J. Whalen*

University of Massachusetts Medical School
Department of Physiology, Worcester, Massachusetts and
*St. Vincent Charity Hospital, Cleveland, Ohio

The ductus arteriosus is a wide muscular artery that connects
the aorta and pulmonary artery allowing blood ejected by the right
ventricle to by-pass the non-functional pulmonary bed in utero.
Shortly after birth, the ductus constricts due to the contraction
of its smooth muscle. Numerous investigators (1,2,3,4) have drawn
attention to the postnatal increase in arterial oxygen pressure as
a stimulus for muscular closure of the ductus arteriosus. Although
other agents may act to constrict the vessel in vivo (1,3,5,6,7,8)
increased oxygen pressure appears to be the major factor responsible for closure of the ductus at birth. The studies described
here represent an attempt to understand the mechanism underlying
the constrictor effect of oxygen on this blood vessel. All of
the studies have been performed on the ductus arteriosus of the
neonatal guinea pig mounted for isometric measurement of force in
an organ bath.

Figure 1 shows typical contractile responses of several ductus
preparations to oxygen, acetylcholine and potassium. As can be
seen, upon increasing the oxygen pressure to 680 mm Hg a pronounced
contraction characterized by a stepwise increase in force was
noted. The O_2 induced contraction is entirely reversed when the
oxygen pressure is returned to 35 mm Hg. Under anaerobic conditions, the addition of acetylcholine or exposure to K^+ substituted
Ringer produces a prompt increase in force which is sustained.
The responses to O_2, K^+ and acetylcholine were obtained from three
different preparations. In a single preparation the response to
oxygen was always greater than the maximum response to either K^+
or acetylcholine. This is quite different from other smooth
muscles where transition from anaerobic to aerobic conditions

123

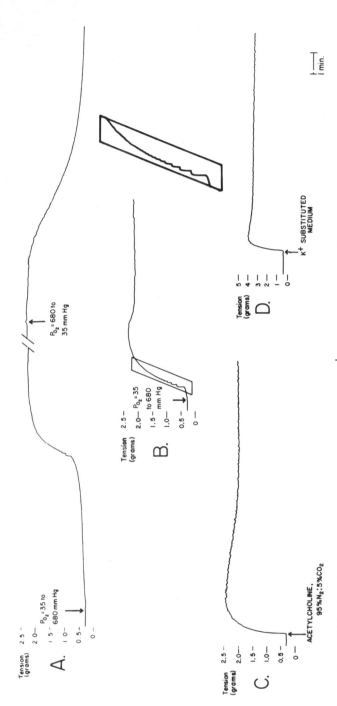

Figure 1. Effect of oxygen, acetylcholine, and K^+ on muscle tension of ductus arteriosus. Parts A–D are polygraph records of muscle tension for 4 different preparations. Changes in PO_2 and K^+ were accomplished by rapid replacement of solution in organ bath. Preparations A and B differed in following way: A had been in organ bath for 20 min. only at low PO_2; B had been in organ bath for several hours, and had contracted and relaxed several times in response to changes in PO_2. Inset in B is a X2 enlargement of tension record during rapid phase of oxygen response; note stepwise tension increments which become smaller but occur with greater frequency as response progresses. Acetylcholine (20 μg/ml) was rapidly injected into organ bath at arrow in C; effects of acetylcholine and K^+ were studied while PO_2 was maintained at 0 mm Hg. In 4 examples shown, tension developed in response to supramaximal levels of acetylcholine or K^+ was greater than responses to oxygen; also at supramaximal concentration. However, in any one preparation the maximal response to oxygen was always greater than that to K^+ or acetylcholine.

yields a slight contractile response which is a small fraction of
the response to K^+ or excitatory transmitters. The steady state
relationship between tension and P_{O_2} for several ducts is shown
in Figure 2.   In these experiments the lumen was perfused with
the bath solution to prevent stagnation of the fluid therein.   As
can be seen the range of maximum sensitivity occurred between 0
and 100 mm Hg, and as P_{O_2} was increased beyond 200 mm Hg no further
increase in force was noted.

     The response to oxygen appears to result from a direct effect
of oxygen on the smooth muscle cells. This conclusion is based on
several lines of evidence. For one, antagonists to all transmitters
known to cause excitation of the ductus fail to blunt the response
to oxygen (3,9). Secondly, nervous reflexes are ruled out by the
finding that local anaesthetics and tetrodotoxin have no inhibitory
effect on the response to oxygen (9). Finally, when the vessel is
subject to gradients of oxygen pressure it responds as if it was
sensing the P_{O_2} within the media, which is composed only of smooth
muscle cells (9). Since the ductus arteriosus is a predominantly
muscular artery (10) and since the response to oxygen occurs by
a direct effect on the smooth muscle cells, this vessel represents
a fortuitous system in which to investigate the biochemical basis
for the response of a tissue to oxygen.

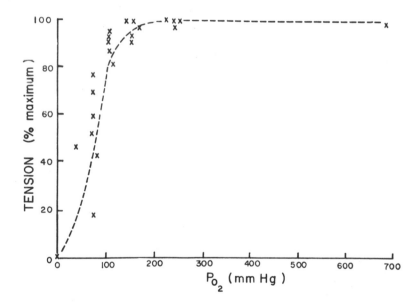

Figure 2.   Effect of P_{O_2} on muscle tension of double-perfused ductus arteriosus. P_{O_2} was varied simultaneously in fluid perfusing
the vessel lumen and organ bath. Each point represents steady-
state tension for a given P_{O2} of a single preparation.

Studies with some inhibitions of the normal respiratory chain (Table 1) suggested that the effects of oxygen might result from increased flux through the cytochrome chain. As can be seen, 1mM cyanide or 0.6 mM chlorobutanol selectively abolished the contractile response to oxygen whereas the response to other stimuli such as acetylcholine or K^+ persisted albeit at a slightly reduced level. These results suggest the involvement of a normal mammalian respiratory chain in the response to oxygen. However, inhibitors such as NaCN are far from specific and thus other studies have been performed to evaluate the involvement of the cytochromes in the response to O_2. In order to assess the possible involvement of cytochrome a_3 in the response of the ductus to oxygen, since it is the usual terminal oxidase in other mammalian cytochrome chains, 10% O_2 and 85% CO were bubbled through the organ bath. In the presence of carbon monoxide, which is known to bind to cytochrome a_3 in other tissues thereby preventing its interaction with oxygen, the normal contractile response to 10% O_2 was inhibited by 30% on the average while the response to other contractile agonists remained unchanged. Of particular interest was the finding that the CO-induced inhibition of the ductus was relieved by illumination quite in line with the known ability of light to dissociate the CO-cytochrome a_3 complex (11, 12). In order to clearly pinpoint the site of CO-inhibition the effectiveness of light of equal intensity but variable wavelength in reversing the CO-inhibition was tested. Figure 3 shows the relative effectiveness of monochromatic light in reversing the CO-inhibition of the O_2 response. Light at all wavelengths between 410 and 460 nm reversed the inhibition thereby allowing for contraction; however, the maximal photoactivated contraction was obtained between 425 and 430 nm. The average action spectrum is quite similar to that for this individual ductus exhibiting its peak between 420 and 425 nm, slightly lower than for this individual preparation. The observed spectrum is quite similar to that from photodissociation of CO from cytochrome a_3 (11,12) which has its peak at 430 nm. The photoactivated contraction might therefore be understood as being due to the photoinduced dissociation of CO from cytochrome a_3 which is then free to react with O_2 thereby increasing force in some manner.

In order to more fully characterize the cytochrome system in the ductus and to directly determine the relationship between cytochrome a_3 redox state and the oxygen induced contraction spectrophotometric techniques were applied to the intact tissue. Anaerobic-aerobic difference spectra exhibited peaks at 430 and 445 nM characteristic of cytochromes $a-a_3$ and b respectively (14). The only atypical aspect of the spectra was the relatively greater amount of cytochrome b in the ductal tissue when compared to skeletal muscle (13). However, the relative abundance of cytochrome b was also noted in the guinea pig aorta, although it was not seen in taenia coli (13). Since cytochrome a_3 appears by spectral observations to be present in the ductus we directly tested for the

Table 1. Effect of inhibitors of oxidative phosphorylation on response of ductus arteriosus to oxygen and acetylcholine.

Inhibitor	No. of Exp.	% Inhibition of Response to		P	Effect on Oxidative Phosphorylation (Ref.)
		Oxygen	Acetylcholine (peak/ steady state)		
NaCN, 1 mM	7	77 ± 7	4 ± 3/ 8 ± 4	>.001	Inhibits e^- transfer between cytochrome a_3 and O_2 (15)
Chlorobutanol, 0.6 mM	4	98 ± 1	36 ± 14/ 44 ± 15	>.01	Inhibits e^- transfer between NADH-linked fp. and cytochrome b (16)
Pentachlorophenol, 50 µM	4	92 ± 5	26 ± 15/ 15 ± 15	>.01	Uncouples oxidative phosphorylation (17)
2,4-Dinitrophenol, 0.5 mM	4	81 ± 7	11 ± 8/ 10 ± 6	>.001	Uncouples oxidative phosphorylation (18)
Oligomycin, 60 µM	4	65 ± 13	7 ± 4 4 ± 4	>.001	Inhibits the reaction: $X \sim I + P_i \rightleftarrows X \sim P + I$ [*] (19)

Percent inhibition was calculated from the tension increment in response to O_2 or acetylcholine with and without inhibitor present. Degree of inhibition is mean ± SE. The extent of inhibition of the peak and steady-state tension increments in response to acetylcholine is given separately. P values are calculated for the difference between inhibition of the oxygen response and inhibition of either the peak or steady-state response to acetylcholine, whichever was larger. [*] $X \sim I$ and $X \sim P$ are hypothetical high-energy intermediates of oxidative phosphorylation as defined by Jöbsis (14).

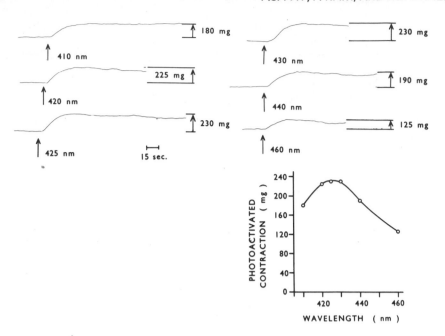

Figure 3. Effect on a ductus arteriosus of illumination with monochromatic light in presence of 85.5% CO and 9.5% O_2. Upper part
of figure shows actual records of increase in tension on illumination with light of different wavelengths. Responses were elicited
in order going from 410 to 460 nm. Numbers at right of each
record indicate amplitude of light-induced tension increment at
its peak. Graph in lower right shows amplitude of these photoinduced contractions plotted as a function of wavelength. Band
width of "monochromatic" light was 3.3 nm.

involvement of this enzyme in the contractile response to oxygen
by simultaneously monitoring cytochrome a_3 redox state and the
tension exerted by the smooth muscle within the ductus arteriosus
following changes in oxygen pressure. The experiments were performed utilizing a dual-wavelength micro-spectrophotometer. The
ductus was illuminated alternatively by pulses of light at 445 nm,
the absorption maximum for reduced cytochrome a_3, and at 465 nm,
used as reference wavelength, to correct for non-specific changes
in light absorption. If the primary site of O_2 interaction is
cytochrome a_3, one would expect that changes in tension induced by
oxygen should always be preceded by changes in the oxidation state
of cytochrome a_3. Secondly, one would also predict that in the
steady state, over the entire range of oxygen pressures where tension
is sensitive to oxygen, changes in a_3 oxidation state should also
be noted.

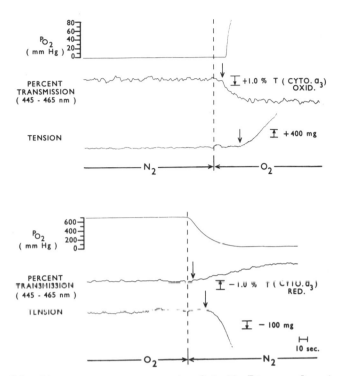

Figure 4. Simultaneous measurement of bath P_{O_2}, and cytochrome a_3 oxidation and tension of a ductus arteriosus preparation. Upper and lower groups of three polygraph records were obtained from same preparation. Uppermost trace in each group registers bath P_{O_2} as monitored with an oxygen electrode. Middle trace in each group indicates cytochrome a_3 oxidation state as measured at 445-465 nm; calibration at right denotes a 1% decrease in optical transmission at 445 nm minus that at 465 nm. Oxidation of cytochrome a_3 results in a decrease in transmission at 445-465 nm. Upper: at dotted line 95% O_2-5% CO_2 was substituted for 95% N_2-5% CO_2 bubbling through tissue chamber. Arrows above optical and mechanical records indicate first noticeable change in these traces after switching gases. Output of P_{O_2} electrode went off scale above 80 mm Hg and record is therefore discontinued above 80 mm Hg. Lower: at dotted line 95% N_2-5% CO_2 was substituted for 95% O_2-5% CO_2 bubbling through bath; coincident with switch in gases, chamber was rapidly rinsed with 3X its volume of Krebs-Ringer bicarbonate saline which had been pre-equilibrated with 95% N_2-5% CO_2 at 37°C. Arrows above optical and mechanical records indicate first noticeable change in these traces after switching to anaerobic conditions.

Results bearing on the first point are shown in Figure 4.
These traces, typical for all 12 ductus preparations studied, show
that a shift from anaerobic to aerobic conditions resulted in an
increase in cytochrome a_3 oxidation which <u>always</u> preceded the O_2
induced force increment. In this particular preparation the onset
of the increase in cytochrome a_3 oxidation preceded the development
of force by 20 seconds. The contraction per se had little or no
effect on the optical signal as judged by experiments in which the
ductus was induced to contract by acetylcholine under anoxic conditions. As may also be seen in Figure 4 a_3 reduction preceded
the first decline in force when this same preparation was returned
to anaerobic conditions. This was seen in all 4 preparations in
which this maneuver was performed. In this particular experiment
the lag between the onset of a_3 reduction and the decline in tension was about 12 seconds. Using similar techniques we have shown the
changes in force induced by oxygen are correlated with changes in
a_3 oxidation over the entire range of force (13). The available
evidence therefore indicates that the first in the sequence of
events underlying the contractile response to O_2 is an interaction
between it and cytochrome a_3.

We have also found that oxygen uptake by the ductus exhibits
the same dependence on P_{O_2} as does muscle tension (9). The similarity of the dependence of both oxygen uptake and muscle tension
on oxygen pressure does not appear to reflect the metabolic cost
of contraction. This follows from the observation that in a ductus
preparation exposed to 5% O_2, in which a measurable force and oxygen uptake were noted, initiation of a further contraction by
acetylcholine produced no further increase in oxygen consumption
(9). These results indicate that cytochrome a_3 oxidation in turn
appears to trigger contraction because it increases the turnover
rate of the cytochrome chain. There is an apparent paradox to the
hypothesis developed thus far. Both Q_{O_2} and tension are sensitive
to changes in oxygen pressure over a much wider range than that
known to affect the cytochrome a_3/cytochrome oxidase system.
Whereas the ductus responds to changes in P_{O_2} between 0 and 200
mm Hg the Km of cytochrome oxidase is usually given as below 1 mm
Hg, P_{O_2} (14,15). This apparent contradiction may be reconciled if
steep gradients for P_{O_2} exist within the wall of the ductus.

As can be seen in Figure 5 measurements of intratissue P_{O_2}
with an ultramicro-oxygen cathode (20) reveal a steep gradient for
P_{O_2} within the wall of the ductus. In these experiments an ultra-
micro oxygen electrode was driven in a series of steps through the
wall of a ductus exposed to 75, 148 and 375 mm Hg while steady-
state isometric force was measured. At the end of every experiment
like this the preparation was fixed in the experimental chamber and
histology performed to enable us to relate the penetration distance
to the three different characteristic layers of the vessel. As may
be seen at 75 and 148 mm Hg, where muscle tension is submaximal, a
portion of the media remains anoxic; only at 375 mm Hg P_{O_2} was

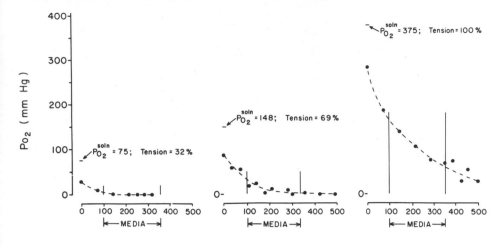

DISTANCE (μm)

Figure 5. P_{O_2} gradients within the wall of a ductus arteriosus exposed to three different P_{O_2}'s in solution. When a steady-state tension response to the P_{O_2}soln was attained, an ultramicro-oxygen electrode was driven in a series of steps through the wall of the ductus. Three such penetrations were made at each P_{O_2}soln. The points show the mean P_{O_2} as a function of distance from the outer surface of the vessel. Note that although the organ bath was vigorously stirred a significant unstirred layer was found near the edge of the vessel as denoted by the drop in P_{O_2} before entering the tissue. The steady-state tension at each P_{O_2}soln is given as a percent of response to 95% O_2. The distance within the vessel corresponding to the media is noted in each trace.

there no anoxic region within the media and at this P_{O_2} maximal muscle tension was produced. At 75 mm Hg P_{O_2}, 39% of the media had a detectable P_{O_2}, whereas at 148 mm Hg the percentage of the wall receiving a detectable amount of oxygen had increased to 81%. This parallels quite nicely the increase in tension observed as P_{O_2} was increased from 0 to 75 and then to 148 mm Hg. In over 70 penetrations in 7 vessels we always found that when submaximal forces were produced some portion of the media remained anoxic. When a maximal response to oxygen was measured there was never any region of the media that remained anoxic. Thus, the presence of steep gradients of P_{O_2} within the wall of the ductus are entirely consistent with the hypothesis that cytochrome a_3 is the primary O_2 sensor underlying the contractile response of the ductus arteriosus to oxygen.

The next question we turned to is how the increased flux through the cytochrome chain triggered by the increased oxidation of cytochrome a$_3$ in turn leads to contraction. The answers here are far less complete. As can be seen from Table 1, agents which prevent the coupling of electron transport to the synthesis of ATP from ADP block the contractile effect of O$_2$ on the ductus. The inhibitory effect of pentochlorophenol or oligomycin on the oxygen induced contraction is quite specific, as seen by the fact that the response to other contractile stimuli such as acetylcholine is largely unaffected. Thus it appears likely that the effect of oxygen on contractile activity is mediated via an increased rate of synthesis of high-energy phosphate compounds. Increased synthesis of ATP somehow causes the ductus to contract. It seems unlikely that this is a direct result of increased availability of ATP to the contractile machinery since the ductus apparently has sufficient ATP under anoxic conditions to contract and maintain tension in response to K$^+$ or acetylcholine. If it can be assumed that contraction of the ductus in response to O$_2$ results from activation of the contractile apparatus by Ca^{+2}, as occurs in other muscles, then it may be that the unique O$_2$ sensitivity of the ductus resides in the step or steps which link oxidative synthesis of ATP and the control of intracellular Ca^{+2}. It is relevant to note here that the step-like manner in which tension increases in response to O$_2$ is characteristically seen in smooth muscle in which propagating action potentials are responsible for the mechanical response. Thus, one might suggest that the increased rate of oxidative phosphorylation causes the increase in intracellular Ca^{+2} as a consequence of an effect on the plasma membrane resulting in propagating action potentials. This possibility remains the subject for further studies.

ACKNOWLEDGEMENTS

This work was supported in part by grants from the National Institutes of Health to Fredric S. Fay (HL 14523) and William J. Whalen (HL 11906). Fredric S. Fay is the recipient of a Research Career Development Award (HL 00048) from the National Institutes of Health. The authors gratefully acknowledge the patience and care of Ms. D. Rusch in the preparation of this manuscript.

References

1. Born, G.V.R., G.S. Dawes, J.C. Mott, and B.R. Rennick. The
    constriction of the ductus arteriosus caused by oxygen and by
    asphyxia in new born lambs. J. Physiol., London 132:304-342,
    1956.
2. Kennedy, J.A., and S.L. Clark. Observations on the physiologi-
    cal reactions of the ductus arteriosus. Am. J. Physiol. 136:
    140-147, 1942.
3. Kovalcik, V. The response of the isolated ductus arteriosus
    to oxygen and anoxia. J. Physiol., London 169:185-197, 1963.
4. Moss, A.J., G.C. Emmanouilides, F.H. Adams, and K. Chuang.
    Response of ductus arteriosus and pulmonary and systemic ar-
    terial pressure to changes in oxygen environment in newborn
    infants. Pediatrics 33:937-944, 1964.
5. Boreus, L.O., T. Malmfors, D.M. McMurphy, and L. Olson. Demon-
    stration of adrenergic receptor function and innervation in the
    ductus arteriosus of the human fetus. Acta Physiol. Scand.
    77:316-321, 1969.
6. Melmon, K.L., M.J. Cline, T. Hughes, and A.S. Nies. Kinins:
    possible mediators of neonatal circulatory changes in man.
    J. Clin. Invest. 47:1295-1302, 1968.
7. Smith, R.W., J.A. Morris, R. Beck, and N.S. Assali. Effect of
    chemical mediators on pulmonary and ductus arteriosus circu-
    lation in the fetal lamb. Circulation 28:808, 1963.
8. Coceani, F. and P.M. Olley. The response of the ductus arter-
    iosus to prostaglandins. Can. J. Physiol. Pharmacol. 51:
    220-225 (1973).
9. Fay, F.S. Guinea pig ductus arteriosus. I. Cellular and
    metabolic basis for oxygen sensitivity. Am. J. Physiol. 221:
    470-479, 1971.

10. Fay, F.S. and P.H. Cooke. Guinea pig ductus arteriosus. II.
    Irreversible closure after birth. Am. J. Physiol. 222:841-
    849, 1972.
11. Warburg, O. and E. Negelein. Über der einfluss der wellenlänge
    auf die verteilung des atmungsferments. Biochem. Z. 193:
    339-346, 1928.
12. Castor, L.N.,and B. Chance. Photochemical action spectra of
    carbon monoxide-inhibited respiration. J. Biol. Chem. 217:
    453-465, 1955.
13. Fay, Fredric S. and Frans F. Jöbsis. Guinea pig ductus arteri-
    osus. III. Light absorption changes during response to O_2.
    Am. J. Physiol. 223(3):588-595, 1972.
14. Jöbsis, F.F. Basic processes in cellular respiration. In:
    Handbook of Physiology. Respiration. Washington, D.C.:
    Am. Physiol. Soc., 1964, sect. 3, vol. I, chapt. 2., p. 63-124.
15. Keilin, D. and E.F. Hartree. Cytochrome and cytochrome oxidase.
    Proc. Roy. Soc., London, Ser B 127:167-191, 1939.

16.   Campbello, A.P., C.H.M. Vianna, D. Brandao, D.O. Voss, and
      M. Bacila. The effect of chlorobutanol on the respiratory
      metabolism and on the normal properties of isolated mito-
      chondria. Bichem. Pharmacol. 13:211-223, 1964.
17.   Weinbach, E.C. The effect of pentachlorophenol on oxidative
      phosphorylation. J. Biol. Chem. 210:545-550, 1954.
18.   Loomis, W.F., and F. Lipmann. Reversible inhibition of the
      coupling between phosphorylation and oxidation. J. Biol.
      Chem. 173:807-808, 1948.
19.   Lardy, H.A., D. Johnson, and W.C. McMurray. Antibiotics as
      tools for metabolic studies. I. A survey of toxic anti-
      biotics in respiratory, phosphorylative and glycolytic sys-
      tems. Arch. Biochem. Biophys. 78:589-597, 1958.
20.   Whalen, W.J., J. Riley, and P. Nair. A microelectrode for
      measuring intracellular PO_2. J. Appl. Physiol. 23:798-801,
      1967.

PROSTAGLANDINS AND THE CONTROL OF MUSCLE TONE IN

THE DUCTUS ARTERIOSUS

F. Coceani, P.M. Olley, I. Bishai, E. Bodach, J. Heaton, M. Nashat, and E. White

Research Institute, The Hospital For Sick Children
Toronto, Canada

For many years it was assumed that the patency of the ductus arteriosus in the foetus is a passive state determined by the haemodynamic balance of the pulmonary and systemic circulations rather than by the action of the smooth muscle in the vessel wall (for a review, see ref. 1). As a result, research focussed upon the events occurring during the immediate postnatal period when the vessel constricts in response to the physiological elevation in blood oxygen tension. The mechanism of the contractile action of oxygen has been the subject of extensive investigation. Several authors (see ref. 1) speculated that oxygen does not act on smooth muscle directly but through the formation of, or the sensitization to, a vasoactive agent. Many different compounds - i.e., acetylcholine, norepinephrine, histamine, bradykinin - were studied, but none of them turned out to be suited to this role (2 - 4). The work of Fay (this volume) represents an original approach to this problem and his findings, while not excluding the occurrence in the tissue of a constrictor agent functionally linked to oxygen, prove that oxygen action is exerted upon cytochrome-dependent oxidative processes. Recent studies on the prostaglandins afford a new perspective to research in this area and suggest that the prenatal patency of the vessel is actively maintained by a local mechanism involving these compounds. Whether prostaglandins are also implicated in the functional closure of the vessel at birth is an open question, and different views on the subject are examined in this article.

PROSTAGLANDINS AND THE PATENCY OF THE DUCTUS ARTERIOSUS

Some years ago, we reported (5) that prostaglandins $(PG)E_1$

TABLE 1

THE RELAXANT EFFECT OF PROSTAGLANDINS, PROSTAGLANDIN ENDOPEROXIDES
AND PROSTAGLANDIN METABOLITES ON THE MATURE LAMB DUCTUS ARTERIOSUS
IN VITRO (P_{O_2} 8-16 mm Hg)

Compound	Threshold (M)
PGE_1	10^{-12} to 10^{-11}
PGE_2	10^{-12} to 10^{-11}
PGH_2	3×10^{-10} to 3×10^{-9}
PGG_2	3×10^{-8} to 3×10^{-7}
15-keto-PGE_1	10^{-7}
15-keto-13,14-dihydro PGE_1	10^{-6}
PGA_1	10^{-6} to 10^{-5}
$PGF_{1\alpha}$	10^{-6} to 10^{-5}
PGD_2	10^{-5}

and E_2 relax the lamb ductus arteriosus in vitro under hypoxic
conditions (P_{O_2} between 10 and 14 mm Hg) while they have little
or no effect on the oxygen-contracted vessel. That finding,
confirmed subsequently by others in a different preparation (6),
suggested a physiological role for E-type PGs in the foetal ductus
and stimulated further investigation.

Our research took several directions. Initially, we examined
(7) the action of several PG compounds (PGs proper, PG endoperoxides and metabolites) on the hypoxic ductus of lambs near
term (133-146 days gestation) and we proved that, with the single
exception of $PGF_{2\alpha}$, they all produced a dose-dependent relaxation.
Table 1 summarizes the results and shows that PGE_1 and PGE_2 are
most active among the compounds tested. An additional finding, not
included in Table 1, was that arachidonic acid, which is the most
common PG precursor in mammals, relaxed the ductus in high doses
(threshold, 3×10^{-6}M). The response to arachidonic acid was

TABLE 2

THE EFFECT OF BLOCKERS OF PROSTAGLANDIN SYNTHESIS AND REDUCED GLUTATHIONE ON THE MUSCLE TENSION OF THE MATURE LAMB DUCTUS ARTERIOSUS IN VITRO

Condition	P_{O_2} of perfusion medium [a]	
	8-16 mm Hg	479-662 mm Hg
Control	3.2 ± 0.4 (16)	9.2 ± 0.3 (17)
Before ETA [b]	3.3 ± 0.5 (7)	—
After ETA (5×10^{-6} to 3×10^{-5}M)	4.1 ± 0.3 (7)*	9.1 ± 0.4 (7)
Before indomethacin	3.8 ± 0.8 (4)	—
After indomethacin (2.8×10^{-5}M)	9.7 ± 0.4 (4)*	12.4 ± 0.3 (3)*
Before ibuprofen	2.6 ± 0.3 (14)	—
After ibuprofen [c] (4.8×10^{-4}M)	6.3 ± 0.3 (14)*	8.3 ± 0.3 (14)
Before GSH	3.3 ± 0.5 (4)	—
After GSH (5×10^{-4}M)	1.8 ± 0.7 (4)*	7.9 ± 0.9 (3)

[a] Values (g) are means $\pm$ S.E., corrected for the initial basal tension. Number of preparations given in parentheses. Asterisk indicates a statistically significant difference from controls (paired t-test or Dunnett's t-test).

[b] 5,8,11,14-eicosatetraynoic acid.

[c] Ibuprofen contracts the hypoxic ductus over a dose range between 2.8×10^{-6} and 4.8×10^{-4}M.

inhibited, partly or in full, by pretreatment with indomethacin, a blocker of PG synthesis. The latter result indicated that arachidonic acid was converted by ductal tissue to a PG compound with relaxant action on the muscle. The foetal ductus contains several PG types, including PGE_1 and PGE_2 (5). $PGF_{2\alpha}$ contracted the ductus at a relatively high concentration (threshold 10^{-7} to $10^{-5}M$) and the possible implications of this finding will be considered in the following section.

An additional line of investigation (8,9) involved the use of drugs which modify the synthesis of PGs in tissues. Table 2 summarizes the results of studies in vitro and shows that all blockers of PG synthesis (indomethacin, ibuprofen and 5,8,11, 14-eicosatetraynoic acid), regardless of their site and mode of action, contracted the hypoxic ductus. The contraction due to indomethacin proved to be particularly marked and it equalled that produced by high PO_2. Tissues pretreated with the blockers developed the usual (ibuprofen and 5,8,11,14-eicosatetraynoic acid) or a stronger (indomethacin) contraction in a high oxygen medium. Interestingly, the same tissues, unlike controls, retained their sensitivity to PGE_2 during the whole period of exposure to high oxygen (8). Unlike the blockers, reduced glutathione (GSH), which favours the synthesis of PGE compounds (10), produced a significant relaxation of the hypoxic ductus. These findings, together with the demonstration of the relaxant effect of arachidonic acid, strongly suggest that an active PG, possibly a PGE, is formed in the hypoxic ductus in spite of the restraint that the low oxygen tension may impose on the synthetic reaction (11,12). Work with another tissue (13) provides direct evidence that some PG is still synthesized in a low oxygen environment. Subsequent experiments in vivo (9, unpublished data) demonstrated that both indomethacin (10 mg/kg) and ibuprofen (20 or 40 mg/kg), given to pregnant ewes close to term, produce marked constriction of the foetal ductus arteriosus in utero. In a recent extension of this work, we showed (14) that the ductus arteriosus of younger lambs (90-124 days gestation) is contracted by ibuprofen in vitro (dose range, 2.8×10^{-6} to $4.8 \times 10^{-4}M$). From this, it is implied that the PG mechanism develops early during foetal life. The lamb ductus is not unique in its response to blockers of PG synthesis. Preliminary results from our laboratory (unpublished data) indicate that the rabbit ductus behaves in an identical manner. In contrast, however, the guinea pig ductus responds marginally, or not at all, to indomethacin or meclofenamate, at least in vitro (unpublished data).

While this work was in progress, several reports have appeared confirming or complementing our data. Sharpe et al. (15, 16) showed that blockers of PG synthesis constrict the ductus of foetal rats and rabbits, while Heymann and Rudolph (17) proved that blood flow across the ductus is substantially reduced in

aspirin-treated foetal lambs. Further, inhibition of PG synthesis
results in constriction, or closure, of patent ductus in the
premature human infant (18; see also ref. 19).

FUNCTIONAL CLOSURE OF THE DUCTUS ARTERIOSUS:
A PROSTAGLANDIN-CONDITIONED PROCESS?

While there is fairly convincing evidence to implicate E-type
PGs in the control of ductus patency, the question of the role of
PGs in the functional closure of the vessel at birth remains a
debatable point. Theoretically, PGs are well fitted to the
function of "messengers" of oxygen action on ductal muscle.
Conversion of polyunsaturated fatty acids to PGs requires molecular
oxygen (11,12). Thus, the postnatal rise in blood oxygen tension
could result in increased PG synthesis throughout the body. Further,
the contractile action of PGs on smooth muscle from various sources,
including vessels, is uniquely dependent on the presence of oxygen
(20 - 24). Experimental data link the oxygen-dependent mechanism to the cytochrome system (20). The relevance of the latter
finding to the model of oxygen action proposed by Fay (this volume)
is obvious. In fact, the remarkable coincidence in the characteristics of the PG and the oxygen action was one of the factors
which prompted us to begin this study (5). Among the PG types
investigated, only $PGF_{2\alpha}$ contracts the ductus arteriosus and could
therefore mediate the action of oxygen. However, results of
experiments with blockers of PG synthesis, and particularly their
inability to reduce the oxygen contraction, are inconsistent with
this idea. Further, effective doses of $PGF_{2\alpha}$ in vitro far exceed
those required with PGE_1 and PGE_2, suggesting a pharmacological
rather than a physiological action of the compound. A possibility
arising from our work is that PGs may participate indirectly in
the action of oxygen. The reduction, or loss, of muscle sensitivity
to the PGEs occurring in vitro under high oxygen, if indicative of
a physiological condition, may be important to the initiation or
persistence of ductus closure. In view of the evidence involving
calcium in the response of vascular smooth muscle to the PGs (25;
see also ref. 26 and 27) this "PGE withdrawal effect" could be
exerted at the step in the sequence proposed by Fay where the
oxidative synthesis of high-energy phosphate compounds is coupled
to the contractile mechanism.

A different view on the role of $PGF_{2\alpha}$ has been formulated by
Elliott and Starling (6,28) on the basis of work on the isolated
ductus of the foetal calf. In brief, these authors reported that
the contractile action of $PGF_{2\alpha}$, although only manifest at high
doses, increases in intensity upon raising the oxygenation of the
medium. Moreover, the oxygen response was inhibited by 7-oxa-13-
prostynoic acid, an antagonist of the PGs in some tissues, and by

pretreatment with blockers of PG synthesis (indomethacin, naproxen). These findings are at variance with those obtained in other species and suggest that $PGF_{2\alpha}$ may mediate the constrictor action of oxygen in the calf. The behaviour of the calf ductus, if confirmed in <u>vivo</u>, would represent a peculiar evolutionary departure.

CONCLUSION

Several lines of evidence implicate E-type PGs in the maintenance of patency of the foetal ductus arteriosus. The PGE mechanism is functional in man, sheep, rat and rabbit, but it is seemingly absent in guinea pig. The role of the PGs in the closure of the vessel at birth is uncertain. Work with different species suggests that as P_{O_2} rises at birth the relaxant effect of PGEs on the ductal muscle decreases. This decreased sensitivity may facilitate the oxygen triggered contraction. The calf ductus is an exception and its closure may be mediated by $PGF_{2\alpha}$. An important fact emerging from this review is that species may differ with regard to the occurrence and possible function of the PGs in the ductus arteriosus. The significance of these differences to the function of the oxygen-sensing mechanism remains a major question for future research.

ACKNOWLEDGEMENTS

Experimental work of the authors was supported by the Ontario Heart Foundation, The Upjohn Company and the Medical Research Council of Canada.

REFERENCES

1. Heymann MA, Rudolph AM: Control of the ductus arteriosus. Physiol Rev 55:62-78, 1975.

2. Kovalčik V: The response of the isolated ductus arteriosus to oxygen and anoxia. J Physiol (Lond) 169:185-197, 1963.

3. Knight DH, Patterson DF, Melbin J: Constriction of the fetal ductus arteriosus induced by oxygen, acetylcholine and norepinephrine in normal dogs and those genetically predisposed to persistent patency. Circulation 17:127-132, 1973.

4. Perin E, Coceani F, Olley PM: Another look at the role of acetylcholine (ACh) in the closure of the ductus arteriosus. Proc Can Fed Biol Soc 17:120, 1974.

5. Coceani F, Olley PM: The response of the ductus arteriosus to prostaglandins. Can J Physiol Pharmacol 51:220-225, 1973.

6. Starling MB, Elliott RB: The effects of prostaglandins, prostaglandin inhibitors, and oxygen on the closure of the ductus arteriosus, pulmonary arteries and umbilical vessels in vitro. Prostaglandins 8:187-203, 1974.

7. Coceani F, Olley PM, Bodach E: Prostaglandins: a possible regulator of muscle tone in the ductus arteriosus. In Samuelsson B, Paoletti R (Editors): Advances in Prostaglandin and Thromboxane Research. New York, Raven Press, 1976, vol 1, pp 417-424.

8. Coceani F, Olley PM, Bodach E: Lamb ductus arteriosus: effect of prostaglandin synthesis inhibitors on the muscle tone and the response to prostaglandin E_2. Prostaglandins 9:299-308, 1975.

9. Olley PM, Bodach E, Heaton J, Coceani F: Further evidence implicating E-type prostaglandins in the patency of the lamb ductus arteriosus. Eur J Pharmacol 34:247-250, 1975.

10. van Dorp DA: Aspects of the biosynthesis of prostaglandins. Progr biochem Pharmacol 3:71-82, 1967.

11. Nugteren DH, van Dorp DA: The participation of molecular oxygen in the biosynthesis of prostaglandins. Biochim Biophys Acta 98:654-656, 1965.

12. Samuelsson B: On the incorporation of oxygen in the conversion of 8,11,14-cicosatrienoic acid to prostaglandin E_1. J Am Chem Soc 87:3011-3013, 1965.

13. Coceani F, Pace-Asciak C, Volta F, Wolfe LS: Effect of nerve stimulation on prostaglandin formation and release from the rat stomach. Am J Physiol 213:1056-1064, 1967.

14. Olley PM, White EP, Bodach E, Heaton J, Coceani F: The contractile response of the developing lamb ductus arteriosus to ibuprofen. 49th Meeting Am Heart Ass (Miami) November 1976.

15. Sharpe GL, Thalme B, Larsson KS: Studies on closure of the ductus arteriosus. XI. Ductal closure in utero by a prostaglandin synthetase inhibitor. Prostaglandins 8:363-368, 1974.

16. Sharpe GL, Larsson KS, Thalme B: Studies on the closure of the ductus arteriosus. XII. In utero effect of indomethacin

and sodium salicylate in rats and rabbits. Prostaglandins 9: 585-596, 1975.

17. Heymann MA, Rudolph AM: Effects of acetylsalicylic acid on the ductus arteriosus and circulation in fetal lambs in utero. Circulation Res 38:418-422, 1976.

18. Friedman WF, Hirschklau MJ, Pitlick PT, Kirkpatrick SE: Pharmacological closure of patent ductus in the premature. Pediat Res 10:312, 1976.

19. Elliott RB, Starling MB, Neutze JM: Medical manipulation of the ductus arteriosus. Lancet 1:140-142, 1975.

20. Coceani F, Wolfe LS: On the action of prostaglandin E_1 and prostaglandins from brain on the isolated rat stomach. Can J Physiol Pharmacol 44:933-950, 1966.

21. Paton DM, Daniel EE: On the contractile response of the isolated rat uterus to prostaglandin E_1. Can J Physiol Pharmacol 45:795-804, 1967.

22. Eckenfels A, Vane JR: Prostaglandins, oxygen tension and smooth muscle tone. Br J Pharmacol 45:451-462, 1972.

23. Chandler JT, Strong CG: The actions of prostaglandin E_1 on isolated rabbit aorta. Arch int Pharmacodyn 197:123-131, 1972.

24. Splawinski JA, Nies AS, Sweetman B, Oates JA: The effects of arachidonic acid, prostaglandin E_2 and prostaglandin $F_{2\alpha}$ on the longitudinal stomach strip of the rat. J Pharmacol Exp Ther 187:501-510, 1973.

25. Wilson WR, Greenberg S, Kadowitz PJ, Diecke FPJ, Long JP: Interaction of prostaglandin A_2 and prostaglandin B_2 on vascular smooth muscle tone, vascular reactivity and electrolyte transport. J Pharmacol Exp Ther 195:565-576, 1975.

26. Kirkland SJ, Baum H: Prostaglandin E_1 may act as a "calcium ionophore". Nature 236:47-49, 1972.

27. Carafoli E, Crovetti F: Interactions between prostaglandin E_1 and calcium at the level of the mitochondrial membrane. Arch Biochem Biophys 154:40-46, 1973.

28. Elliott RB, Starling MB: The effects of prostaglandin $F_{2\alpha}$ in the closure of the ductus arteriosus. Prostaglandins 2: 399-403, 1972.

THE SENSING OF OXYGEN TENSION IN THE PULMONARY CIRCULATION

Alfred P. Fishman
University of Pennsylvania School of Medicine
Cardiovascular-Pulmonary Division
3600 Spruce Street
Philadelphia, Pennsylvania 19104

It now seems settled that acute hypoxia elicits pulmonary vasoconstriction and that the predominant site of constriction is the small muscular pulmonary artery[1-3]. What remains to be resolved is how this vasoconstriction comes about[4].

A considerable research effort over the last 30 years has helped considerably in focusing the question and in relegating to subsidiary roles certain mechanisms that were once considered to be candidates for primary mechanisms[5-6]. For example, pulmonary vasomotor nerves have been discounted as a primary ingredient in the pressor response to acute hypoxia since the response can be elicited in the isolated, perfused lung which is devoid of all nervous connections. Even less of a role is currently envisaged for humoral substances that are carried to it by the blood from afar.

Instead, attention is riveted on the lung itself: the pressor mechanism appears to originate and to exert its effects entirely within the substance of the lungs. And, the search for the intrapulmonary ("local") mechanism has come to a critical fork in the road: is it direct or indirect? Although the current tide has veered towards an indirect intrapulmonary mechanism, as this presentation will indicate, I am more inclined towards a direct mechanism.

In seeking a physiological basis for the pulmonary pressor response to acute hypoxia it seems natural to seek parallels between the responses of the pulmonary circulation and those of the carotid body[7]. For both, acute hypoxia has proved to be the most effective stimulus. Also, for both, acidosis enhances the stimulatory effect

of hypoxia. Not quite as comforting for the analogy is the fact
that for neither the carotid body nor the pulmonary vessels are
the sensing and the transduction mechanisms known. How is a decrease in arterial blood PO_2 or in O_2 delivery (O_2 concentration
x blood flow) translated into contraction of vascular smooth
muscle? How do the responses of systemic resistance vessels to
hypoxia relate to the pulmonary pressor response that hypoxia
elicits in the pulmonary circulation? Unfortunately, extrapolation
is not easy: hypoxia causes a diametrically opposite response in
the systemic circulation; systemic arterioles dilate instead of
constricting.

Comparisons are complicated further by clinical difficulties.
It is no simple matter to isolate smooth muscle of resistance
vessels for study in either circulation. Therefore, most attempts
to examine the hypoxic responses in isolated preparations have had
to be satisfied with extrapolations from the responses of large
vessels, i.e. a large pulmonary artery or aorta, instead of resistance vessels[8-10]. Nevertheless, although progress in dealing
with vascular smooth muscle has been slow, enough insight has been
gained in recent years to provide some basis for considering
whether an indirect or direct intrapulmonary mechanism is the basis
for the pulmonary pressor response to hypoxia.

Indirect Effect as the Basis for the
Pulmonary Pressor Response to Hypoxia?

The popular idea of the mechanism by which acute hypoxia might
elicit pulmonary vasoconstriction indirectly is shown in Figure 1.
In response to alveolar hypoxia, intrapulmonary chemical mediators
are pictured as being released within the lung and reaching pulmonary vascular smooth muscle by diffusion. There the unknown mediator either affects special receptors on, or chemical transmitters
in, the smooth muscle to initiate vasoconstriction. Of all the
cells in the lungs, the mast cell has attracted most attention as
the likely source of the mediator[6,11]. However, other parenchymal
cells, particularly endothelium, have not been excluded as potential
sources. In any event, finding a reasonable source for the mediator
has not been an important conceptual problem since there is sufficient diversity among the cells of the lung to support the idea of
a local reservoir that would release a mediator when prompted to do
so by alveolar hypoxia.

Alveolar hypoxia, i.e. hypoxia induced by airway rather than
by blood, has been the cornerstone of this "indirect" hypothesis:
it is alveolar hypoxia[12-13] that presumably prompts the unidentified cells to release the indefinite mediator. However, the architecture of this hypothesis has been weakened by the demonstration
that hypoxia elicited by blood stream, as well as by alveoli, can

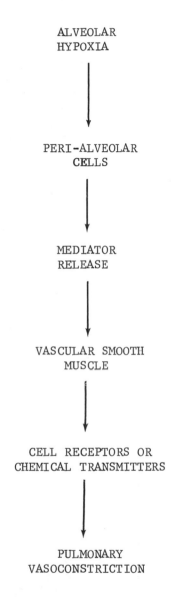

Figure 1. Proposed pathway for indirect action of hypoxia in elic-
           iting pulmonary vasoconstriction.

elicit pulmonary vasoconstriction[14,15]. Indeed, instead of being the unique pathway for inducing pulmonary vasoconstriction, the emphasis on alveolar hypoxia seems to originate in the greater practicality of inducing hypoxia by airway than by the bloodstream in the experimental laboratory.

With respect to mediators, histamine is the favorite. Supporting this notion is a considerable experience in a few laboratories with the use of antihistamines to block the hypoxic pressor response[16]. Further support for this view has been adduced by demonstrating degranulation of periarterial mast cells in the lungs during acute hypoxia[6]. But the blocking effects of the antihistamines are generally recognized to be somewhat imprecise as tools for pharmacologic dissection. Moreover, not all investigators have been equally successful in blocking the hypoxic pressor response by administering antihistamines[17]. Nor has it been shown that degranulation of mast cells is prerequisite for release of histamine in the lungs. The net effect of these and other uncertainties has been the mounting suspicion that histamine may not be the unique mediator of the pressor response to hypoxia.

In turn, uncertainty about histamine has stimulated a search for a more convincing prospect. The prostaglandins[18,19] and angiotensin have their supporters but the ranks seem to be thinning. Serotonin, once a promising candidate, no longer appears to be in the running[3].

Direct Effect as the Basis for the
Pulmonary Pressor Response to Hypoxia?

The equivocal nature of the proposed cells of origin of the mediator, and of its identity, has rekindled interest in the possibility that a direct effect of hypoxia on pulmonary vascular smooth muscle may be the root cause of the pulmonary vasoconstriction. This idea has the attraction of not being dependent on alveolar hypoxia. Instead, the route by which the smooth muscle cell is rendered hypoxic becomes immaterial: either the blood phase or the gas phase will do. Moreover, since the idea of a direct effect allows hypoxia to be induced by bloodstream, it becomes easier to understand the synergistic effects of acidosis and hypoxia in eliciting a pressor response in the pulmonary circulation since most would agree that acidosis affects pulmonary vascular smooth muscle by way of the bloodstream[20,21].

Unfortunately, because of the experimental difficulties inherent in exploring a direct effect of hypoxia on the small pulmonary vessels, the hypothesis remains difficult to put to critical test. As a result, the case for a direct effect rests heavily on exclusion. But there have been flurries of experimental evidence

in favor of a direct effect. For example, the elegant experiments
of Bergofsky and Holtzman led them to consider seriously that elec-
tromechanical events at the surface of the smooth muscle cell might
be affected by hypoxia[6].

Instead of the membrane, Detar and Bohr implicated the energetics of muscular contraction and ATP production in the pressor
response. They showed that hypoxia accelerates ATP production in
pulmonary vascular smooth muscle by enhancing the glycolytic pathway[9,10]. This is in contrast to the depressant effect of hypoxia
that they observed on the oxidative production of ATP in systemic
vascular smooth muscle. From these experiments, the O_2-consuming
pathway emerges as the mechanism sensitive to hypoxia and cytochrome A-3 as a leading candidate for the sensor. The extent of
involvement of other oxygenases is not settled. These experiments
also open the door to providing a common denominator for the dis-
crepant effects of hypoxia on the systemic and pulmonary circulations: vasodilation in the systemic circulation would be explained
as the end-result of a decrease in energy production and in the
level of ATP; the opposite effect would explain the response to
hypoxia in the pulmonary circulation.

McMurtrey et al have returned to the smooth muscle membrane,
focusing on the possible role of calcium as the regulator ion[22].
They have provided evidence that hypoxia can promote the flow of
calcium into the smooth muscle cell where it can activate the contractile machinery. The picture of the calcium ion as the essential element is attractive as a unifying concept since it seems to
account for the seemingly divergent experiences of others, using
blocking agents, anesthetics and competitive inhibitors, as nonspe-
cific effects. Unfortunately, the experiments favoring the calcium
ion also rely heavily on pharmacological antagonists.

Despite the inherent attractiveness of the calcium hypothesis,
it would be premature to consider the matter settled. Nonetheless,
it does seem reasonable to conclude that even though a direct effect has not been proved as the basis for the pulmonary pressor response to hypoxia, the theoretical bases for such a mechanism remain plausible[23].

Concluding Comments

The intensity of the search of recent years for a unique chemical mediator that is responsible for the pressor response to acute
hypoxia appears to be waning. The loss of research drive in this
direction seems to stem from the inconclusive nature of the evidence
that has been marshalled for the hypothesis that a chemical mediator
is involved as the primary mechanism. As enthusiasm for the idea
of a chemical mediator wanes, interest is shifting once again to a

direct effect of hypoxia as the likely basis for the pressor response. The theoretical framework for a direct effect is strong
and experimental evidence is accumulating to support this view.
By de-emphasizing the need for "alveolar" hypoxia and by resorting
to the biochemical and biophysical techniques of the muscle physiologist, the way has been reopened to full exploration of the direct, as well as indirect, pathways that may be involved in the
hypoxic pressor response in the pulmonary circulation and to the
vasodilation elicited by hypoxia in the systemic circulation.

REFERENCES

1. Von Euler US, Liljestrand G: Observations on the pulmonary
    arterial blood pressure in the cat. Acta Physiol Scand 12:
    301-320, 1946.

2. Fishman AP: Dynamics of the pulmonary circulation. In
    Hamilton WF, Dow P (Editors): Handbook of Physiology, Section
    2, Circulation, vol 2. Washington, American Physiological
    Society, 1963, pp 1667-1743

3. Bergofsky EH: Mechanisms underlying vasomotor regulation of
    regional pulmonary blood flow in normal and disease states.
    Am J Med 57:378-394, 1974.

4. Fishman AP: Hypoxia on the pulmonary circulation. Circ Res
    38:221-231, 1976.

5. Szidon JP, Fishman AP: Autonomic control of the pulmonary cir-
    culation. In Fishman AP, Hecht HH (Editors): The Pulmonary
    Circulation and Interstitial Space. Chicago, University of
    Chicago Press, 1969, pp 239-268

6. Bergofsky EH, Holtzman S: A study of the mechanisms involved
    in the pulmonary arterial pressor response to hypoxia. Circ
    Res 20:506-519, 1967.

7. Torrance RW: The idea of a chemoreceptor. In Fishman AP,
    Hecht HH (Editors): The Pulmonary Circulation and Interstitial
    Space. Chicago, University of Chicago Press, 1969, pp 223-237

8. Somlyo AP, Somlyo AV: Vascular smooth muscle. II. Pharma-
    cology of normal and hypertensive vessels. Pharmacol Rev 22:
    249-353, 1970.

9. Detar R, Bohr DF: Oxygen and vascular smooth muscle contrac-
    tion. Am J Physiol 214:241-244, 1968.

10. Detar R, Bohr DF: Contractile responses of isolated vascular smooth muscle during prolonged exposure to anoxia. Am J Physiol 222:1269-1277, 1972.

11. Kay JM, Grover RF: Lung mast cells and hypoxic pulmonary hypertension. Prog Respir Res 9:157-164, 1975.

12. Lloyd TC Jr: Role of nerve pathways in the hypoxic vasoconstriction of lung. J Appl Physiol 21:1351-1355, 1966.

13. Hauge A: Conditions governing the pressor response to ventilation hypoxia in isolated perfused rat lungs. Acta Physiol Scand 72:33-44, 1968.

14. Daly I de B, Michel CC, Ramsay DJ, Waaler BA: Conditions governing the pulmonary vascular response to ventilation hypoxia and hypoxaemia in the dog. J Physiol (Lond) 196:351-379, 1968.

15. Hauge A: Hypoxia and pulmonary vascular resistance: the relative effects of pulmonary arterial and alveolar PO$_2$. Acta Physiol Scand 76:121-130, 1969.

16. Hauge A, Staub NC: Prevention of hypoxic vasoconstriction in cat lung by histamine-releasing agent 48/80. J Appl Physiol 26:693-699, 1969.

17. Silove ED, Simcha AJ: Histamine-induced pulmonary vasodilatation in the calf; relationship to hypoxia. J Appl Physiol 35:830-836, 1973.

18. Said SI, Voshida T, Kitamura S, Vreim G: Pulmonary alveolar hypoxia: release of prostaglandins and other humoral mediators. Science 185:1181-1183, 1974.

19. Vaage J, Hauge A: Prostaglandins and the pulmonary vasoconstrictor response to alveolar hypoxia. Science 189:899-900, 1975.

20. Harvey RM, Enson Y, Betti R, Lewis ML, Rochester DF, Ferrer MI: Further observations on the effect of hydrogen ion on the pulmonary circulation. Circulation 35:1019-1027, 1967.

21. Barer GW, McCurrie JR: Pulmonary vasomotor responses in the cat: the effect and interrelationship of drugs, hypoxia and hypercapnia. Q J Exp Physiol 54:156-172, 1969.

22. McMurtry IF, Reeves JT, Grover RF: Inhibition by verapamil of pulmonary vasoconstrictive response to alveolar hypoxia. Physiologist 17:285, 1974.

23. Souhrada JF, Dickey DW: Effect of substrate on hypoxic response of pulmonary artery. J Appl Physiol 40:533-538, 1976.

THE SENSING OF OXYGEN TENSION IN THE PULMONARY CIRCULATION—

DISCUSSION

Norman C. Staub

University of California, San Francisco
Cardiovascular Research Institute
San Francisco, CA 94143

I think the reason I was invited to participate in this symposium was that I collaborated with Anton Hauge in some experiments suggesting histamine as the mediator by which reduced alveolar oxygen tension was sensed in the pulmonary circulation[1]. I am not going to defend histamine or any other mechanism, but will inquire as to how we can learn the truth about this fascinating problem that has led reputable scientists on a merry chase for decades. Dr. Fishman's review[2] covers all the essential issues. My brief comments will be confined to stating my approach to the problem, assembling the scattered results of our laboratory's work which bear on the issue, and describing an interesting new lead. I will even mention histamine briefly.

BIOLOGICAL SIGNIFICANCE

When I last reviewed this field[3] I began by discussing the possible adaptive significance (survival of the fittest) of pulmonary vasoconstriction in response to decreased alveolar oxygen tension. I believe that it is our view on this matter that directs our experimental approach to the problem. I was convinced then and still am that the significance of the pulmonary vasoconstrictor response to acute and chronic alveolar hypoxia is to be sought not in terms of total body hypoxia, either in the fetus or the adult, but rather in the local regulation of perfusion to ventilation within the lung.

When small areas of the lung are involved even slight constrictor responses become very effective in shunting flow to other parallel units[4]. Thus, according to this view, the constrictor mechanism is to be sought within the lung and in small

blood vessels. It must be sensitive to relatively modest decreases
in lung tissue oxygen tension because, even in a completely
unventilated terminal respiratory unit, the tissue oxygen tension
is unlikely to be much less than that of the mixed venous blood,
namely 30-40 torr.

SITE OF HYPOXIC VASOCONSTRICTION

Figure 1 is a model of the anatomy of the lung. A knowledge
of the relation of the blood vessels to the airway and alveolar gas
space is critical. The pulmonary veins, which receive blood from
several terminal respiratory units, are unlikely candidates for the

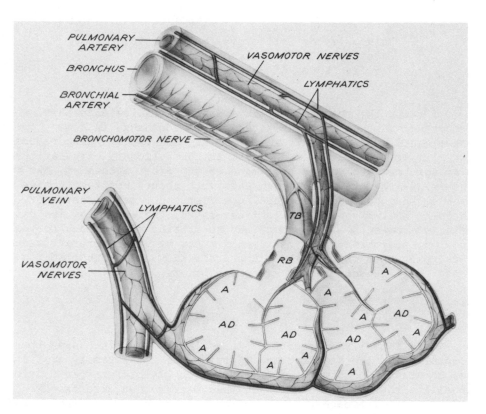

Figure 1. Lung model showing simplified, but anatomically correct
interrelations among the structural elements of the lung. Note the
close relationship of each pulmonary artery to airway it accompanies
and to the terminal respiratory unit it supplies. The veins do not
have such specificity. A terminal respiratory unit consists of a
respiratory bronchiole (RB) and its distal subdivisions of alveolar
ducts (AD) and alveoli (A). A terminal bronchiole (TB) is also shown
(From Staub, Human Pathology 1:419-432, 1970.)

constrictor sites if only one terminal unit becomes hypoventilated.
Although some data continues to be interpreted as consistent with
venous constriction during hypoxia[5], the overwhelming mass of
evidence indicates the active constrictor sites are in small muscular
pulmonary arteries.

Dr. Fishman has reviewed much of this evidence. A few recent
additional bits of information include the failure of Hyman and
Kadowitz[6] to find venous constriction in sheep during acute alveolar
hypoxia. In our own laboratory, Bland[7] followed lung lymph and
protein flow for up to 48 hr in unanesthetized sheep breathing 10%
O_2(Figure 2). Since the lung lymph flow is very sensitive to changes
in microvascular pressure, as we have recently demonstrated[8], Bland's
finding of no change in lung lymph flow in these animals is clear
evidence against venous constriction and for a purely arterial
constrictor site. Pulmonary vascular resistance was increased in

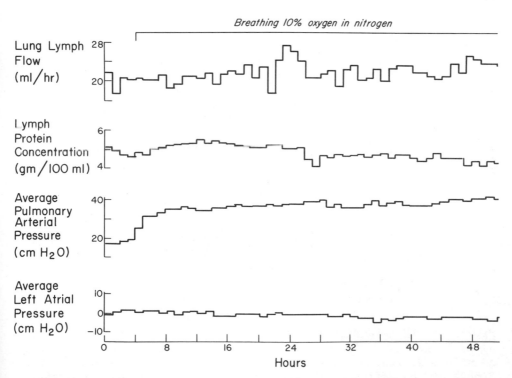

Figure 2. Evidence that the hypoxic pulmonary vasoconstrictor
response is proximal to the fluid exchange vessels. Lung lymph
flow remained constant during 48 hr of alveolar hypoxia although
average pulmonary arterial pressure doubled.[7]

these animals and pulmonary artery pressure was nearly twice
baseline level; yet none was transmitted to the fluid exchange
sites. In addition, Vreim and Staub[9] found no differences in
pulmonary capillary blood volume in cats during air breathing
compared to 10% oxygen breathing.

Kapanci and associates[10] suggested that the pulmonary
capillaries are the site of the hypoxia-induced resistance change.
They believe that "contractile interstitial cells" are stimulated
by hypoxia and contract and compress the capillary network. There
is no evidence to support this hypothesis. Indeed, there is no
evidence that lung volume or compliance is affected by any level of
alveolar hypoxia which, of course, must occur if the alveolar walls
are contracted.

Lauweryns[11] suggested that the neuro epithelial bodies in the
small airways secrete vasoactive substances into the pulmonary
venous system during hypoxia. This is also an unlikely mechanism

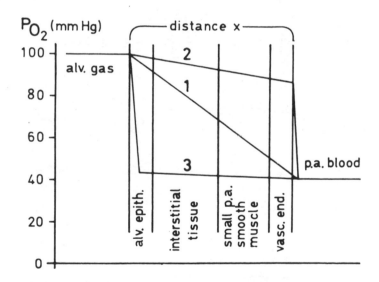

Figure 3. Three different theoretical oxygen tension profiles from
alveolar gas to blood in small pulmonary arteries. Profile 1 shows
a uniform diffusion resistance, all within the tissues; in profile
2 most of the diffusion resistance is within the blood; in profile
3 the resistance is in the alveolar epithelium.[12]

for the vasoconstrictor response because it lacks specificity when
the constrictor site is in the pulmonary arteries.

Figure 3 is a model used by Hauge[12] as part of a study to try
to determine whether the hypoxia receptors were closer to the
alveolar gas than to the pulmonary arterial blood. The model shows
that unless we are absolutely sure of the oxygen tension profile
through the intervening tissue, we cannot make a categorical answer.

Although I had obtained preliminary qualitative evidence in
1961 that oxygen diffused directly through the wall of the pulmonary
arteries[13], it is only recently that we have begun to quantify the
process[14]. We believe that oxygen tension throughout the walls of
the small pulmonary arteries is approximately that of the surrounding
alveolar gas, that is, closest to profile 2.

This explains the relatively trivial effect of lowering mixed
venous oxygen tension on the hypoxic vasoconstrictor response, as
well as the counteracting effects of an artificially high blood gas
tension. Naturally, given my view that the value of the hypoxic
response is for local regulation of perfusion to ventilation, I
would not expect blood gas tensions to be of importance anyway.

Unfortunately, profile 2 does not afford any assistance in
localizing the site of action of low oxygen tension since all of
the tissues in the pathway are at nearly the same tension.

HOW DOES DECREASED OXYGEN TENSION CAUSE VASOCONSTRICTION?

Figure 4, modified from Johansson[15] shows the vascular smooth
muscle stimulus-response profile. Where along this pathway does
decreased oxygen tension act? There are certain restrictions on
any selected mechanism, namely, 1) the response begins at a
relatively high level of alveolar oxygen tension (11% inspired O_2
as shown in Figure 5); 2) the response comes and goes quickly
(Figure 6) and is sustained (Figure 2).

A.   Innervation

Dr. Fishman has discussed the possible role of autonomic
innervation extensively. Although recent evidence suggests that
sympathetic nervous system stimulation does increase pulmonary
vascular resistance substantially[16], I agree with his conclusion
that it is unlikely to be primarily involved in the hypoxic
vasoconstrictor response.

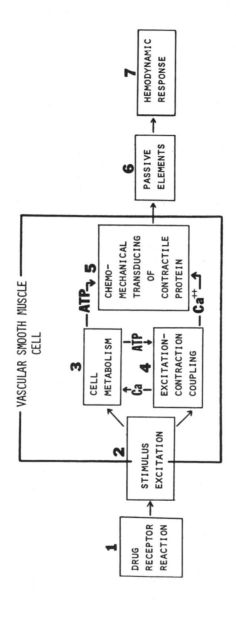

ADAPTED FROM JOHANSSON, 1974

Figure 4. Scheme illustrating the major events that link the application of a stimulus to the final vascular response[15].

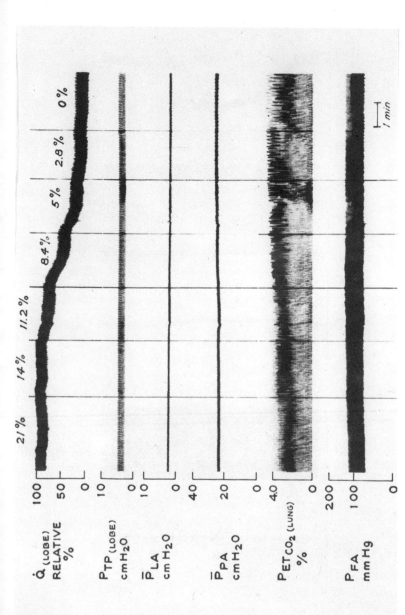

Figure 5. Dose-response relationship between decreasing inspired oxygen concentration and lobar blood flow in the left lower lobe of an anesthetized, open thorax cat. The gas mixture used to ventilate the lobe was changed at the vertical bais (approximately every two min). The recordings from above downward are lobar blood flow as a percent of the air-ventilation flow; lobe transpulmonary pressure, average left atrial and pulmonary artery pressures; lung end tidal CO_2 which increased as flow shifted away from the hypoxic lobe, and femoral artery pressure[1].

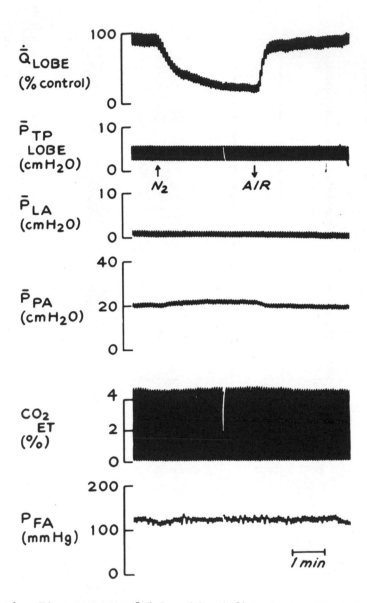

Figure 6.   Time course of lobar blood flow in response to low oxygen ventilation.   Records and symbols same as in Figure 5[1].

B.   Direct Action of Oxygen

If oxygen has a direct effect on the contractile response,
where along the pathway shown in Figure 4 would it act? Again, Dr.
Fishman is correct in saying there is no evidence for a direct
action of oxygen on the contractile machinery itself. Is there a
direct effect via cell energy metabolism? This is a reasonable
possibility, but we need answers to two questions. First, would
the effect be rapid enough to fit the known time course of the
hypoxic vasoconstrictor response (Figure 6)? If the lung's cells
can readily adapt to anerobic metabolism, how is it that the
vasoconstrictor response can persist unaltered for long periods
(Figure 2)? Does the pulmonary vascular smooth muscle lack this
capability for anerobic metabolism? Second, the response begins
at a relatively high tissue oxygen tension; well above the levels
that are known to interfere with cellular energy production
(Figure 5). Have lung cell energy systems adapted to high oxygen
levels? The oxygen tension in lung tissue is the highest in the
body.

The same restrictions apply to any cell membrane receptor
affected by the presence or lack of oxygen molecule itself.

C. Mediators

So many investigators have been frustrated in their search for
a specific mediator, I can't blame Dr. Fishman for favoring a more
direct action. What evidence is there for a mediator?

An exciting new approach was reported by Benumoff and
associates[17]. They found that right duct lymph obtained from
hypoxic dogs constricted an isolated pulmonary artery strip, whereas
lymph taken during hyperoxia did not. In other experiments, they
found that suffusion fluid from isolated, perfused cat lungs also
caused vasoconstriction indicating that the material was locally
released in the lung (Benumoff, personal communication). They have
not identified the substance. Hara and Said[18] confirmed the presence
of a smooth muscle contracting substance in hypoxic dog lung lymph.

I was and still am attracted by Hauge's histamine mediator
hypothesis[19;12]. Even if incorrect, it provided new impetus for
investigations by setting up a specific hypothesis to attack. In
spite of the attractive location of the majority of lung mast cells
adjacent to pulmonary arteries, I admit that the weight of evidence
is not nearly so favorable towards histamine as it once was.
Nevertheless, it is still possible that the action of exogenous
histamine and the failure to block the hypoxic vasoconstrictor
response with histamine inhibitors in some experiments is not quite
the same as the action of locally produced or released histamine
adjacent to or within the pulmonary vascular smooth muscle.

SUMMARY

The view that the hypoxic pulmonary vasoconstrictor response is an adaptive mechanism to adjust perfusion to ventilation leads to certain predictions about the site of the vasoconstrictor response which have been overwhelmingly confirmed, namely, that it is confined to the small muscular pulmonary arteries. It also leads to predictions about the nature of the vasoconstrictor mechanism as an effect of altered oxygen tension locally within the lung.

I believe the available evidence still favors one or more mediators rather than a smooth muscle cell oxygen receptor or an effect of low oxygen on smooth muscle energy metabolism.

I certainly hope the riddle will be solved soon. I also hope that histamine is somehow involved.

REFERENCES

1.   Hauge A, Staub NC: Prevention of hypoxic vasoconstriction in cat lung by histamine-releasing agent 48/80. J Appl Physiol 26:693-699, 1969.

2.   Fishman AP: Hypoxia on the pulmonary circulation - How and where it acts. Circulation Res 38:221-231, 1976.

3.   Staub NC: Respiration. Annual Rev of Physiol 31:173-202, 1969.

4.   Kato M, Staub NC: Response of small pulmonary arteries to unilobar hypoxia and hypercapnia. Circulation Res 21:426-439, 1966.

5.   Wagner WW Jr, Latham LP: Pulmonary capillary recruitment during airway hypoxia in the dog. J Appl Physiol 39:900-905, 1975.

6.   Hyman AL, Kadowitz PJ: Effects of alveolar and perfusion hypoxia and hypercapnia on pulmonary vascular resistance in the lamb. Am J Physiol 228:397-403, 1975.

7.   Bland RD, Demling RH, Selinger SL, Staub NC: Effects of alveolar hypoxia on lung fluid and protein transport in unanesthetized sheep. Circulation Res in press, 1976.

8.   Erdmann AJ III, Vaughan TR Jr, Brigham KL, Woolverton WC,
      Staub NC: Effect of increased vascular pressure on lung fluid
      balance in unanesthetized sheep.   Circulation Res 37:271-284,
      1975.

9.   Vreim CE, Staub NC: Indirect and direct pulmonary capillary
      blood volume in anesthetized, open-thorax cats.   J Appl Physiol
      34:452-459, 1973.

10.   Kapanci Y, Assimacopoulos A, Irle C, Zwahlen A, Gabbiani G:
      Contractile interstitial cells in pulmonary alveolar septa: A
      possible regulator of ventilation-perfusion ratio?   J Cell
      Biol 60:375-392, 1974.

11.   Lauweryns JM, Cokelaere M: Hypoxia-sensitive neuro-epithelial
      bodies.   Intrapulmonary secretory neuroreceptors modulated by
      the CNS.   Z Zellforsch Mikrosk Anat 145:521-540, 1973.

12.   Hauge A: Hypoxia and pulmonary vascular resistance.   The
      relative effects of pulmonary arterial and alveolar Po_2.
      Acta Physiol Scand 76:121-130, 1969.

13.   Staub NC: Gas exchange vessels in the cat lung.   Fed Proc
      20:107(abs.), 1961.

14.   Conhaim RL, Staub NC: Reflection microspectrophotometric
      evidence for precapillary oxygenation in pulmonary arteries of
      quick-frozen cat lungs.   Physiologist 18:173(abs.), 1975.

15.   Johannson B: Determinants of vascular reactivity.   Fed Proc
      33:121-126, 1974.

16.   Kadowitz PJ, Joine PD, Hyman AL: Influence of sympathetic
      stimulation and vasoactive substances on the canine pulmonary
      veins.   J Clin Invest 56:354-365, 1975.

17.   Benumof JL, Mathers J, Wahrenbrock EA: The pulmonary
      interstitial compartment and hypoxic pulmonary vasoconstriction.
      Physiologist 18:138(abs.), 1975.

18.   Hara N, Said SI: Pulmonary lymph: Smooth-muscle contracting
      activity and its increase during hypoxic ventilation in dogs.
      Clin Res 24:385A, 1976.

19.   Hauge A: Role of histamine in hypoxic pulmonary hypertension
      in the rat.   Circulation Res 22:371-383, 1968.

CIRCULATORY EFFECTS OF TISSUE OXYGEN TENSION SENSORS

Robert M. Berne and Rafael Rubio

Department of Physiology, University of Virginia

Charlottesville, VA 22901

There is no disagreement that in practically all tissues hypoxia results in vasodilation and in muscle such as the heart hypoxia is undoubtedly the most potent physiological vasodilator. The unresolved question, and one that has attracted the attention of investigators for many years is the mechanism whereby an inadequate oxygen supply for the tissue needs elicits relaxation of the smooth muscle of the resistance vessels. In 1925 Hilton and Eichholtz[1] performed experiments with the dog heart-lung preparation in which they carried out a series of interventions such as reducing the oxygen content of the arterial blood, adding lactic acid, CO_2 or cyanide to the arterial blood and changing to fresh blood after prolonged coronary perfusion that had resulted in progressive coronary vasodilation. On the basis of their findings they concluded that there were not significant amounts of "vasodilator metabolites" liberated from the myocardium and implied that the impressive inverse relationship between blood oxygen levels and coronary blood flow was due to a direct effect of oxygen lack. Similar conclusions about a direct effect of oxygen lack as a stimulus to vasodilation have been proposed by Smith and Vane[2] in isolated superfused strips of rat aorta and by Crawford et al[3] in the intact dog hind limb and Carrier et al[4] in small isolated perfused arteries obtained from dog skeletal muscle. No one has gone so far as to postulate the existence of an "oxygen receptor" but by the same token the supporters of a direct effect of PO_2 on the contractile state of vascular smooth muscle have not discarded the possibility of its existence. Chemoreceptors, responsive to reductions in PO_2 are well recognized, but there is no evidence to indicate that they are present in the arteries or arterioles of organs like the heart, and if present, can evoke vascular resistance changes via local neural circuits. Gellai et al[5] have shown that with

strips of rabbit aorta caused to contract by acetylcholine, there was
no difference in the contractile response with oxygen tensions
between 10 and 100 mm Hg in the bathing solution (Fig. 1B). Furthermore, from studies on strips of hog carotid arteries, Pittman and
Duling[6] extrapolated their observations to 10 μ arterioles and
proposed that the vascular smooth muscle cells would be unaffected
by oxygen tensions greater than 2-6 mm. Hg. These authors[6] suggest
that experiments purporting to show a direct relationship between
PO_2 and the contractile state of vascular smooth muscle in strips
of aorta or large arteries may be misleading because of the long
diffusion distance and the possibility that the innermost cells
are hypoxic even at high levels of PO_2 in the bathing solution.
Since in vivo studies[7] indicate that the vascular smooth muscle
of the resistance vessels is normally exposed to PO_2 levels of
20-70 mm. Hg., it is difficult to see how oxygen tension per se can
play a direct role in the control of vascular resistance.

The direct effect of PO_2 on vascular resistance has also been
studied in the hind limb by comparing the changes in conductance
under conditions of active hyperemia with those observed when
the hind limb was perfused with venous blood that produced
comparable levels of PO_2 in the effluent blood from the perfused

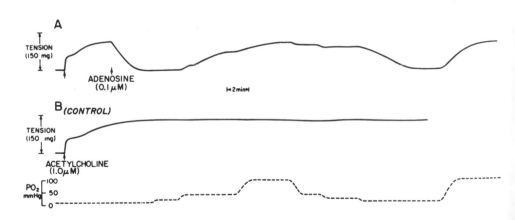

Fig. 1 Effects of PO_2 on contractile tension in helical coronary
arterial strip. A: In the presence of a low concentration of
adenosine, contractile tension was directly related to PO_2 in the
bath. B: In the absence of adenosine, contractile tension was not
affected by changes in PO_2 between 10 and 100 mm. Hg. (Reproduced
from Circulation Research 32:279, 1973 by permission of the American
Heart Association.)

limb[8]. These experiments showed that during active hyperemia
the blood flow increase was more than threefold greater than when
the vascular bed was perfused with venous blood. With active
hyperemia the effluent blood PO_2 averaged 25 mm. Hg. whereas during
venous blood perfusion it averaged 23 mm. Hg. Other studies on
smooth muscle from turkey gizzard suggested that hypoxia could
conceivably act locally by inhibition of APTase activity brought
about by increments in smooth muscle AMP and inorganic phosphate
secondary to hypoxia-induced impairment of ATP regeneration[9].
However, no evidence for ATPase inhibition by AMP or inorganic
phosphate was observed when purified actomyosin from hog carotid
arteries was used[10]. These experiments[10] and those of Ross et al[8]
also do not support the concept that hypoxia induces relaxation
of vascular smooth muscle by a direct influence on the muscle
itself either by means of an oxygen receptor or by interference
with metabolic processes in the tissue.

Stimulated by the early report of Hilton and Eichholtz[1],
we performed experiments in 1957 to determine the effect of arterial
PO_2 on coronary vascular resistance in the open chest dog under
conditions that permitted perfusion of the left coronary artery
at any desired pressure with normoxic or hypoxic blood[11]. When the
left coronary artery was perfused with hypoxic blood (about 14
vol %) and an adequate oxygen supply to the myocardium was maintained
by increasing coronary perfusion pressure, coronary dilation did
not occur, whereas perfusion with hypoxic blood at control pressure
resulted in an increase in coronary blood flow (Fig. 2). In these
experiments coronary vasodilation only occurred when coronary sinus
blood oxygen levels reached a critically low value of 5.5 vol %
or less. Similar conclusions were reached by Guz et al[12] from
studies done on isolated rabbit hearts perfused with different
concentrations of bovine hemoglobin solutions but of the same PO_2.
In these experiments[12] coronary flow varied inversely with oxygen
supply suggesting that oxygen availability and not PO_2 influences
coronary resistance. These results and those obtained with
reactive hyperemia, where the duration of the reactive hyperemia
paralleled that of the coronary occlusion suggest that arterial
PO_2 is not of primary importance in the control of coronary
resistance. In the reactive hyperemia experiments the coronary
venous blood was about fully saturated with oxygen after release
of either short (15 sec.) or long (120 sec.) occlusions. Therefore
the smooth muscle of the arterioles was presumably exposed to the
same PO_2 after short and long coronary occlusions and a mechanism
other than PO_2 per se must be invoked to account for the prolonged
reactive hyperemia after the release of long occlusions.

Since observations discussed up to this point failed to
indicate a direct effect of oxygen on coronary vasculature, we
looked for other possible mediators for the dilation observed when

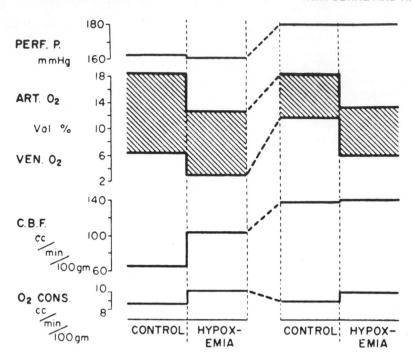

Fig 2.   Effect of hypoxemia on coronary blood flow at two different perfusion pressures.   (Reproduced by permission from J. Clin. Invest. 36:1101, 1957.)

oxygen supply fell short of the myocardial requirements. We sought the presence of a stabile vasodilator substance by infusing coronary sinus blood from hypoxic hearts, reoxygenating it and infusing it into a test coronary artery[13]. No vasodilation was produced by this reoxygenated coronary sinus blood. Nevertheless, we examined the possibility that potassium release from the hypoxic myocardium might be involved in the coronary dilation, but were unable to confirm this hypothesis[14]. Studies by Scott et al[15] confirmed this observation but their data suggested that perhaps the initial dilation could be attributed to potassium. These same investigators also showed that changes in osmolarity that can occur with increased contractile activity cannot account for active hyperemia. With respect to pH changes secondary to hypoxia or ischemia, produced by increasing tissue concentrations of lactic acid or CO_2, the vasodilation observed is small relative to the effects of physio-logical stimuli such as increased cardiac work or hypoxia alone, and consequently can at best be considered to be a minor contributing factor. Finally, the prostaglandins which are potent vasodilators are released during cardiac anoxia, but studies by Block et al[16] have conclusively demonstrated that blockage of prostaglandin synthesis with indomethacin did not block anoxia-induced coronary flow in isolated perfused rabbit hearts nor did exogenous prostaglandin mimic the flow changes produced by anoxia.

Among the various possible mediators of coronary dilation secondary to ischemia or hypoxia is the nucleoside, adenosine. Adenosine is formed by hydrolysis of AMP by 5'-nucleotidase, which is located at the myocardial cell margins, and hence adenosine can readily reach the interstitial fluid and the resistance vessels without being deaminated to inosine (which is not vasoactive) by intracellular adenosine deaminase[17]. We have found that adenosine is present in normal myocardium and can show a threefold increase in a matter of 5 seconds after interruption of the blood supply to the rat heart[18]. It also increases to a similar degree when the inspired gas of the rat is changed from room air to 10% O_2 in N_2[19]. Furthermore, experiments on isolated perfused guinea pig hearts illustrate the close relationship between oxygen content of the perfusion medium and 1) the coronary flow, 2) the tissue adenosine concentration and 3) the release of adenosine into the perfusate (Fig. 3). As the oxygen content of the perfusion medium was reduced there was little change in flow or adenosine production and release until the per cent oxygen was reduced to about 30%. With further reduction in the oxygen supply to the isolated heart there was an abrupt and striking parallel increment in coronary flow and adenosine production and release. Although this parallelism between coronary flow and myocardial adenosine levels during hypoxia is suggestive of a cause and effect relationship, it certainly does not document a dependency of coronary vascular smooth muscle relaxation on the cardiac adenosine concentration.

Adenosine levels are also enhanced in the heart under more physiological conditions. For example, with increased cardiac work produced by thoracic aorta constriction in the open chest rat, the myocardial adenosine content is significantly increased despite the increased coronary perfusion pressure induced by the aortic constriction[21]. Also, fluid introduced into the pericardial sac of the open chest dog showed a significant increase in the adenosine levels with stellate ganglion stimulation[22] or simulated exercise produced by repetitive electrical stimulation of the motor nerves to the limb muscles (unpublished observations).

Ischemia or hypoxia also results in the formation of adenosine in several other tissues, such as brain, skeletal muscle, kidney and lung. In brain, adenosine is increased several fold within 2-3 sec. of ischemia and is capable of inducing marked vasodilation of

CORONARY FLOW AND ADENOSINE FORMATION

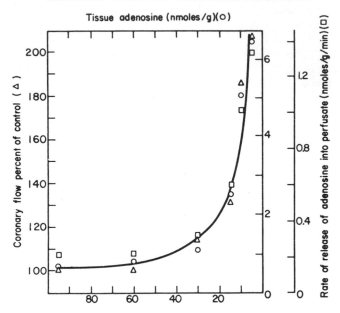

Fig. 3   Parallelism between coronary flow, tissue adenosine levels
and rate of release of adenosine observed at different levels of
PO_2 of the perfusion medium.   Abscissa: per cent oxygen in gas
phase of perfusion medium.   Ordinates: Coronary flow as per cent of
that observed with 95% O_2 in perfusion medium (Δ), tissue adenosine
levels (O) in nmoles/g and rate of release of adenosine into the
perfusate (□) in nmoles/q/min.   (Reproduced with modification by
permission from J. Mol. Cell. Cardiol. 6:561, 1974.)

the vessels[23].   Hypoxia also produces a large increment in cerebral
adenosine levels (Fig. 4) as does arterial hypotension, hypocapnia
and electrical stimulation of the brain[24].   A major difference
between heart and brain is that adenosine does not readily cross
the blood-brain barrier, and when it is released into the cerebrospinal fluid it is not lost to the tissue and can be reincorporated
into intracellular nucleotides.   Recent evidence indicates that in
skeletal muscle, as in the case of heart and brain, adenosine
probably plays an important role in the control of blood flow under
physiological conditions as well as with ischemia and hypoxia[25,26].
However, the role of adenosine in kidney and lung remains to be
elucidated.

The mechanism of action of adenosine on vascular smooth muscle
and the means whereby its production is matched to tissue oxygen

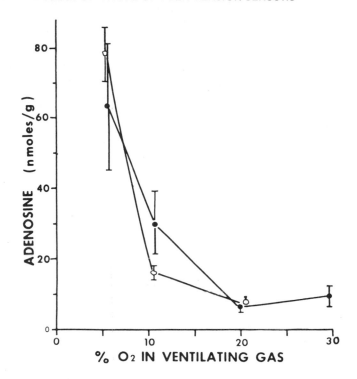

Fig. 4   Increase in brain adenosine levels produced by lowering
per cent O_2 in respired gas below 20%. Increase in per cent O_2 above
20% did not change adenosine levels (filled circles). Open circles
represent brains that were stimulated at 30 Hz, 10V, 3 ms whereas
filled circles represent brains that were not electrically
stimulated. Each point represents average of 5 (●) and 10 (O)
observations. Ventilation was kept constant at 60/min. tidal volume
= 5 ml. (Reproduced by permission from Am. J. Physiol. 228:1896,
1975.)

levels have not been established. Norepinephrine or potassium-
contracted strips of hog carotid arteries relax with physiological
concentrations (10^{-6} M) of adenosine and at pharmacological concentrations 10^{-3} M) produce significant increases in cyclic AMP[27].
Despite the need for 10^{-3} M adenosine in the bathing solution to
induce changes in cyclic AMP, it is conceivable that such a
mechanism is involved in vascular smooth muscle relaxation since the

adenosine deaminase activity of the strips and the bathing solution
(leached out adenosine deaminase) is so great that adenosine added
to the bath is very rapidly deaminated and the small amount of
adenosine produced by vascular smooth muscle strips subjected to
anoxia is undetectable[28].

Another possible mechansim of action of adenosine on vascular
smooth muscle is by interference with calcium uptake and its
utilization by the contractile machinery. Studies on isolated
guinea pig atrium have revealed that the calcium current is abolished
by the addition of adenosine (10^{-6}M) to the superfusion fluid and
is immediately restored upon the addition of adenosine deaminase[29].
Whether adenosine in some manner blocks calcium activation of
vascular smooth muscle remains to be determined.

Gellai et al[5] have suggested that adenosine and oxygen tension
work in concert to produce relaxation of helical strips of rabbit
coronary arteries (Fig. 1A). They found that adenosine became
much more effective in eliciting relaxation of the strips if the PO_2
of the bathing solution was reduced; the lower the PO_2 the lower the
adenosine concentration necessary to induce relaxation. They
concluded that the control of coronary resistance is possibly
caused by alterations in PO_2 at constant adenosine levels. This
interpretation is open to criticism since it is known that adenosine
concentrations vary inversely with the tissue oxygen supply, and
under physiological conditions, such as with increased cardiac
work, the myocardial oxygen demands are increased whereas the
arterial, and presumably the arteriolar, PO_2 levels are unchanged.

To date, our hypothesis has been that in the presence of an
inadequate oxygen supply for tissue needs that there is net
degradation of adenosine nucleotides with increases in AMP (the
substrate for 5'-nucleotidase) and a resultant dephosphorylation
of AMP to adenosine which in turn mediates metabolic vasodilation.
This concept is supported by studies on preparations that range
from intact animals[22] to cultured heart cells[30]. Implicit in this
idea is that the oxygen supply to the mitochondria is limiting and
this is difficult to square with the facts that 1) there is no
impairment of oxidative phosphorylation of mitochondria at PO_2 of
1 mm Hg or less, and 2) that the PO_2 of the intracapillary blood is
about 15-20 mm Hg or more. Since the capillaries lie in close
proximity (ca 6 μ) to the myocardial cells, the gradient between
capillary and mitochondrion is large, (ca 3 mm.Hg./μ) and such a
steep gradient of PO_2 is hard to conceptualize on an anatomical
basis.

It is quite conceivable that adenosine formation is not
solely linked to inadequate PO_2 at the subcellular level but to
the metabolic machinery of the cell. Recent studies by Gorczynski
and Duling[31] in the hamster cremaster muscle preparation have

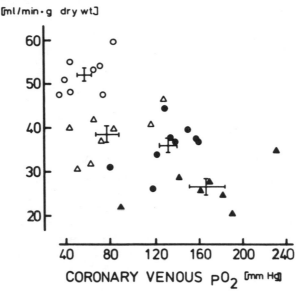

Fig 5. Relationship between coronary flow and coronary venous PO_2. Open symbols = low arterial PO_2, closed symbols = high arterial PO_2; triangles = low work load, circles = high work load; crosses = mean ± standard error of mean. (Reproduced by permission from Pflügers, Arch. 361:197,1976.)

demonstrated that there is dissociation between arteriolar dilation and PO_2 of the muscle when the muscle is stimulated to contract: onset and cessation of dilation closely paralleled contraction whereas the PO_2 decrease showed some latency in onset and persisted after termination of stimulation. Furthermore arterioles in very close proximity to contracting muscle dilated but showed no change in intravascular PO_2.

In concordance with these observations are studies by Müller-Ruchholtz and Neill[32] who examined the relationship between coronary flow, cardiac work and venous PO_2 at low and high work loads in the isolated perfused guinea pig heart. As illustrated in Figure 5, coronary flow was greater at low that at high coronary venous PO_2 However the increase in coronary flow secondary to an increased work load was not consistently associated with a decrease in venous

PO_2. Although venous PO_2 may not provide a true reflection of tissue PO_2 because of some counter current O_2 exchange between adjacent coronary arteries and veins, the data nevertheless suggest that increased metabolic activity may result in vasodilation (possibly by adenosine release) in the absence of significant decreases in tissue PO_2. In these experiments [32] the creatine phosphate : creatine ratio showed a significant inverse correlation with coronary flow with low and high work loads at high arterial PO_2.

In conclusion, there is little evidence for an oxygen sensor in the coronary vasculature, and possibly other vascular beds. The mediator of vasodilation in ischemia, hypoxia or enhanced metabolic activity of the tissue appears to arise in the parenchymal tissue rather than the vascular smooth muscle and evidence suggests that an important metabolic mediator is the nucleoside, adenosine. Whether the release of vasodilator quantities of adenosine are solely related to inadequate tissue oxygen supply is unsettled since some conditions have been observed where vasodilation occurs in response to increased tissue metabolic activity with apparently adequate oxygen availability.

REFERENCES

1. Hilton R, Eichholtz F: The influence of chemical factors on the coronary circulation. J. Physiol. (Lond.) 59:413-425, 1925.
2. Smith DJ, Vane JR: Effects of oxygen tension on vascular and other smooth muscle. J. Physiol. (Lond.) 186:284-294, 1966.
3. Crawford DG, Fairchild HM, Guyton AC: Oxygen lack as a possible cause of reactive hyperemia. Am. J. Physiol. 197: 613-619, 1959.
4. Carrier O Jr., Walker JR, Guyton AC: Role of oxygen in auto-regulation of blood flow in isolated vessels. Am. J. Physiol. 260:951-954, 1964.
5. Gellai M, Norton JM, Detar R: Evidence for direct control of coronary vascular tone by oxygen. Circ. Res. 32:279-289, 1973.
6. Pittman RN, Duling BR: Oxygen sensitivity of vascular smooth muscle 1. In vitro studies. Microvas. Res. 6:202-211, 1973.
7. Duling BR: Microvascular responses to alterations in oxygen tension. Circ. Res. 31:481-489, 1972.
8. Ross J Jr., Kaiser GA, Klocke FJ: Observations on the role of diminished oxygen tension in the functional hyperemia of skeletal muscle. Circ. Res. 15:473-484, 1964.
9. Honig CR: Control of smooth muscle actomyosin by phosphate and 5' AMP. Possible role in metabolic autoregulation. Microvasc. Res. 1:133-146, 1968,

10. Herlihy JT, Murphy RA: Absence of a direct effect of phosphate or 5' AMP on the contractile proteins of hog carotid arteries. Circ. Res. 28:434-440, 1971.

11. Berne RM, Blackmon JR, Gardnèr TH: Hypoxemia and coronary blood flow. J. Clin. Invest. 36:1101-1106, 1957.

12. Guz A, Kurland GS, Freedberg AS: Relation of coronary flow to oxygen supply. Am. J. Physiol. 199:179-182, 1960.

13. Jelliffe RW, Wolf DR, Berne RM, Eckstein RW: Absence of vasoactive and cardiotropic substances in coronary sinus blood of dogs. Cric. Res. 5:382-387, 1957.

14. Driscol TE, Berne RM: Role of potassium in regulation of coronary blood flow. Proc. Soc. Exptl. Biol. & Med. 96:505-508, 1957.

15. Scott JB, Radawski D: Role of hyperosmolarity in the genesis of active and reactive hyperemia. Circ. Res. (Suppl. 1) 28:26-32, 1971.

16. Block AJ, Feinberg H,Herbaczynska-Cedro K, Vane JR: Anoxia-induced release of prostaglandins in rabbit isolated hearts. Circ. Res. 36:34-42, 1975.

17. Rubio R, Berne RM, Dobson JG Jr.: Sites of adenosine production in cardiac and skeletal muscle. Am. J. Physiol. 225:938-953, 1973.

18. Berne M, Rubio R, Duling BR, Wiedmeier VT: Effects of acute and chronic hypoxia on coronary blood flow. Adv. in Cardiol. 5:56-66, 1970.

19. Berne RM, Rubio R: Adenine nucleotide metabolism in the heart. Circ. Res. (Suppl. III) 34:109-120, 1974.

20. Rubio R, Wiedmeier VT, Berne RM: Relationship between coronary flow and adenosine production and release. J. Mol. Cell Cardiol. 6:561-566, 1974.

21. Foley DH, Herlihy JT, Thompson CI, Rubio R, Berne RM: Relationship between cardiac work and levels of myocardial adenosine. Fed. Proc. 35:348, 1976.

22. Watkinson WP, Foley DH, Rubio R, Berne RM: Adenosine production by canine myocardium during stellate ganglion stimulation. Circulation (In Press).

23. Berne RM, Rubio R, Curnish RR: Release of adenosine from ischemic brain: effect on cerebral vascular resistance and incorporation into cerebral adenine nucleotides. Circ. Res. 35:262-271, 1974.

24. Rubio R, Berne RM, Bockman EL, Curnish RR: Relationship between adenosine concentration and oxygen supply in rat brain. Am. J. Physiol. 228:1896-1902, 1975.

25. Dobson JG Jr., Rubio R, Berne RM: Role of adenine nucleotides, adenosine and inorganic phosphate in the regulation of skeletal muscle blood flow. Circ. Res. 29:375-384, 1971.

26. Bockman EL, Berne RM, Rubio R: Adenosine and active hyperemia in dog skeletal muscle. Am. J. Physiol. 230:1531-1537, 1976.

27. Herlihy JT, Bockman EL, Berne RM, Rubio R: Adenosine relaxation of isolated vascular smooth muscle. Am. J. PHysiol. 230: 1239-1243, 1976.

28. Van Harn GL, Rubio R, Berne RM: Adenine nucleotide metabolite
     formation in vascular smooth muscle during hypoxia. The
     Physiologist 19:398, 1976.
29. Schrader J, Rubio R, Berne RM: Inhibition of slow action
     potentials of guinea pig atria by adenosine. J. Mol. Cell.
     Cardiol. 7:427-433, 1975.
30. Mustafa SJ, Berne RM, Rubio R: Adenosine metabolism in cultured
     chick-embryo heart cells. Am. J. Physiol. 228:1474-1478, 1975.
31. Gorczynski RJ, Duling BR: The role of O_2 lack in contraction
     induced arteriolar vasodilation in hamster striated muscle.
     Fed. Proc. 35:448, 1976.
32. Müller-Ruchholtz ER, Neill WA: The mechanism of coronary
     hyperemia induced by increased cardiac work. Pflugers Arch.
     361:197-199, 1976.

BIOASSAY AND PHARMACOLOGIC EVALUATION OF THE ADENOSINE HYPOTHESIS

Francis J. Haddy

Department of Physiology
Uniformed Services University of the Health Sciences
Bethesda, Maryland 20014

Our approach to the mechanism of hypoxic, ischemic, and exercise dilation has differed from that of Berne and Rubio. We have mainly used bioassay and pharmacological techniques. The data[1] generated by these techniques support the adenosine hypothesis for regulation of blood flow in cardiac and skeletal muscle and in addition suggest a contributory role for AMP in cardiac hypoxic dilation.

CARDIAC MUSCLE

In 1965, we reported that, in the dog, release of coronary occlusion of short duration results in the appearance in coronary sinus blood of a vasoactive substance which has the bioassay characteristics of adenosine and AMP[2]. Our technique was to perfuse another organ with coronary sinus blood at a constant rate while measuring perfusion pressure. We first used the forelimb as the bioassay organ and found that release of coronary artery occlusion produced dilation in the forelimb having roughly the time course of the reactive hyperemia in the heart. We next used the kidney[2] as the bioassay organ because previous studies in our laboratory and in the laboratory of Thurau[3] had shown that the response of kidney to intra-renal injection of adenosine or AMP is unique, namely vasoconstriction rather than vasodilation. We found that release of coronary artery occlusion also produced renal constriction and this too had a time course similar to the reactive hyperemia in the heart (advantages of bioassay are that it immediately indicates whether substances are released in vasoactive quantities and allows correlation of the temporal sequence of their appearance to the vascular response in the donor organ).

In 1971 we improved the renal bioassay system by removing
the kidney from the body and continually infusing a vasoconstrictor
agent into the renal artery.[4] Removal from the body decreased the
lag time of the system by allowing us to place the kidney nearer
the heart and increased its stability by eliminating neural influences. Infusion of a vasoconstrictor increased the sensitivity of
the renal vascular bed to adenosine and AMP and in addition allowed
us to assay for dilator agents. Using this system, we confirmed
our 1965 findings[2] and also showed that the renal constrictor responses to release of coronary occlusion are not influenced by
adrenergic blockade of the kidney.[4] Thus, as suspected from the
dilator responses in the forelimb,[5] the renal constrictor responses
do not result from catecholamine release by the heart.

Working with Schrader and Gerlach in East Germany, the release
of adenosine and its degradatives, inosine and hypoxanthine, from
the isolated perfused guinea pig heart was measured during reactive
hyperemia, hypoxic hyperemia, and autoregulation with a new sensitive radio-assay.[5] In brief, cardiac adenine nucleotides were labeled
for 35 minutes with (8-^{14}C)-adenine. They then served as precursors
for the formation of labeled adenosine, inosine and hypoxanthine
which were continuously released into the effluent perfusate. Coronary flow increased when the oxygen tension in the perfusate was
lowered and this was accompanied by enhanced appearance of labeled
adenosine in the effluent. Reactive hyperemia following 15, 30,
and 60 sec. of cardiac ischemia was also paralleled by a progressive
increase in the release of labeled adenosine. Furthermore, changes
in coronary resistance in the course of flow-autoregulation correlated linearly with the release rate of labeled adenosine from the
myocardium, resistance decreasing as release rate increased. In all
cases, release of labeled hypoxanthine paralleled that of labeled
adenosine whereas during hypoxia and autoregulation (over the lower
pressure range) the release of labeled inosine increased more steeply
than did labeled adenosine. Thus the myocardium released (^{14}C)-
adenosine at an enhanced rate whenever oxygen delivery was reduced.
The findings are entirely compatible with the adenosine hypothesis
for regulation of coronary blood flow.

We encountered some problems however. Working with Bünger
and Gerlach, we were able to show that theophylline, in concentrations without effect on cardiac rate or contractility, competitively inhibits the coronary dilation produced by exogenous adenosine in this preparation.[6] At the highest concentrations of theophylline which we were able to use, inhibition ranged from 30 to
60% depending on the concentration of adenosine. However, like
other investigators, we could not inhibit hypoxic hyperemia or
reactive hyperemia with theophylline (unpublished observation).
We also were unable to inhibit autoregulation with this agent

(unpublished observation). Here then is the major objection to the adenosine hypothesis (we were also unable to inhibit these responses with ouabain in concentrations which block the dilation produced by exogenous potassium[7]). We were aware however that this negative finding is not necessarily incompatible with a role for adenosine in regulation of coronary blood flow. We discussed the possibility that increased hydrogen ion concentration during ischemia and hypoxia interferes with the ability of theophylline to competitively inhibit adenosine vasodilation. We also discussed the possibility that ischemia and hypoxia produce adenosine concentrations exceeding those which are blocked by the limited amount of theophylline given to the heart (the amount is limited by side effects such as tachycardia and increased contractility).

We therefore readdressed the problem in our Michigan State laboratories. We confirmed the observation that theophylline does not[8] block reactive hyperemia in the isolated perfused guinea pig heart. In this same preparation, adenosine vasodilation and inhibition of this vasodilation by theophylline were not less at a low pH (produced by increasing the carbon dioxide tension of the perfusate). We therefore rejected our "hydrogen ion interference" hypothesis.

In the meantime, Oswald showed that theophylline also competitively inhibits the renal vasoconstriction response to adenosine.[9] We therefore returned to our improved canine bioassay system and administered very large amounts of theophylline to the bioassay kidney, producing concentrations far exceeding those that have been used in the heart.[10,11] This completely blocked the renal constrictor response to intrarenal injection of large amounts of adenosine. We found that the same was true for AMP. Furthermore, in the absence of theophylline, hypoxia localized to the heart (with a lung interposed in the coronary perfusion line) produced vigorous constriction in the kidney which had essentially the same time course as the dilation of the coronary vascular bed. This constriction was greatly reduced during theophylline infusion. Unfortunately, since theophylline blocks AMP as well as adenosine, the technique does not allow differentiation between adenosine and AMP.

We also brought Hashimoto's adenosine autoblockade[12] to bear on the problem. An interesting but unexplained feature of the renal response to adenosine is that during intraarterial _infusion_ at a high rate the increased resistance gradually disappears and then the kidney no longer responds to bolus injection of adenosine (but responds in an exaggerated fashion to norepinephrine or sympathetic nerve stimulation).[12] Thus adenosine infusion produces a type of self-antagonism. We examined this phenomenon in some detail[10,11] and found that the adenosine infusion also blocks the constrictor response to AMP but has no effect on the dilator responses to ADP and ATP.

Adenosine autoblockade converted the large renal constrictor responses seen on release of coronary occlusion and during cardiac hypoxia to small dilator responses.[10,11] The large constrictor responses promptly reappeared on stopping the adenosine infusion, as did the constrictor responses to adenosine and AMP. Unfortunately this technique also fails to allow differentiation between adenosine and AMP.

It was then anonamously suggested to us that adenosine deaminase might allow such differentiation since this enzyme degrades adenosine but not AMP. After a number of trials we found that 1)lengthening the circuit between coronary sinus and kidney to 200 cm (thereby increasing the lag time from 5 to 30 sec.), 2)placing the circuit tubing in a water bath at 37°C, and 3)infusing the adenosine deaminase into the coronary artery (rather than into the renal artery) provided a preparation in which intracoronary injection of adenosine was without effect on the kidney whereas intracoronary injection of AMP still produced renal constriction.[11] In this preparation, adenosine deaminase completely eliminated the renal constrictor response to cardiac ischemia but only reduced the renal constrictor response to cardiac hypoxia by 40% (adenosine deaminase was without effect on the dilator responses of the coronary vascular bed to adenosine, AMP, cardiac ischemia and cardiac hypoxia).[11] These findings suggest that the agent seen in coronary sinus blood on release of ischemia is adenosine but that both adenosine and AMP appear during cardiac hypoxia.

We still cannot state with certainty that these agents act at the level of the coronary arteriole during reactive hyperemia and hypoxic hyperemia. ATP injected into the coronary artery is degraded in a single pass through the heart[4,11,13-15] and the degradation products include AMP[13] and adenosine.[14] Thus while the agents in coronary sinus blood appear to be adenosine in the case of reactive hyperemia and adenosine and AMP in the case of hypoxic hyperemia it is possible that the vasodilating agents at the coronary arteriolar level include ATP and ADP as well as AMP and adenosine. One might ask whether this is the reason why reactive dilation in the coronary vascular bed was not influenced by intracoronary infusion of adenosine deaminase. An answer in the negative is probably correct since the infusion also failed to influence the coronary responses to exogenous adenosine. It seems more likely that the failure of adenosine deaminase to block reactive coronary vasodilation is related to the short exposure time of adenosine to adenosine deaminase at the arteriolar level.

Why doesn't theophylline, an inhibitor of the vasodilating actions of adenosine and the adenine nucleotides in heart,[6] block cardiac reactive hyperemia, hypoxic hyperemia, and autoregulation when it is given to heart? Two possibilities can be offered for this apparent contradiction. Since the inhibition is of the

competitive type[6] and only a limited amount can be given to heart,
it is possible that the concentration of theophylline used is not
great enough to substantially inhibit the amounts of adenosine and
adenine nucleotides liberated. It also seems likely that several
different vasoactive agents and the myogenic response act in concert
to produce myocardial blood flow regulation. We have, for example,
previously reported increased hydrogen and potassium ion concentrations and increased osmolality in coronary sinus blood during the
reactive hyperemia which follows the release of a 30 second occlusion
of the left common coronary artery in the dog.[16] All of these changes
are in the direction to produce cardiac vasodilation (and could
explain the dilation we observed in the autoblocked bioassay kidney
during cardiac reactive hyperemia and hypoxic dilation), as is the
change in vascular transmural pressure during the occlusion (Bayliss
response). Thus selective inhibition of adenosine and/or AMP by
theophylline administration might not substantially affect the overall response.

SKELETAL MUSCLE

In our 1965 study,[2] we showed that exercise of hindlimb skeletal
muscle in the dog is also associated with release of a substance or
substances into femoral venous blood which has the bioassay characteristics of adenosine and/or AMP. This finding was confirmed in
1971 utilizing the improved bioassay system.[4] That same year, Dobson
et al[17] and Berne et al[18] reported that ischemic exercise of rat and
dog skeletal muscle is associated with increased tissue levels of
AMP and adenosine, but that only adenosine appears in the venous
effluent. Increased tissue levels of adenosine and AMP in rat
skeletal muscle were again reported by Rubio et al[19] in 1973. In
this paper they also point out that the adenosine hypothesis for
regulating skeletal muscle blood flow is inconsistent with the fact
that in skeletal muscle adenine nucleotide degradation occurs primarily via inosinic acid formation, with only a small production of
adenosine. However, they point out that in skeletal muscle from
rats and guinea pigs 5'-nucleotidase (the enzyme that degrades AMP
to adenosine) activity is found in endothelium and in localized
skeletal muscle cells in close proximity to blood vessels. This
strategic position with respect to the blood vessels is consistent
with the adenosine hypothesis and could explain the observation that
only small amounts of adenosine are found in whole tissue and effluent during ischemic exercise. Recently Collingsworth et al[20] reported
that AMP does not appear in the effluent from exercising canine gracilis muscle (perfused at constant flow with modified Ringer's solution) unless the stimulation parameters are such as to activate the
sympathetic nerves. Since adenosine is a potent dilator of the
skeletal muscle vascular bed, all of these observations suggest that
this agent may well participate in the vasodilation seen in skeletal
muscle during exercise at constant flow or under ischemic conditions.

We recently brought theophylline to bear on the problem in the canine gracilis muscle perfused at constant flow[21], [22] We found that the vasodilator responses to intraarterial injections of adenosine and AMP were completely blocked during intraarterial infusion of theophylline. Again the rate of infusion exceeded that which can be used in the heart. The vasodilator responses to ATP and acetylcholine were unaffected. Under this condition, exercise dilation was much attenuated, as judged by the magnitude, area, and duration of the response. The degree of exercise, as judged by contractile force and venous Po_2, was not affected by theophylline. Thus it appears that adenosine in fact plays a role in the exercise dilation seen at constant flow in the gracilis muscle of the dog. Additional experiments must be conducted to determine whether this is also the case at natural flow.

Other observations also indicate a need for more study. Both chemical[17], [18] and bioassay[2], [4] analysis of the venous effluent from the muscle mass of the canine hindlimb indicate that the blood contains adenosine only during severe or ischemic exercise. Venous blood from the canine gracilis muscle (perfused at constant flow) develops enhanced vasodilator activity only during moderate to high frequency exercise[23] and this enhanced vasodilator activity can be completely abolished by correcting the fall in P_{O_2} and pH[24] In this experiment, the gracilis venous effluent is perfused at constant flow through the resting contralateral gracilis muscle. Low frequency faradic stimulation of the gracilis nerve of the first muscle produces slight dilation in that muscle but this is not accompanied by dilation in the second resting muscle[23] Dilation with a time course similar to that in first muscle is seen during higher frequency stimulation[23] but this dilation can be completely abolished by inserting a permeator in the line connecting the two muscles and correcting P_{O2} and pH back to the levels seen prior to exercise[24] While these findings are not incompatible with the adenosine hypothesis (the adenosine may not have reached the second muscle in vasodilating concentrations), they do indicate a need for critical evaluation of the contribution of adenosine to the hyperemia seen under natural conditions of exercise.

REFERENCES

1. Berne RM: Cardiac nucleotides in hypoxia: possible role in regulation of coronary blood flow. Am. J. Physiol. 204:317-322, 1963.

2. Scott JB, Daugherty RM, Dabney JM, Haddy FJ: Role of chemical factors in regulation of flow through kidney, hindlimb, and heart. Am. J. Physiol. 208:813-824, 1965.

3. Thurau K: Renal hemodynamics. Amer. J. Med. 36:698-719, 1964.

4. Scott J, Chen W, Radawski P, Anderson D, and Haddy F: Bioassay evidence for participation of adenosine and the adenine nucleotides in local blood flow regulation. Proc. Intl. Union Physiol. Sci. 9:504, 1971.

5. Schrader J, Haddy FJ, Gerlach E: Release of (^{14}C) adenosine from the guinea pig heart during autoregulation. In Harris P, Bing RJ, Fleckenstein A (Editors): Recent Advances in Studies on Cardiac Structure and Metabolism. Baltimore, University Park Press, 1976, vol 7, pp 171-175.

6. Bünger R, Haddy FJ, Gerlach E: Coronary responses to dilating substances and competitive inhibition by theophylline in the isolated perfused guinea pig heart. Pflügers Arch. 358:213-224, 1975.

7. Bünger R, Haddy FJ, Querengässer A, Gerlach E: Studies on potassium induced coronary dilation in the isolated guinea pig heart. Pflügers Arch. 363:27-31, 1976.

8. Merrill GF, Haddy FJ, Dabney JM: Effects of pH and theophylline on the coronary response to adenosine. Physiologist 18:317, 1975.

9. Oswald H: Renal effects of adenosine and their inhibition by theophylline in dogs. Nauyn-Schmiedeberg's Arch. Pharmacol. 288:79-86, 1975.

10. Scott J, Nyhof R, Anderson D, Swindall B, Ely S, Haddy F: Possible explanation for failure of theophylline to block hypoxic coronary dilation; further support for the adenosine hypothesis. Fed. Proc. 34:415, 1975.

11. Scott JB, Chen WT, Swindall BT, Dabney JM, Haddy FJ: Bioassay evidence indicating a role for adenosine in cardiac ischemic dilation and for AMP and adenosine in hypoxic dilation. Circul. Res. In press.

12. Hashimoto K and Kobubun H: Adenosine-catecholamine interaction in the renal vascular response. Proc. Soc. Exptl. Biol. and Med. 136:1125-1128, 1971.

13. Liu PK, Selleck BH, Chou CC: Release of adenine nucleotides during reactive hyperemia in guinea pig heart. Fed. Proc. 35: 349, 1976.

14. Bear HP, Drummond GI: Catabolism of adenine nucleotides by the isolated perfused rat heart. Proc. Soc. Exptl. Biol. and Med. 127:33-36, 1968.

15. Stowe, DF, Sullivan TE, Dabney JM, Scott JB, Haddy FJ: Role of ATP in coronary flow regulation in the isolated perfused guinea pig heart. Physiologist 17:339, 1974.

16. Scott JB, Radawski D: Role of hyperosmolarity in the genesis of active and reactive hyperemia. Circ. Res. 28(Suppl. I):26-32, 1971.

17. Dobson JG, Rubio R, Berne RM: Role of adenine nucleotides, adenosine, and inorganic phosphate in the regulation of skeletal muscle blood flow. Circul. Res. 29:375-384, 1971.

18. Berne RM, Rubio R, Dobson JG, Curnish RR: Adenosine and adenine nucleotides as possible mediators of cardiac and skeletal muscle blood flow regulation. Circul. Res. 28 (Suppl I):115-119, 1971.

19. Rubio R, Berne RM, Dobson JG, Jr.: Sites of adenosine production in cardiac and skeletal muscle. Am. J. Physiol. 225:938-953, 1973.

20. Collingsworth A, Selleck B, Chou C, Scott J: Outflow of AMP from dog gracilis muscle during vasoconstriction produced by norepinephrine. Fed. Proc. 35:720, 1976.

21. Tabaie H, Scott J, Haddy F: Reduction of exercise dilation by theophylline. Physiologist 18:415, 1975.

22. Tabaie HMA, Scott JB, Haddy FJ: Reduction of exercise dilation by theophylline. Proc. Soc. Exptl. Biol. Med. In press.

23. Radawski DP, Hoppe W, Haddy FJ: Role of vasoactive substances in active hyperemia in skeletal muscle. Proc. Soc. Exptl. Biol. Med. 148:270-276, 1975.

24. Stowe DF, Owen TL, Anderson DK, Haddy FJ, Scott JB: Interaction of O_2 and CO_2 in sustained exercise hyperemia of canine skeletal muscle. Am. J. Physiol. 229:28-33, 1975.

Mechanism of Oxygen Sensing

in Tissues

Chairman: S. Lahiri

INTRODUCTORY REMARKS: OXYGEN LINKED RESPONSE OF CAROTID CHEMORECEPTORS

Sukhamay Lahiri

Department of Physiology and Department of Medicine
(Cardiovascular-Pulmonary Division), University of
Pennsylvania, Philadelphia, Pa. 19174, U.S.A.

Recognition of oxygen in the animal organism is a fundamental
phenomenon in biology. There are various examples of physiologic
responses to small changes in oxygen pressure in the range of
normal P_{O_2} at sea level. We have already had glimpses of these
chemoreception functions in the previous sessions of the symposium.
In mammals the outstanding examples are provided by the microscopic organs along the aortic and carotid arteries known as
peripheral arterial chemoreceptors. Their oxygen reception
function is well seen in the stimulation of breathing due to
hypoxia. It is well known that a decrease in arterial P_{O_2} results
in an increase in breathing if the nervous connections of the
receptors with central nervous system are intact. This is shown
in figure 1. After denervation of these receptors a similar intensity of hypoxia results in decreases of ventilation. Thus decreases in alveolar and arterial P_{O_2} show simultaneous dual effects
on ventilation: the net effect in intact animal being stimulation
of ventilation. Regardless of the mechanisms involved these results
clearly demonstrate oxygen sensitive property in more than one
system.

In this session, however, we are concerned with the arterial
chemoreceptors. Ever since the discovery of carotid and aortic
bodies numerous attempts have been made to understand the mechanism
of chemoreception but it remains still a goal rather than an
accomplishment. Studies of the reflex ventilatory effects of
hypoxia, provided some clue to the chemoreceptor activity but
ventilation is too remote from the chemoreceptors for studying its
mechanism. A direct recording from the afferent fibers of carotid
body provided a closer window to the chemoreceptors. But, as you

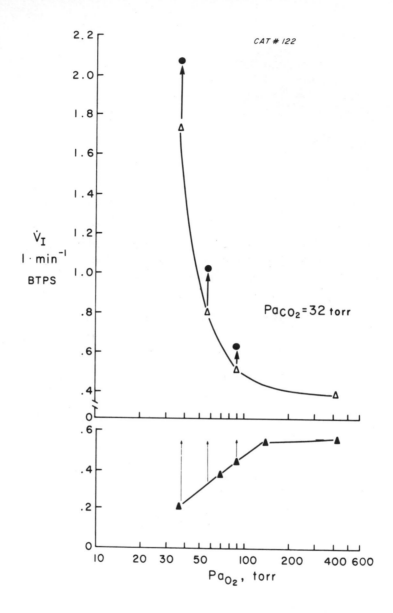

Figure 1: Cat, α–chloralose anesthesia. Effects of changes in
arterial P_{O_2} on ventilation ($\dot{V}_I$) at a maintained arterial P_{CO_2}
before (upper panel) and after (lower panel) bilateral section of
carotid sinus nerves. Hypoxia increased ventilation before and
depressed it after denervation. The arrows indicate the amount of
depression. The dual effects of hypoxia indicate two aspects of
oxygen sensors.

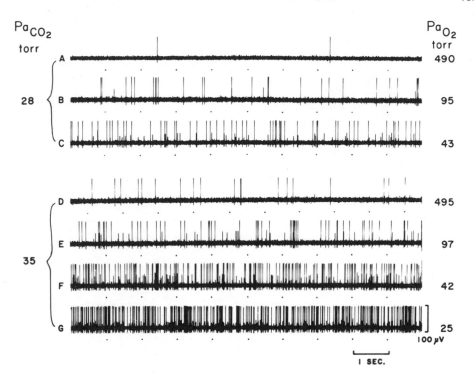

Figure 2: Cat, α-chloralose. Effects of hypoxia and hypercapnia
on the activity of carotid chemoreceptors. Both hypoxia and
hypercapnia stimulated carotid chemoreceptor activity (with
permission of the editor, Respiration Physiology).

will see later, it is not quite close enough, because it is not
known of what the receptor consists. Nonetheless, the activity of
afferent fibers has been used as a tool to look into the nature
of chemoreception. My function here is to illustrate some salient
aspects of carotid chemoreceptor excitation.

P_{O_2} and P_{CO_2}-H^+ interaction

Figure 2 shows the relationship between arterial blood gases
and carotid chemoreceptor activity. A single fiber response is
illustrated here. It is noteworthy that a varying spike interval
is a characteristic of the chemoreceptor discharge. These data
show that a decrease of arterial P_{O_2} from 500 torr to 95 torr

caused more than a ten-fold increase in its activity. Thus an
exquisitely sensitive mechanism is available in the carotid body
for detection and transduction of the changes in P_{O_2} even in the
absence of so to speak arterial hypoxia. In the hypoxic range the
activity is increased further in a hyperbolic or presumably sigmoid
fashion. The hyperbolic response to hypoxia is also a characteristic of other organs and tissues, such as pulmonary arterial
vessels, red blood cells production, etc.

Another feature of the receptor is that an increase in
arterial P_{CO_2} from the normal value of 28 torr to 35 torr caused
about ten-fold increase in its activity in hyperoxia. The effect
of CO_2 is increased dramatically by hypoxia. These and similar
data[1-3] bring out the important point that hypercapnia and hypoxia
show stimulus interaction. A more complete set of results on a
single afferent carotid chemoreceptor fiber in cat is shown in
figure 3.

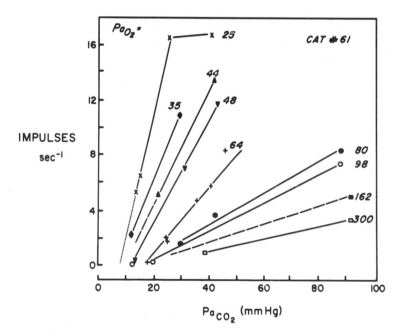

Figure 3: Cat, α-chloralose anesthesia. Response of a single
carotid chemoreceptor afferent fiber to changes in arterial P_{CO_2}
at several levels of arterial P_{O_2}. The combined effects of hypoxia
and hypercapnia were more than additive (with permission of the
editor, Respiration Physiology).

An interaction between the two stimuli can also be seen in the threshold of activity. The receptors can be made silent completely by lowering arterial P_{CO_2} at an appropriate P_{O_2}. This is shown in figure 4. The animal was passively hyperventilated to lower $PaCO_2$ at a relatively high PaO_2. The hyperventilation was terminated at the arrow but the chemoreceptor remained silent for about 22 seconds until a threshold arterial blood gas stimulus (PaO_2 and $PaCO_2$) was reached.

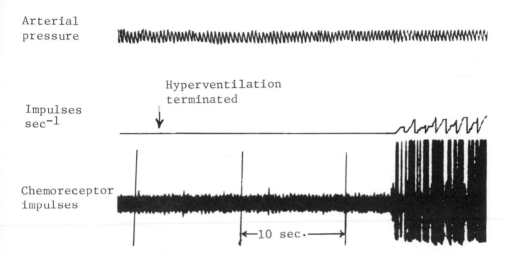

Figure 4: Cat, α-chloralose. Silence and activation of carotid chemoreceptors by a combination of arterial P_{CO_2} and P_{O_2}. Hypocapnia due to passive hyperventilation with 100% O_2 silenced the receptor. During apnea the chemoreceptors were activated due to an increase in arterial P_{CO_2} and a decrease in P_{O_2}.

The relationship between threshold arterial P_{O_2} and P_{CO_2} shows interaction between the two stimuli: a low PaO_2 lowered $PaCO_2$ threshold as shown in figure 5. The lowering of $PaCO_2$ threshold is more than predicted by a simple linear relationship with PaO_2 threshold. I expect Dr. Torrance will talk about the convergence of the two stimuli.

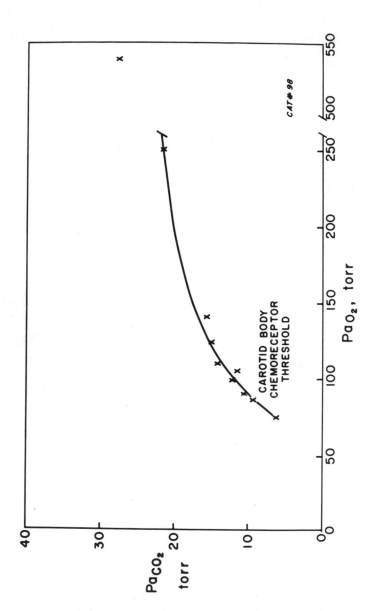

Figure 5: Cat, α-chloralose. Relationship between arterial P_{O_2} and P_{CO_2} threshold for carotid chemoreceptors. A decrease in Pa_{O_2} decreased the Pa_{CO_2} threshold showing convergence of the two stimuli.

It is important to point out here that much of the effect of CO_2 is presumably due to a concomitant change in $[H^+]$.

These results are reminiscent of a reversible binding of O_2 by hemoglobin, and the effect of H^+ on this combination: the Bohr effect.   Using maximal activity as maximal O_2 desaturation, the chemoreceptor activity can be expressed as receptor O_2 saturation as a function of P_{O_2}.   The resemblance of this relationship to O_2-hemoglobin equilibrium is striking[4].   Thus there is an indication that the receptor showed allosteric properties of a polymeric chromophore protein.   The Hill coefficient, nH, of the receptor O_2 saturation curves was greater than 1.   Thus there seemed to be a cooperative effect of oxygen chemoreception.

P_{O_2} and temperature

The well known effect of temperature on hemoglobin O_2 equilibrium is also seen in the receptor activity.   The receptor activity with the change in P_{O_2} at a constant pH is shown in figure 6.   A decrease of temperature from 38° to 30° C decreased the activity considerably.   Also, the effect of temperature change increased as the hypoxic stimulus was increased.   A part of the effect of cooling on the rate of discharge of afferent fibers is certainly due to an effect on the nerve fibers per se.   A decrease in temperature increases duration and refractory period of spikes[5]. As a result the sufficiently close action potentials generated at the receptor may not all be propagated at a lower temperature. Chances of such missing impulses would certainly increase with the increase of stimulation.   Thus the observed greater decrease of discharge rate with an increased hypoxic stimulus during cooling could be explained at least in part.   The idea can be verified by examining the pattern of response to hypercapnic stimulus.

These results can also be expressed as receptor O_2 saturation which again resembles hemoglobin-oxygen equilibrium curves.   The temperature coefficient is as great as that seen for human blood. Cooling also raised threshold stimulus profoundly.   Previously Paintal[6] and Eyzaguirre[7] looked at the effect of temperature on aortic and carotid chemoreceptors respectively.   In agreement with Eyzaguirre these data suggest that the response of the receptors depends on chemical rather than a direct mechanical distortion of nerve endings and subsequent transduction.

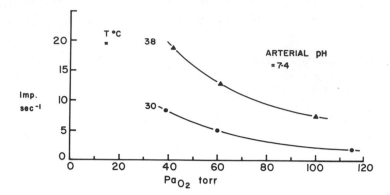

<u>Figure 6</u>: Cat, α-chloralose, Effect of change of temperature on
the response of carotid chemoreceptors to changes in PaO$_2$ at a constant arterial pH of 7.4. A decrease of temperature from 38° to
30° C caused a great decrease in the activity. Since cooling increases pH and since increases in pH causes a decrease in the activity of carotid chemoreceptors the uncorrected effect of temperature would be even greater.

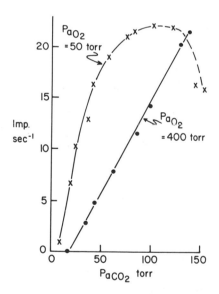

<u>Figure 7</u>: Cat, α-chloralose. Stimulus saturation of carotid
chemoreceptor activity. At low levels of PaCO2 a change of PaO2
from 400 torr to 50 torr showed stimulus interaction. However,
at high levels of hypercapnia the response leveled off during
hypoxia. At one level of hypercapnia there was no difference
between hypoxia and hyperoxia. A greater strength of hypercapnia
diminished the activity.

Stimulus Saturation

Another property of the chemoreceptors is that various combinations of arterial P_{O_2} and P_{CO_2} can produce a relative saturation of activity. A single fiber response is shown in figure 7. At low levels of arterial P_{CO_2} hypoxic stimulus needed to excite chemoreceptors was also low. This is consistent with the observation discussed previously and with the notion of synergism. At a fixed arterial P_{O_2} the maximal activity was obtained as arterial P_{CO_2} was increased. At this level of activity a further increase in hypercapnia or hypoxia did not stimulate the fiber any further. The maximal steady state activity indicated saturation of receptor sites by the stimulus. That the limitation was not in the fiber itself could be shown by a transient increase in activity by the administration of acetylcholine. There was a lack of a sustained maximal activity during hypoxic hypercapnia. This suggests that the failure presumably occurred at the level of transduction.

P_{O_2} and excitation by drugs

There are metabolic and non-metabolic drugs which are known to stimulate carotid chemoreceptors in the cat[8]. It could be argued that the agents which interact with some metabolic aspects of O_2 would show dependence of their effect on arterial or receptor P_{O_2}. On the other hand, the effect of non-metabolic drugs may not depend on P_{O_2}. HCN is known to react with a host of metaloproteins and other enzymes and interfere with oxidation reduction as well as binding and use of molecular O_2[9]. NaCN is commonly used to stimulate peripheral chemoreceptors. Unlike HCN, acetylcholine, another stimulating agent, is not known to influence oxygen metabolism directly. Comparison of the effects of these two drugs are shown in figure 8. The activity of carotid chemoreceptors in the cat is plotted against arterial P_{O_2}. The top panel shows the effect of NaCN at various levels of steady-state arterial P_{O_2}. Slugs of 40 μg NaCN were administered through the femoral vein under maintained conditions of arterial blood gases. The effect of the particular dose of NaCN was negligible at a high arterial P_{O_2} but the effect increased progressively as PaO_2 was decreased.

The lower panel shows the effect of acetylcholine. Acetylcholine in 40 μg slugs stimulated the chemoreceptors but the effect was not augmented by hypoxia.

The difference between the effects of cyanide and acetylcholine is quite clear. The results are apparently consistent with the idea that a stimulus interaction with PaO_2 is in some way linked with oxygen metabolism in the carotid body.

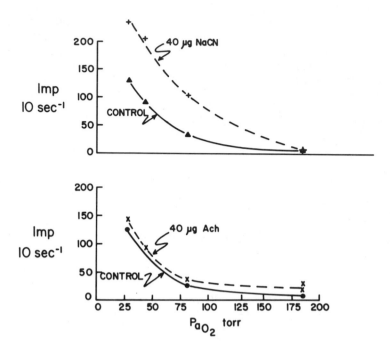

Figure 8: Cat, α-chloralose. Effects of cyanide and acetylcholine on the response of carotid chemoreceptors to changes in PaO2. Cyanide and P_{O_2} showed an interactive effect and acetylcholine an additive effect.

It is appropriate to note here that HCN does not show inter-active effect with CO_2-H^+ stimulus but hypoxia does show inter-action with CO_2-H^+. Thus HCN does not act like a hypoxic stimulus. Rather, HCN simply added to and increased the effect of CO_2-H^+.

Like CO_2-H^+, HCN in high concentrations elicited chemoreceptor response at a high P_{O_2}, and the dose response relationship was linear which ultimately reached a plateau. As P_{O_2} was decreased the concentrations of cyanide needed to elicit a response and to reach the plateau diminished. It is interesting to note that the extracellular concentrations of cyanide (10-20 μ molar) required to stimulate carotid chemoreceptors is rather small. The intra-cellular concentrations would be smaller than that used in most enzymic studies[9]. Also, the speed of the effect seems to be too fast compared to its rate of reaction with cytochrome oxidase[10].

P_{O_2} and osmolarity effects

Many sensory receptors behave like mechanoreceptors. Accordingly Paintal[5] proposed that the mechanism of excitation of peripheral chemoreceptors is a distortion of afferent nerve endings. A change in osmolarity in the environment of the receptors is a possible way of testing the hypothesis, although a change in osmolarity can induce a variety of cellular changes. Recently Eyzaguirre and his colleagues[11] reported that the activity of carotid chemoreceptor afferents are extremely sensitive to small changes in osmolarity of the bathing fluid. He, I believe, does not ascribe this effect to mechanoreceptor property, and will present some new data on this topic in a while. What I would like to present at this time is to show that the osmolarity effect is dependent on PaO_2. A change in osmolarity was induced by intravenous (femoral) administration of 3 ml of 2.5 molar sucrose solution during hypoxia and hyperoxia. The results are shown in figure 9. Clearly the effect was most pronounced during steady-state hypoxia. From the beginning of the administration of sucrose solution to the emergence of the effect there was a lag period of about a minute. This lag period and the dependence of the effect on arterial P_{O_2} are striking and do not seem to be consistent with the notion of mechanoreception. Movement of water according to the osmotic gradient is expected to occur during a single passage through the capillaries and achieve osmotic equilibrium passively. The delay in showing the effect was far too long for it to be mechanical. Also, the effect was not evident on barofibers in the sinus nerve whenever we looked for it. All this information seems to suggest that some intermediate steps are involved in the process of osmotic excitation. In steady state increase of osmolarity from 305 to 314 mosmoles per liter plasma there was a steady increase in chemoreceptor activity which was P_{O_2} dependent. The effect could have occurred through ionic changes including H^+ at the receptor site. It is also possible that a conformational change of the receptor occurred which in turn influenced O_2 binding by the receptor. Changes in the structure of neuromuscular junctions caused by variations in osmotic pressure have been reported[12].

Osmotic excitation has been reported for mechanoreceptors like muscle spindle. Unlike carotid chemoreceptors, however, the activity of the spindle was increased by both hypotonic and hypertonic solutions, and showed adaptation. The change in tonicity employed to elicit a response was rather large (50 to 500 percent). On the other hand, carotid chemoreceptors behaved like hypothalamic osmoreceptors which responded to small changes in tonicity (less than 10 percent), and did not show adaptation[14]. A direct effect of osmotic pressure cannot, however, be ruled out totally. It is possible to argue that gas exchange in the carotid body causes redistribution of molecular species across the membranes of cells and

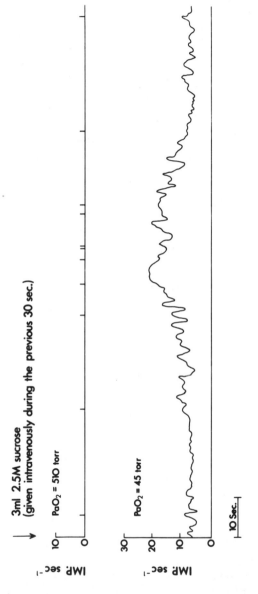

Figure 9:   Cat, α-chloralose. Dependence on PaO2 of the effect of sucrose
            administration on the activity of carotid chemoreceptors. An
            increase in plasma osmolarity stimulated carotid chemoreceptor
            activity after a delay, and the effect was greater during hypoxia.

organelles resulting in small changes in local osmotic pressure.
This osmotic effect may lead to the excitation process.

It is interesting to note that we found several carotid
afferent fibers which showed profound responses to increases in
plasma tonicity but little response to blood gas changes. These
afferent fibers may have synaptic terminals into the hypothalamic
area linking carotid body with yet another function of osmoregu-
lation and homeostasis.

Hypothesis

The basic question is one of recognition of oxygen by the
receptor tissue, and whether CO_2-H^+ and oxygen converge on the
same mechanism. Cytochrome oxidase is a natural candidate because
it has the potential mechanism for detection as well as transduction. This possible mechanism assumes particular importance
at this symposium because of the presence of so many experts on
cytochrome oxidase.

Mills and Jöbsis[15] proposed that the chemoreception at the
carotid body occurs through cytochrome oxidase with low affinity
for O_2. In vitro studies have shown that 1 torr P_{O_2} at the mitochondrial level is more than sufficient to maintain cytochrome
oxidase fully functional[16], and it is generally thought that mitochondrial P_{O_2} is kept well above 1 torr during arterial hypoxia
compatible with life. It is known that oxygen uptake is not
impaired in resting man sojourning and living at high altitude[17],
although his carotid chemoreceptors are stimulated due to hypoxia.
Thus a variety of cytochrome oxidase with low affinity for O_2 is a
necessary requirement because carotid body chemoreceptors are excited by small changes in arterial P_{O_2} far above the normal P_{O_2} of
about 100 torr at sea level. The assumption here was that the
carotid chemoreceptor tissue P_{O_2} paralleled closely the perfusate
P_{O_2} in their preparation. Dr. Whalen who will speak here this
morning provided support for this contention. In their published
papers Whalen and Nair[18] gave P_{O_2} values which ranged from 1 to
86 torr at an arterial P_{O_2} of 80–100 torr in the cat breathing
room air at sea level. Some of their very low values kept the
possibility open that the cytochrome oxidase with high O_2 affinity
might as well be reduced, and one need not postulate the participation of another cytochrome oxidase. It is possible that the P_{O_2} at
a particular site in the carotid body fluctuates with time even at
a constant arterial P_{O_2}, and activation of the chemoreceptors occurs
according to this fluctuation and reduction of cytochrome oxidase.
Whalen and Nair noted such fluctuation and very steep gradients
from one site to another. I hope Dr. Whalen gives us more information on this point. In this context we must not forget the work of
Dr. Lübbers and his colleagues. The data of Acker et al[19] are not

exactly the same as those of Whalen and Nair. Indeed, they reported lower values of carotid body tissue P_{O_2} at a given arterial
P_{O_2}. Also, unlike Whalen and Nair, they reported an increase in
tissue P_{O_2} from the periphery to the center of the carotid body
in the cat. According to their experience carotid chemoreceptor
P_{O_2} may be low enough to reduce the usual cytochrome oxidase with
high affinity for oxygen. There is thus uncertainty about receptor P_{O_2}, and therefore uncertainty about the mechanism of
chemoreception by cytochrome oxidase.

The notion that cytochrome oxidase reduction is the first
step in chemoreception is nonetheless attractive but the hypothesis
does not explain the effect of CO_2-H^+ and its interaction with the
hypoxic stimulus. Nor is the explanation for the dependence of
cyanide effect on P_{O_2} obvious. However, such a competitive
effect of cyanide with oxygen did not follow from the known properties of cytochrome oxidase[9], and therefore some other mechanism
of chemoreception seems to be indicated.

Cyanide is a highly reactive compound and is known to react
with a variety of heavy metal proteins and enzymes and other
organic molecules. However, a consistently reproducible pattern of
response of chemoreceptors suggests a rather specific action of
cyanide in the mechanism of chemoreception. Binding of cyanide
with hemoproteins is well known, and it is not unreasonable to
consider hemoprotein molecule as a candidate for the recognition
function for oxygen. Cytochrome oxidase is partly a hemoprotein,
and the balance of evidence suggests that the oxidized form of
cytochrome oxidase has a greater affinity for oxygen than the reduced form[20]. Thus cyanide is expected to show a greater effect
at a higher P_{O_2} when more cytochrome oxidase is oxidized. But the
observation is contrary to this expectation. However, a conceivable
explanation may be that a ratio of cyanide to oxidized cytochrome
oxidase is the determining factor. At a high level of P_{O_2} the
ratio is small for a given dose of cyanide. With increasing hypoxia
there is a progressive increase in the ratio and the excitatory
effect.

The observations on the activity of chemoreceptors also suggest
that a hemoprotein with a distinct Bohr effect is a possible candidate. The protein receptor could be a cellular membrane component
or an enzyme which reacts with molecular O_2. A conformational
change resulting from this reaction initiates the process of chemoreception which is followed by transduction. A hemoprotein showing
Bohr proton effect usually shows Haldane molecular CO_2 effect.
Whether molecular CO_2 has an effect on the activity of chemoreceptor
is not clear[21]. It is clear, however, that CO_2-H^+ has a pronounced
effect which indicates that an ionizable group may be involved in
the process of chemoreception. A similar hypothesis for chemo-

reception in aplysia has been discussed by Dr. Chalazonitis in the last session.

An interesting comparison between cytochrome oxidase and Bohr hypotheses can be made by looking into the effect of CO_2-H^+ on carotid body tissue P_{O_2}. According to Bohr hypothesis tissue P_{O_2} would increase during hypercapnia at a constant arterial P_{O_2} whereas it would decrease if a reduction of cytochrome oxidase is involved. Dr. Whalen tells me that carotid body tissue P_{O_2} is somewhat increased during hypercapnia at a constant PaO_2.

The convergence of hypoxic and CO_2-H^+ stimulus seems to suggest that there is a single mechanism for chemoreception. According to Torrance[22] the ultimate stimulus is $[H^+]$ which is manipulated by P_{O_2} sensitive bicarbonate pump. The hypothesis apparently does not address itself to the question of P_{O_2} sensing.

There is also a suggestion that oxygen and CO_2-H^+ may work through independent mechanisms[3,23]. The argument is that the oxygen effect is expected to be abolished at a hyperbaric state, and CO_2-H^+ stimulation under such conditions is free from oxygen influence. The data on hyperbaric effect on carotid chemoreceptors are meager. The only information we have is in an abstract by Hall et al[23]. They studied the whole sinus nerves in the cat at 1 and 3.5 atmospheres absolute, and used analysis of variance to distinguish between the effects. Increases in P_{CO_2} in O_2 at 3.5 atmospheres increased the activity but it is not clear if the responses were the same at 1 and 3.5 atmospheres. Also it would be important to know the effect of high pressure per se. The study should be repeated with identifiable chemoreceptor fibers.

Hyperbaric oxygenation and chemoreceptor stimulation is an interesting question particularly in view of the observation that oxygen uptake of the carotid body is one of the highest in the body, although not particularly rich in mitochondria. Its oxygen consumption, however, is not increased by its activity. Its increased activity is rather associated with a decreased oxygen consumption. Torrance[24] discussed some aspects of the problem more recently.

The activity of afferent fibers certainly tell us about the behavior of chemoreceptors but it does not tell us what they consist of, where they are located and how the chemoreception and transduction take place. In order to gain answers to these questions it is obviously necessary to probe the carotid body more closely. The speakers of this session will certainly tell us more about the inside story of the chemoreceptors.

Acknowledgment. Supported in part by the USPHS grant HL-08805. The author is grateful to Mrs. Carol Siegrist, Dr. R.G. DeLaney and Mr. A. Mokashi for their help.

References

1. Eyzaguirre C., Lewin J.: Chemoreceptor activity of the carotid body of the cat. J. Physiol. (London) 159:222-237, 1961.

2. Hornbein, T.F., Griffo, Z.J., Roos, A.: Quantitation of chemo-receptor activity: interaction of hypoxia and hypercapnia. J. Neurophysiol. 24:501-508, 1961.

3. Fitzgerald, R.S., Parks, P.: Effect of hypoxia on carotid body chemoreceptor response to carbon dioxide in cats. Respir. Physiol. 12:218-229, 1971.

4. Lahiri, S., DeLaney, R.G.: Stimulus interaction in the responses of carotid body chemoreceptor single afferent fibers. Respir. Physiol. 24:249-266, 1975.

5. Tasaki, I., Spyropoulos, C.S.: Influence of changes in temper-ature and pressure on the nerve fiber. In: Influence of Tem-perature on Biological Systems. (Ed.) F.H. Johnson. American Physiological Society, Washington, D.C., 1975, pp. 201-220.

6. Paintal, A.S.: The responses of chemoreceptors at reduced tem-peratures. J. Physiol. (London) 217:1-18, 1971.

7. McQueen, D.S., Eyzaguirre, C.: Effects of temperature on car-otid chemoreceptor and baroreceptor activity. J. Neurophysiol. 37:1287-1296, 1974.

8. Krylov, S.S., Anichkov, S.V.: The effect of metabolic inhibitors on carotid chemoreceptors. In: Arterial Chemoreceptors. (Ed.) R.W. Torrance, Blackwell Scientific Publications, Oxford, 1968, pp. 103-113.

9. Dixon, M., Webb, E.C.: Enzymes. Academic Press, New York, 1964, pp. 315-359.

10. Forster, R.E.: The diffusion of gases in the carotid body. In: Arterial Chemoreceptors. (Ed.) R.W. Torrance, Blackwell Scientific Publications, 1968, pp. 115-132.

11. Gallego, R., Eyzaguirre, C.: Effects of osmotic pressure changes on the carotid body of the cat in vitro. Federation Proc. 35: 404, 1976.

12. Clark, A.W.: Changes in the structure of neuromuscular junctions caused by variations in osmotic pressure. J. Cell Biol. 69:521-538, 1976.

13. Ottoson, D., Shepherd, G.M.: Transducer properties and integrative mechanisms in the frog's muscle spindle. In: Principles of Receptor Physiology. (Ed.) W.R. Lowenstein, Springer-Verlag, Berlin, 1971, pp. 442-499.

14. Verney, E.B.: The antidiuretic hormone and the factors which determine its release. Proc. Roy. Soc. Ser. B 135:25-106, 1947.

15. Mills, E., Jöbsis, F.F.: Mitochondrial respiratory chain of carotid body and chemoreceptor response to changes in oxygen tension. J. Neurophysiol. 35:405-428, 1972.

16. Chance, B.: Cellular oxygen requirements. Federation Proc. 16:671-680, 1957.

17. Lahiri, S.: Physiological responses and adaptations to high altitude. In: Environmental Physiology, MTP International Review of Science, Physiology Series One, Vol. 7. (Ed.) D. Robertshaw, Butterworths, London, 1974, pp. 271-312.

18. Whalen, W.J., Nair, P.: Microelectrode measurements of tissue P_{O_2} in the carotid body of the cat. In: Oxygen Supply. Theoretical and Practical Aspects of Oxygen Supply and Microcirculation of Tissue. M. Kessler, D.F. Bruley, L.C. Clark, Jr., D.W. Lübbers, I.A. Silver, J. Strauss, Urban and Schwarzenberg, München, 1973, pp. 236-237.

19. Acker, H., Lübbers, D.W., Purves, M.J.: Local oxygen tension field in the glomus caroticum of the cat and its change at changing arterial P_{O_2}. Pflügers Arch. 329:136-155, 1971.

20. Wikstrom, M.K.F., Harmon, J.H., Ingledew, W.J., Chance, B.: A reevaluation of the spectral potentiometric and energy linked properties of cytochrome c oxidase in mitochondria. FEBS Letters 65:259-277, 1976.

21. Biscoe, T.J.: Carotid body: Structure and function. Physiol. Rev. 51:437-495, 1971.

22. Torrance, R.W.: An amendment to Winder's acid receptor hypothesis of the sensitivity of arterial chemoreceptors to hypoxia. J. Physiol. (London) 244:64P, 1975.

23. Hall, P., Matsuyama, Y., Williams, K.R., Gelfand, R., Lambertsen
     C.J.: Effect of oxygen at 0.2, 1, and 3.5 atm abs on carotid
     chemoreceptor discharge in the cat at various levels of carbon
     dioxide. Federation Proc. 26:379, 1967.

24. Torrance, R.W.: Arterial Chemoreceptors. In: Respiratory
     Physiology, MTP International Review of Science, Physiology
     Series One, Vol. 2. (Ed.) J.G. Widdicombe, Butterworths,
     London, 1974, pp. 247-271.

CONVERGENCE OF STIMULI IN ARTERIAL CHEMORECEPTORS

R.W. TORRANCE

University Laboratory of Physiology

Oxford, England

A single chemoreceptor fibre of the carotid sinus nerve responds both to hypoxia and to hypercapnia/acidity of the arterial blood. These reactions have been well brought out by such recent studies as those of Lahiri[1] which he has illustrated in a figure in his paper at this symposium. If reactions to CO_2 are presented as a series of CO_2 response curves at various intensities of hypoxia, the curves appear as a fan of approximately straight lines which have a steeper slope the more intense the hypoxia. It is when there is some degree of hypoxia that the effects of CO_2 become marked in the steady state, as Neil[2] has always emphasised, but if the P_{CO_2} of the arterial blood is changing, the effects of CO_2 on discharge are more striking, for adaptation of the response to a sudden change of P_{CO_2} is marked, particularly in hyperoxia. Thus if a receptor is discharging at some steady initial level and the Pa_{CO_2} is suddenly raised, the discharge immediately rises along a steep transient response curve and then adapts down to lie upon the steady state curve. Adaptation to CO_2 may be so striking in a minority of chemoreceptor fibres that they seem to be little sensitive to CO_2 in the steady state and this marked adaptation may account for assertions that have been made that the response to CO_2 is trivial when in fact one of this group of fibres does show a good response to a changing P_{CO_2}. Hence the behaviour of some chemoreceptors resembles that of a completely adapting mechanoreceptor, the Pacinian corpuscle. It responds at the start of a maintained mechanical stimulus but then it adapts quickly to silence. One does not regard it as any the less a mechanoreceptor.

Thus we have a receptor, the arterial chemoreceptor, which responds both to hypercapnia and to hypoxia. The response to hypercapnia is prompt and adapts whilst that to hypoxia is slower and does not adapt. For the hypercapnic stimulus the receptor behaves like a lead network and for the hypoxic one like a lag network. These terms give more precise descriptions of its behaviour than the more common ones, the static and the dynamic response. Its discharge is affected by changes in a stimulus but it is not itself strictly sensitive to the rate of change of that stimulus.

Since the same single afferent fibre does conduct impulses in response to each of two stimuli, the stimuli must somehow each act and then converge to give impulses in that fibre. It is therefore interesting to consider how these actions and this convergence might take place. What ideas are conceivable depends naturally upon what structures are present within the carotid body. In simplest outline, it contains a set of cells, the Type I cells which look as if they secrete something, perhaps a neurotransmitter, and so act as a presynaptic element to the sensory nerve endings which lie against them. The Type I cell and the nerve ending are enveloped by a Type II cell which is rather like a glial or Schwann cell. With even so simple an array of structures as this, a large variety of possible models of action and convergence can be imagined and I shall enumerate some of them. Very few of them have however been put out in the literature with a degree of precision which is adequate for them to be tested.

(1) The Bohr Hypothesis supposes that a protein combines with O_2 and that its affinity for O_2 is affected by P_{CO_2}/pH in much the same way that the affinity of haemoglobin for O_2 is affected. It is conceivable that this protein controls some ionic channel in the same sort of way that a neurotransmitter does, so that depolarisation of a membrane takes place by a membrane conductance change when P_{O_2} falls or P_{CO_2} rises. Thus in a simple version of the hypothesis a generator potential is set up at the nerve terminal and nerve impulses result when the protein is not combined with O_2 (Lahiri & Delaney)[1].

(2) The Haldane Hypothesis. Equally plausibly one might suppose that a carbamino compound of a protein is formed to a degree that is affected by local P_{CO_2} but that the affinity of the protein for CO_2 is affected also by local P_{O_2} and pH, as in the formation of carbamino haemoglobin. Impulses arise when the molecule changes but here it is when the molecule is combined with CO_2 whereas in the Bohr hypothesis it is when the molecule is not combined with O_2. Travis[3] considered such a hypothesis of a receptor for molecular CO_2 which could be blocked by acetazolamide.

(3) In contrast, one can suppose that O_2 and CO_2 do not so much affect the state of a molecule as affect the rate at which

a process procedes.   Thus Biscoe[4] has developed the idea that a
fine nerve ending will depolarise if O_2 is not available for
pumping out of it any sodium that leaks in. CO_2 might converge
with hypoxia by disturbing the relation between P_{O_2} and the rate
of sodium pumping.   Alternatively CO_2 or acidity might act by a
quite distinct mechanism to contribute to the generator potential
and so to nerve impulses.   Thus the convergence here would take
place at a membrane potential by the interaction of a variable
O_2 dependent ion pump and a variable pH dependent membrane
conductance.

(4) The acid receptor hypothesis. An alternative approach
supposes that convergence takes place at a stage before any event
which might be called neurophysiological takes place and before
any nervous tissue has been involved. Winder,[5] in 1937, supposed
that this was at the level of the pH somewhere within the carotid
body.   Arterial P_{CO_2} naturally affected this space but hypoxia
did also because in hypoxia lactic acid was formed and entered the
space.   Thus a single nervous mechanism was postulated and it was
sensitive only to acidity.   More recently Torrance[6] has amended
this early hypothesis in the sense that hypoxia leads to failure
of an active mechanism of the Type II cell which tends to
stabilise the pH in a space around an acid receptor in the cleft
between the Type I and Type II cells, keeping it more alkaline
than the blood, so that again the acid receptor is excited by
hypoxia.

(5) Now we should consider how the seemingly neurosecretory
Type I cells of the carotid body might fit into these various
ideas. We have already considered some ways in which CO_2 and
hypoxia might act. Each stimulus might act at a different cell
and there are many possible combinations. The nerve ending
might itself sense acidity but hypoxia might affect the Type I cell
which would then act upon the nerve ending through release of a
neurotransmitter. The reverse may be true, with the nerve ending
itself sensitive to hypoxia as Biscoe[4] suggests and the Type I
cell responding to hypercapnia and acting upon the nerve ending
through a neurotransmitter. If there is no direct action of a
stimulus upon the nerve ending and it only responds to
neurotransmitters, a further array of possibilities exists
(i) that hypoxia and CO_2 converge at a neurosecretory cell which
acts upon the nerve ending through a single neurotransmitter.
(ii) that a single cell type releases two distinct transmitters,
one for each stimulus (and thus incidentally contravenes Dale's Law.)
(iii) that there are two types of cell, each with its own
sensitivity and transmitter, one reacting to CO_2/pH and the other
to hypoxia.

If convergence occurs at an extracellular pH (4) this pH

might be sensed by the nerve ending directly or else by a single cell which releases a single transmitter. Similarly it can be supposed that the molecules of the Bohr (1) and the Haldane (2) hypotheses exist in Type I cells which act upon the nerve endings through a neurotransmitter.

Recently attention has been focussed upon dopamine which is present in the Type I cells and may be an inhibiter of chemoreceptors. If it is involved in the basic process of chemoreception and not merely in the control of the sensitivity of chemoreceptors by efferent nerve fibres or reciprocal synapses, excitation must be produced by a reduction in its rate of release by whatever excitatory stimulus it is that uses it. One can fit in an inhibitory transmitter in all those places at which an excitatory transmitter has already been considered merely by inverting the relation between stimulus and rate of secretion.

In enumerating these possible ways of convergence, I have made little reference to phasic control of the receptor by glossopharyngal and sympathetic efferents or by reciprocal synapses, though it may be that the Type I cells are principally important as mediators of this control. Alternatively, Type I cells may be concerned in somehow maintaining the sensitivity of the nerve endings. Pearse[7] continues to emphasise that these cells are members of his APUD group of cells, most of which have been shown undoubtedly to secrete polypeptide hormones. The thyroid C cells secreting calcitonin are an example. The APUD cells have nevertheless many of the histochemical characteristics which have been taken to suggest that the Type I cell is dopaminergic. In this context, the recent finding of Barker & Smith[8] that small polypeptide hormones can produce longlasting effects on voltage dependent ion conductances of some nerve membranes is very interesting: the Type I cell might release a polypeptide which has such an effect on the membrane of the nerve ending near to it.

At the symposium, a particular acid receptor hypothesis was described which will account for much of the behaviour of chemoreceptors but it has already been put out elsewhere[6,9,10] and so it is not repeated here.

REFERENCES

1. Lahiri S, Delaney RG: Stimulus interaction in the responses of carotid body chemoreceptor single afferent fibres. Respir.Physiol. 24: 249–266, 1975.

2. Neil E: Panel discussion. In Hatcher JD, Jennings DB (Editors): Cardiovascular and Respiratory Effects of Hypoxia. Basel, Karger, 1966, p 171.

3. Travis DM: Molecular CO_2 is inert on carotid chemoreceptor: demonstration by inhibition of carbonic anhydrase. J. Pharmacol. Exp. Ther: 178 : 529-540, 1971.

4. Biscoe TJ: Carotid Body: Structure and Function. Physiol.Rev. 51: 437-495, 1971.

5. Winder CV: On the mechanism of stimulation of carotid gland chemoreceptors. Am.J. Physiol. 118: 389-398, 1937.

6. Torrance RW: An amendment to Winder's acid receptor hypothesis on the sensitivity of arterial chemoreceptors to hypoxia. J. Physiol. 244: 64-66P, 1975.

7. Pearse AGE, Polak JM, Rost FWD, Fontaine J, LeLievre C, LeDouarin N: Demonstration of the neural crest origin of Type I (APUD) cells in the avian carotid body, using a cytochemical marker system. Histochimie 34: 191-203, 1973.

8. Barker JL, Smith TG: Peptide regulation of neuronal membrane properties. Brain Research 103: 167-170, 1976.

9. Torrance RW: Arterial Chemoreceptors. In Widdicombe JG (Editor) Respiratory Physiology, International Review of Science Physiology, Series one Vol.2, pp 247-271, 1974.

10. Torrance RW: A New Version of the Acid Receptor Hypothesis of Carotid Chemoreceptors. In Paintal AS, (Editor): Morphology and Mechanisms of Chemoreceptors. Delhi, Vallabhbhai Patel Chest Institute 1976, pp 131-135.

INTRACELLULAR STUDIES OF CAROTID BODY CELLS: EFFECTS OF TEMPERA-

TURE, "NATURAL" STIMULI AND CHEMICAL SUBSTANCES

C. Eyzaguirre, Margarita Baron & R. Gallego

Dept. of Physiology, Univ. of Utah College of Medicine

Salt Lake City, Utah 84132

The carotid body consists of clusters of small cells which have received several names such as epithelioid, glomus, chemo-receptor, etc., in addition to a network of nerve fibers and capillaries. The glomus cells, more recently, have been designated as type I and are surrounded by another type of cell which has been designated as sustentacular, capsular, satellite or type II.

Glomus (type I) cells are intimately apposed to nerve endings, provided by the terminal branches of the carotid nerve, a branch of the glossopharyngeal nerve. Recent evidence has corroborated an old observation of de Castro indicating that they are sensory fibers.[1,2] Thus, it is possible that the glomus cell-sensory nerve ending complex forms a "chemoreceptor synapse" as suggested by de Castro,[3] based exclusively on morphological evidence.

The mechanisms involved in chemoreception have attracted the attention of a number of investigators in the past three decades and the problems encountered have been far more complex than expected at first. In fact, these receptors are not specific to one form of stimulation. They are readily activated by low pO_2, high pCO_2 and low pH. In addition, the receptors respond to a number of chemical agents such as cholinomimetic substances, cate-cholamines, salts such as KCl, and agents that alter tissue metabo-lism such as cyanide. The variety of effective stimuli makes it extremely difficult to think of a unified mode of action, thus, a number of hypotheses have been developed in an effort to understand the basic mechanisms of receptor activation. These hypotheses vary from some that have been more or less well tested to others which, scientifically, could be classified as either good or bad ideas without any, or little, experimental evidence.

Work done in this laboratory for the past fifteen years has favored the idea of a chemoreceptor synapse; the glomus cells would be the presynaptic elements of the junction and the nerve endings, apposed to them, would be the postsynaptic element of this complex. These ideas are based on relatively indirect experimental evidence where, in the majority of cases, nerve discharges have been recorded from the carotid nerve. The receptors have been stimulated by a variety of means and many pharmacological substances have been used in an effort to modify the discharge thus obtained. These studies have suggested the possibility of a cholinergic mechanism being important in the genesis of chemoreceptor discharges. In addition, the receptor or generator potential, produced in the nerve endings during stimulation, has been recorded by using oil or air gaps _in vivo_ and _in vitro_. The study of receptor potentials has revealed some interesting features of the nerve endings in terms of ionic mechanisms involved in their production and the response of these structures to pharmacological agents.[4,5]

These studies have contributed to our knowledge of the problems involved, but have not solved the final questions: 1) do we have a chemoreceptor synapse?; 2) if so, where is the primary site of stimulus action?; are these sites located in the nerve endings or do the cells (type I or II) contribute significantly to the generation of sensory discharges?; 3) what is the mechanism of action of these diverse stimuli in setting up action potentials in the nerve fibers? These questions are extremely complex and cannot be discussed in detail in this article. However, it is clear that one of the main problems in trying to find an answer lies in the fact that there is no information as to the membrane properties of carotid body cells, either type I or II. Thus, one of the present aims of this laboratory is to obtain information about these cells and to see if their electrophysiological behavior can be correlated with the generation of the sensory nerve discharges.

In these studies, the carotid body of the cat was removed from the animal and placed _in vitro_ in mammalian saline[6] at 36-37° which was allowed to flow through the chamber at 1-3 ml/min. The nerve discharges were recorded from the carotid nerve with a suction electrode and the preparation was ready for intracellular recording. This was done with glass micropipettes (10-40 MΩ) filled with 3M KCl and advanced through the organ with a micromanipulator. Thus, simultaneous records of intracellular activity, nerve discharges and bath temperature (monitored with a thermistor probe placed very close to the organ) were routinely obtained in every experiment. Penetrations of the carotid body were blind and it was necessary to identify the cells impaled with the microelectrode. This was done by ejection of 6% Procion Navy Blue from the recording micropipette (once it was firmly lodged inside a cell) by passing hyperpolarizing current (2-4 nA) through the microelectrode. This procedure stained the impaled cells as shown in Fig. 1. In the majority of impalements (90%) these cells showed to be type I. In some instances, however, cells possibly being type II and an occasional glomerulus (cluster of small cells) were stained. Nevertheless, we feel confident that the majority of the observations reported here refer to behavior of type I cells.

One of the most striking characteristics shown by the cells was their extreme sensitivity to temperature.[6] The membrane potential (MP) and input resistance (R_O) showed marked fluctuations with variations in temperature which were far in excess of what could be predicted from the Nernst equation. Thus, extreme care had to be taken when measuring some of the membrane constants in these preparations. The temperature of the bathing solution had to remain fixed at a certain level.

The membrane potential of 499 type I cells (measured at 36-37°) showed values of from 10-55 mV with a mean of 19.8 mV ± 0.4 s.e.m.

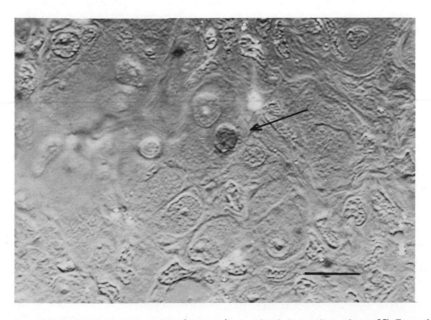

Fig. 1. Glomus type I cell (arrow) marked by ejecting 6% Procion Navy Blue from recording micropipette. Notice intense staining of nucleus. There is an unstained type I cell immediately adjacent to the previous one. Interference contrast (Nomarski) optics. Cal., 10 µ.

These values are low if one compares them with those obtained in
excitable tissues. Part of this may be due to slight injury of
the cell membrane (induced by the microelectrode) since these cells
are small, usually not larger than 10 μ in fresh preparations.
However, as shown later, this may also be due to the ionic species
involved in the maintenance of the membrane potential. The input
resistance (R_O) of these cells varied between 10 and 170 MΩ. The
mean value obtained from 405 cells was 42.2 MΩ ±1.6 s.e.m. These
values are large, probably due to the small size of these cells.
In fact, calculating R_m from the mean R_O value gives 132.5 Ω cm^2
which is, in fact, low compared to excitable cells. Again, this
may be due to the small size of the cells. The membrane capacity
(C_m) studied in 20 cells gave a mean of 5.5 μF/cm^2 ± 0.3 s.e.m.
which is in line with values obtained by others using excitable
tissues.[7] Both R_O and C_m were directly proportional to the membrane
potential values. Thus, cells yielding large membrane potentials
also had large R_O and C_m values and vice versa. These correlations
may have been due, at least in part, to cell damage during penetration with the microelectrode. Damage would produce a "leaky"
membrane that would allow a limited flow of ions between extra- and
intracellular compartments that, otherwise, would be better separated. In fact, the input resistance did not appear to be voltage
dependent. Passive displacement of the membrane potential in either
direction by currents injected through the recording microelectrode
did not induce clear changes in R_O. This may indicate that glomus
cells are not electrically excitable in the classical sense.

     Effects of temperature. Glomus cells proved to be extremely
sensitive to temperature changes. Thus, a drop in temperature
from, say, 37°C to 30°C induced marked cell depolarization and a
loss of input resistance. These changes were accompanied by a great
reduction in the frequency of the sensory discharges.[6] The sensitivity of different cells to temperature varied accordingly with
the state of the preparation and the initial MP and R_O values. Thus,
cells showing large MP and R_O values showed a greater change in
these parameters than cells that showed lower initial values. Also,
the speed of the temperature change was important. The faster the
cooling the larger were the effects. In addition, glomus cells
showed a dynamic response to cooling; the effects of temperature
were larger at the beginning of the cooling period since "adaptation" followed this initial change.

     A good way of obtaining an overall view of impedance (resis-
tance) values of membranes is to construct current-voltage (I-V)
curves since resistance measurements employing only a single current
pulse may be misleading. In fact, a number of membranes show variations depending on the intensity and polarity of the applied pulses
because of rectification. Also, if input impedance varies because
of changes in temperature, as in this case, I-V curves constructed

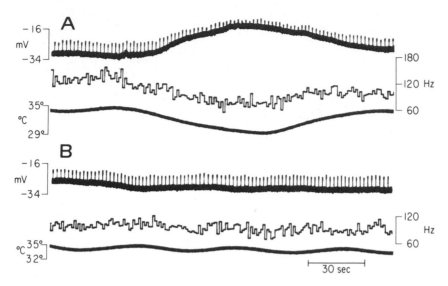

Fig. 2. A, effect of cooling on MP, R_0 and sensory discharge frequency. Upper trace, MP is reduced from 34 to 16 mV; R_0 falls from 30 to 12 MΩ; middle trace, sensory discharge frequency falls from about 120 to 70/sec; lower trace, temperature drops from 35 to 29°C. B, taken immediately after A, shows recovery of the preparation when temperature returns to baseline levels.

before and after cooling give a good overall picture of these changes (Fig. 3).

In order to analyze the influence of different ions on the temperature effects, it was necessary to see whether or not depolarization by cooling had a reversal or equilibrium potential. For this purpose, the membrane potential of the cells was displaced (by currents injected through the microelectrode) in either direction.

A systematic analysis made in 24 cells showed that indeed there was a reversal potential for cooling effects at about -7 mV. These results indicated that, perhaps, there was a simultaneous increase in conductance to more than one ionic species during a drop in temperature. Thus, ionic substitution experiments were conducted.

Removal of sodium ions from the bathing medium at normal (i.e., 37°C) temperature induced cell hyperpolarization of about 4mV and an increase in R_0 of about 25 MΩ. These changes still occurred in the cold (i.e., 30°C). However, in Na-free solutions, cooling was less effective in inducing cell depolarization although it induced larger resistance changes. These results indicate that,

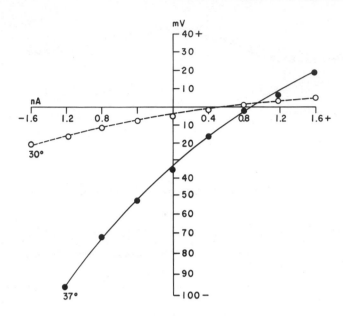

<u>Fig. 3</u>.   Current-voltage (I-V) curves constructed at 37°C (filled circles and solid line) and at 30°C (open circles and broken line). Notice marked decrease in input resistance at low temperature. Also, membrane rectification seen at normal temperature is less marked in the cold (see also Baron & Eyzaguirre[6]).

probably, Na ions are important in the maintenance of the cell membrane potential at normal and low temperatures. However, the large resistance drop induced by cooling in 0 Na may indicate that in the absence of this ion, movements of other ions are facilitated. The larger change in resistance and the smaller depolarization by cooling in sodium-free solutions, may be telling us that, under these conditions, an increased K conductance may occur. However, it must be realized that this suggestion is at present purely speculative since, as shown later, there is no evidence that K ions contribute significantly to the membrane potential of these cells. However, K ions may move more freely if external sodium is removed.

Ca and Mg ions proved important in the maintenance of MP and R_O in these cells. Thus, removal of calcium from the bathing medium induced cell hyperpolarization of 3-4 mV and an unstable input resistance at normal temperatures. In the cold, lack of Ca still induced cell hyperpolarization and an increase in input resistance of 4 to 5 $M\Omega$. This is interesting since at low temperatures the instability in input resistance observed at normal temperatures

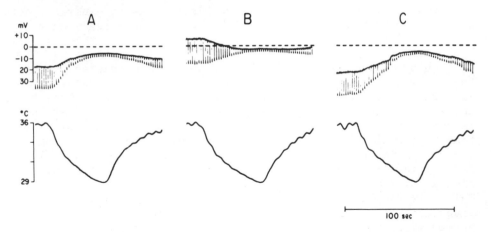

Fig. 4. Equilibrium or reversal potential of the response to cooling. Preparation kept at 36°C and periodically cooled to about
29°C. Upper traces, changes in MP and R_o induced by cooling
applied at three membrane potential levels. Lower traces, temperature changes recorded close to the carotid body. In A, the cell
had a resting potential of −17 mV and an input resistance of 90 MΩ.
Cooling reduced these values to −5 mV and 12 MΩ. In B, the MP was
displaced in a depolarizing direction by outward steady current
to +6 mV and R_o increased to 100 MΩ. Cooling repolarized the cell
to −2.5 mV and resistance fell to 10 MΩ. In C, the membrane potential was driven to −24 mV by inward steady current (90 MΩR_o) and
cooling reduced these values to −8 mV and 10 MΩ. During cooling
the equilibrium or reversal potential appears to be about −4 mV
(from Baron & Eyzaguirre[6]).

seems to disappear. One interpretation of this phenomenon is
that, probably, lack of calcium creates some membrane instability
which allows other ions to move across the cell membrane. This
possibility seems to disappear when the temperature is lowered.

     Bathing the preparations with an excess (10.8 mM) of Ca or
Mg ions induced cell depolarization of about 4 mV in either case
and a decrease in input resistance. The effects of Ca were more
pronounced than those of Mg. At low temperatures only an excess
of calcium changed (in the same direction) MP and R_o. Mg ions
were ineffective in the cold.

     The effects of calcium on glomus cells, namely, cell hyper-
polarization in 0 Ca and depolarization in high calcium are quite

different from what happens in excitable tissues in general. Nerve
and muscle cells are usually depolarized and their resistance
becomes low in calcium-free media.[8]

Chloride ions proved to be important in the maintenance of
the MP of glomus cells. Thus, reducing the external chloride to
11.2 mM induced cell depolarization of about 8 mV and a loss of
input resistance of about 23 MΩ. These effects remained at low
temperatures. Cooling effects were more marked in low chloride
than in normal solutions in terms of membrane potential changes.
Changes in input resistance due to cold were more marked in low
Cl only in 55% of the cases. These experiments show that Cl ions
play a role in maintaining the membrane potential of these cells.
This, perhaps, is not too unusual since chemosensitive neurons of
invertebrates, such as Aplysia, operate through changes in chloride
permeability during chemical stimulation provided by CO_2.[9]

Glomus cells showed remarkable insensitivity to changes in
external K. Thus, removal of this ion from the bathing solution
did not change significantly either MP or R_0 of these cells.
Also, adding an excess of potassium (46.9 mM total concentration)
only induced some changes in MP and R_0 which could be accounted
for by the inevitable reduction of Na ions in the bathing solution.
Reducing Na was necessary, as shown later, to keep constant the
osmolarity of the bathing fluid. Likewise, total replacement of
Na (154 mM) with K ions induced MP and R_0 changes that were exclusively due to the removal of sodium ions. These observations are
in disagreement with previous ones by Goodman and McCloskey[10] who
have reported cell depolarization during superfusion with isotonic
KCl (150 mEq/l). The reasons for these discrepancies are not
entirely clear. Furthermore, we have reported[11] effects of K on
carotid body cells studied in tissue slices. Now we feel (as shown
later) that cell depolarization in high potassium and hyperpolarization in low K were entirely due to osmotic effects. In fact,
in those experiments 0 K was achieved simply by removing KCl from
the bathing solution while high K was obtained by adding KCl to
the medium with no further precautions. These solutions were,
respectively, about 3.5% hypo- and hyperosmotic. It is very likely
that under those conditions, with great exposure of the cells to
the bathing medium, small changes in osmolarity may have marked
effects on their membrane potential.

Ouabain (5 x 10^{-5} M) was applied for fairly long periods of
time. This glycoside was used to investigate whether or not there
is a Na pump operating in these cells. This could be the case
since ouabain induced cell depolarization at normal temperatures
and this effect was potentiated during exposure of the cells to
cold. However, it is felt that at the present time this evidence
is still too incomplete to postulate the presence of such a pump.

That the activity of glomus cells is highly dependent on temperature is not too surprising since the carotid body tissue has a high metabolism which is reflected in its high oxygen consumption.[12] Admittedly, it is not known which are the elements responsible for this phenomenon; but, the chances are that high O_2 consumption would be located either at the glomus or sustentacular cell level. The other elements in the carotid body (nerve fibers, blood vessels, supporting tissue, etc.,) are likely to behave more conventionally. Thus, the great dependence of the membrane potential and input resistance of glomus cells on temperature makes them good candidates to be the site of this high metabolic activity. Admittedly, there is no experimental evidence to dismiss out of hand the role of sustentacular cells in this process and they may be important also. This problem will not be solved until metabolic studies are conducted on suspensions of cells isolated by differential centrifugation or another suitable method, such as tissue culture. This is probably difficult but it should not prove to be an impossible task.

Effects of "natural" and chemical stimuli. A number of agents, which are known stimuli for chemoreceptors, have been tried.

In 10 preparations bathed with saline equilibrated with 50% O_2 in N_2, the cells were impaled with the recording microelectrode and the nerve discharges were simultaneously recorded. After baselines were obtained, saline equilibrated with pure N_2 was allowed to flow through the preparation for 15 to 20 min. N_2 induced an appreciable increase in sensory discharge frequency, but, there was no significant change in either MP or R_o. Thus, two important membrane parameters seemed to be unaffected by oxygen lack. Likewise, MP and R_o were not significantly changed by superfusing the preparations (10 cells) with a total bath concentration of NaCN 5-50 mg/1. However, the nerve discharges underwent a very marked increase during the action of CN. The hyperpolarizing effect of NaCN on cells in tissue slices[11] is most likely due to an increase in pH induced by the salt applied directly on the slice in a small chamber (also see below).

Acetylcholine (10-100 mg/1) was tried on 7 preparations and, again, there was a marked increase in sensory discharge activity without concomitant changes in either MP or R_o.

CO_2 had interesting effects. This agent was applied in concentrations of 6% CO_2 in 50% O_2 and 44% N_2. When the pH of the external saline was buffered to 7.43 (identical to that of the control solution containing 50% O_2 in N_2), there was an increase in the frequency of the sensory discharges but no changes in either MP or R_o in 27 trials. However, when (in 50 trials) pH of the bathing medium was allowed to fall to 6.0-6.6, there was a more

marked increase in sensory discharge frequency, a mean cell depolarization of 3.6 mV ± 0.4 s.e.m. (p < 0.01) and no significant changes
in input resistance. Thus, the effects of CO_2 on the membrane potential appeared to be due exclusively to the fall in external pH.
This was further tested by bathing the preparations in an acid
medium (pH 6.5-6.8) which also induced cell depolarization (n = 27)
by a mean of 3.4 mV ± 0.3 s.e.m. (p < 0.001) although, again in
this case, the input resistance did not change significantly. Conversely, when pH of the bathing solution was allowed to increase
to 8.2-8.5, there was an increase in membrane potential by a mean
of 2.9 mV ± 0.3 s.e.m. (p < 0.001) and no significant changes in R_o.

These experiments indicate that H ions do have an important
role in maintaining the cell membrane potential. It is puzzling,
however, that MP changes were not accompanied by R_o changes. The
reason for this apparent paradox is unknown and is at present under
investigation.

In 22 instances, flow of the bathing solution was interrupted
and this invariably produced a marked increase in sensory discharges
as has been shown repeatedly in in vitro studies. Most often, but
not invariably, interruption of flow induced marked cell depolarization (mean ΔMP = 15 mV ± 2.5 s.e.m.; p < 0.001) and a loss of
input resistance (mean ΔR_o = 49 MΩ ± 9.3 s.e.m.; p < 0.001). It is
not known what mechanisms are involved in these effects of lack of
flow. However, the phenomenon, when present, had a reversal or
equilibrium potential (about 0 to -8 mV) which may indicate simultaneous changes in permeability to more than one ion.

Osmolarity effects. When one works with ionic substitution
experiments it is important to control the total osmolarity of the
test solutions and this was done by using an osmometer (freezing
point method). Using some of these solutions, it became clear
that the carotid body in vitro is quite sensitive to osmotic changes.
Thus, this case of serendipity prompted us to begin a systematic
analysis of this phenomenon which may have physiological implications.

When osmolarity of the test solution was increased by 50%, by
adding sucrose, Na-glutamate or glycerol, the membrane   potential
and input resistance of the cells decreased markedly. These effects
were observed even with increases in osmolarity as low as 5%. Using
more hyperosmotic solutions (15% or more), the cells depolarized
slowly to values close to 0 mV in a few minutes. This change was
concomitant with a decrease in R_o to very low values. The cells
remained depolarized for the duration of the flow of the hyperosmotic solution (up to 15 min); when the control solution was
again allowed to flow, MP and R_o slowly recovered to control levels.
Using more hyperosmotic solutions, exaggerated the effects already

mentioned. Thus, increasing osmolarity by 30–50%, there was a more rapid and pronounced fall in both MP and R_O. Recovery was slower after the more hypertonic solutions and, sometimes, it took a long time if the exposure to the hyperosmotic medium was more prolonged than usual.[13]

Hypo-osmotic solutions were first prepared by removing all or part of the Na-glutamate from the control solution. This bathing medium had the disadvantage that part of the normal Na content was reduced. To avoid this problem, control solutions were made with a lower than normal sodium content (with less Na-glutamate) and osmolarity was brought to normal levels (305 mOsm/l) by addition of sucrose. Test solutions were then made hypo-osmotic by removing or reducing the sucrose content without changing the ionic composition of the medium.

Hypo-osmotic solutions induced a clear increase in both MP and R_O. These effects were observed with a decrease in osmolarity as low as 5% of the control. More hypo-osmotic solutions (10 to 33% of the control) induced greater increases in both MP and R_O. After exposing the preparations to hypo-osmotic solutions, a return to the control medium induced a slow recovery toward baseline levels. The fact that similar changes were observed by reducing either the Na-glutamate or sucrose content of the bathing medium indicates that these changes were due to differences in osmotic strength and not to a reduction of sodium ions.[13] Furthermore, it seems that the increase in MP and R_O induced by hypo-osmotic solutions far exceeds similar changes induced by total removal of sodium ions. This point is still under investigation and quantitative data are forthcoming and will be presented elsewhere.

Osmotic changes seem to modify cell permeability to some ions. At present we do not know what ionic species are involved in this phenomenon. It may be that osmolarity variations change the membrane configuration, with consequent permeability changes; also, it is possible that this effect may be partly due to movements of water across the cell membrane that may modify the intracellular concentration of some crucial ionic species.

Conclusions

Results presented here are the beginning of an extensive study being carried out in this laboratory regarding the properties of carotid body cells. They indicate that certain ions such as Na, Ca, Mg and Cl contribute to the maintenance of both MP and R_O. But, they alone or in combination cannot be the exclusive elements involved in these processes. In fact, H ions are also important since the cell membranes seem to be somewhat permeable to hydrogen.

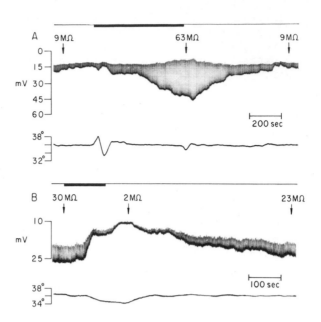

Fig. 5. Response of carotid body cells to changes in osmolarity.
Upper records in A and B, membrane potential and input resistance
recorded intracellularly from two different cells. Resistance
measured by passing 0.4 nA depolarizing current pulses at 0.2/sec
through recording micropipette in A. In B, 0.2 nA current pulses
were delivered at 0.5/sec. Lower records in A and B, temperature
changes recorded near the carotid body. In A, a 22% hypo-osmotic
solution (reduced sucrose) was passed for 9.5 min, marked by horizontal black bar above upper trace. Notice hyperpolarization from
15 to 45 mV and increase in R_O from 9 to 63 MΩ. In B, a 30% hypertonic solution (excess sucrose) is applied for 2 min (horizontal
black bar above upper trace). Notice marked depolarization from
26 to 10 mV and the decrease in input resistance from 30 to 2 MΩ.
Changes in temperature are due to arrival of new solution into
chamber and partially contribute to changes in MP and R_O, especially
in B. (From Gallego & Eyzaguirre.[13])

The latter, however, may only have an indirect role in modulating
the permeability of the membrane to other ionic species. But,
until more evidence is available it is impossible to reach definite
conclusions.

    A number of questions, posed at the beginning of this presen-
tation, still remain unresolved. For instance, acidity, flow

interruption and hyperosmolarity induce cell depolarization and an increase in sensory discharge frequency. An increase in temperature has the same effect on the sensory discharges but it induces cell hyperpolarization and an increase in input resistance. Other agents such as CO_2 (at normal pH), NaCN, ACh and N_2, which are good stimuli of these receptors, do not change appreciably either the membrane potential or input resistance of the carotid body (most likely type I) cells. It may be that stimuli that do not ostensibly act on glomus cell membranes may have a different primary locus for their action (type II cells or nerve endings). Alternatively, it is possible that, if the type I cells are the primary transducer elements in the carotid body, this action may not necessarily involve changes in MP and R_O. This assumption may entail a situation similar to that observed at the neuromuscular junction where osmotic changes induce acetylcholine release from the nerve endings without changes in either membrane potential or input resistance.[14] However, one must keep in mind that, even when ACh is released from the carotid body cells during stimulation and this agent is very effective in inducing nerve ending depolarization,[15] the evidence suggesting that ACh is a "transmitter" agent in these receptors is not entirely conclusive.[16]

In summary, these studies have shown that glomus (type I) cell membranes have some interesting characteristics, that the cells are exquisitely sensitive to temperature and osmolarity changes and that they do respond to variations of extracellular pH. But, their role as primary transducer elements for a variety of stimuli is still uncertain. Nevertheless, one should keep in mind that carotid body cells (type I or II) do seem to have an important role in the generation of chemosensory discharges. Thus, Verna, Roumy and Leitner[17] and also Zapata, Stensaas and Eyzaguirre[18] have shown that apposition of nerve endings to carotid body cells is essential to have normal chemosensory function. The crucial question is, how is this done? Is it release of a "transmitter" substance, or is it conditioning of the nerve endings to become chemosensitive? Or, is it through mechanical deformation of the endings through "contraction" of type II cells?[19] Obviously, we do not know the answers to these questions[18] which makes these problems the more fascinating and challenging.

ACKNOWLEDGEMENTS

This work was supported by grants NS 05666 and NS 07938 from the U.S. Public Health Service. The technical assistance of Messrs. P. Lenoir, J. Fisher and R. Perry is gratefully acknowledged. Dr. Margarita Baron was an NIH International Fellow from the Department of Physiology and Biochemistry, Universidad Complutense de Madrid, Spain. Dr. Roberto Gallego was a Fellow of the Program of Cultural Cooperation between the U.S.A. and Spain.

REFERENCES

1. Hess, A., Zapata, P. Innervation of the cat carotid body: normal and experimental studies. Fedn. Proc. 31:1365-1382, 1972.

2. Fidone, S.J., Stensaas, L.J., Zapata, P. Sensory nerve endings containing "synaptic" vesciles: an electron microscope auto-radiographic study. J. Neurobiol. 6:423-427, 1975.

3. Castro, de F. Sur la structure de la synapse dans les chemo-cepteurs: leur mécanisme d'excitation et rôle dans la circu-lation sanguine locale. Acta physiol. Scand., 22:14-43, 1951.

4. Eyzaguirre, C., Nishi, K. Further study on mass receptor potential of carotid body chemosensors. J. Neurophysiol., 37: 156-169.

5. Eyzaguirre, C., Nishi, K. Effects of different ions on resting polarization and on the mass receptor potential of carotid body chemosensors. J. Neurobiol.,1976 (in press).

6. Baron, M., Eyzaguirre, C. Thermal responses of carotid body cells. J. Neurobiol., 6:521-527, 1975.

7. Hubbard, J.I., Llinás, R., Ouastel, D.M.J. Electrophysiological analysis of synaptic transmission. Baltimore, The Williams & Wilkins Co., 1969.

8. Shanes, A.M. Electrochemical aspects of physiological and pharmacological action in excitable cells. Pharmacol. Rev., 10:59-273, 1958.

9. Brown, A.M. Effects of CO_2 and pH on neuronal membranes. Fedn. Proc., 31:1399-1403, 1972.

10. Goodman, N.W., McCloskey, D.I. Intracellular potentials in the carotid body. Brain Res., 39:501-504, 1972.

11. Eyzaguirre, C., Fidone, S., Nishi, K. Recent studies on the generation of chemoreceptor impulses. In Purves, M.J. (Editor): The Peripheral Arterial Chemoreceptors. Cambridge University Press, 1975, pp. 175-194.

12. Daly, M. de B., Lambertsen, C.J., Schweitzer, A. Observations on the volume of blood flow and oxygen utilization of the carotid body in the cat. J. Physiol., 125:67-89, 1954.

13. Gallego, R., Eyzaguirre, C. Effects of osmotic pressure changes on the carotid body of the cat in vitro. Fedn. Proc., 35:404, 1976.

14. Hubbard, J.I., Jones, S.F., Landau, E.M. An examination of the effects of osmotic pressure changes upon transmitter release from mammalian motor nerve terminals. J. Physiol., 197:639-657, 1968.

15. Eyzaguirre, C., Zapata, P. The release of acetylcholine from carotid body tissues. Further study on the effects of acetylcholine and cholinergic blocking agents on the chemosensory discharge. J. Physiol., 195:589-607, 1968.

16. Torrance, R.W. Arterial chemoreceptors. In Widdicombe, J.G. (Editor): Respiratory Physiology, MTP International Review of Science, London: Butterworths, 1974, pp. 247-271.

17. Verna, A., Roumy, M., Leitner, L.-M. Loss of chemoreceptive properties of the rabbit carotid body after destruction of the glomus cells. Brain Res., 100:13-23, 1976.

18. Zapata, P., Stensaas, L.J., Eyzaguirre, C. Axon regeneration following a lesion of the carotid nerve: electrophysiological and ultrastructural observations. Brain Res., 1976 (in press).

19. Paintal, A.S. Mechanism of stimulation of aortic chemoreceptors by natural stimuli and chemical substances. J. Physiol., 189:63-84, 1967.

TISSUE PO$_2$ IN THE CAT CAROTID BODY AND RELATED FUNCTIONS*

W. J. Whalen and P. Nair

St. Vincent Charity Hospital

Cleveland, Ohio   44115   U.S.A.

The mechanism by which chemoreceptors sense changes in arterial oxygen and carbon dioxide remains a mystery (Biscoe[1], Butler[2], Howe[3], Whalen[4]). In an effort to shed some light on this question we have measured tissue PO$_2$ (TPO$_2$) polarographically in the carotid body under a variety of conditions.

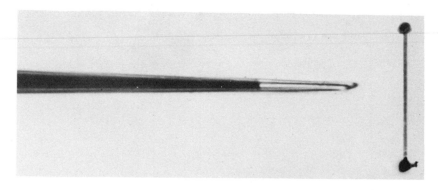

Figure 1: Micro O$_2$ electrode. The calibration bar represents 20μ.

The micro O$_2$ electrode used (Whalen[5]) has a long tapering point (Figure 1). The recessed glass tip is bevelled and measures 3-4μ at the beginning of the bevel. It is thus capable of intracellular recording. The O$_2$ current is less than 1×10^{-12} Amps/mmHg. Thus, O$_2$ consumption by the electrode is negligible, and there is no stir-sensitivity. Response time is less than a

---
* Supported in part by USPHS grants nos. HL 13134 and HL 12703.

second.   Under usual conditions the sensitivity is of the order
of 1 mmHg, and gradients over s distance of a few microns can be
detected (Ganfield[6]).

We have used cats, which usually weighed between 1 and 2 Kg,
anesthetized with pentobarbital (40 mg/Kg).   As described previously (Whalen[7]), the carotid body (CB) is carefully exposed, and
warmed (36-38° C) saline equilibrated with air or N_2 (normally air)
allowed to flow over it.   The cat is kept warm (36-39° C) and usually artificially ventilated to control arterial blood gasses and pH.

In our earlier work (Whalen[4]) the electrode was inserted into
the CB in steps of 50-100μ to a depth of about 600μ.   The O_2 pro-

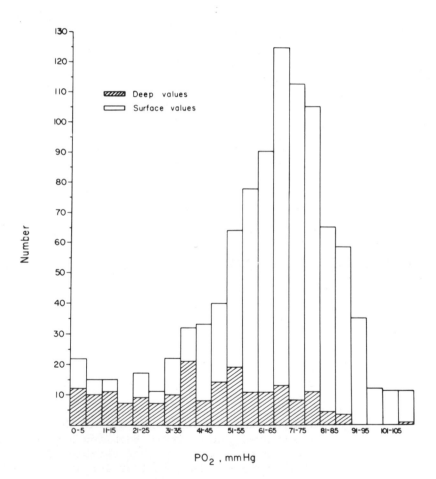

Figure 2:   Frequency distribution of 1071 TPO_2 values from 29 cats.
Surface = outer 200μ of CB.

files thus obtained under normal conditions revealed very few steep gradients and almost no TPO_2 values below 5 mmHg. A frequency distribution is shown in Figure 2. As can be seen values in the core of the CB tended to be lower. Even when the cats were given low O_2 and/or high CO_2 to breathe no more than 5% of the TPO_2 values were below 5 mmHg (Figure 3). Since chemoreceptor discharge would be expected to be near maximum under these circumstances we tentatively concluded that the PO_2 threshold for discharge must be high.

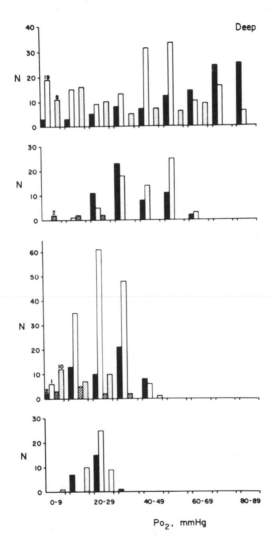

Figure 3: Frequency distribution of TPO_2 values deeper than 200μ into the CB grouped according to the arterial PO_2; from above down = 70–89, 50–69, 30–49, <30. Shadings further subdivide the data (see Whalen[4]).

In subsequent work we found that when the O_2 electrode was only 50-100µ beneath the surface of the CB, the TPO_2 was not affected
by the O_2 in the external environment (Whalen[7]). However, when
blood flow was reduced or stopped, TPO_2 varied with the external
PO_2 even when the tip was deep in the CB. We concluded that the
apparent barrier to O_2 diffusion was due to the normally rapid
blood flow which provided an enormous "sink" for the external O_2
(cf. Acker[8]). In this same study we also noted that when the arterial pressure of the cat was reduced to 50-60 mmHg, TPO_2 fell significantly; most impressively if the hematocrit was low. The fall
was at least partly due to sympathetic nerve activity since it was
blocked by phentolamine.

More recently, we have superfused the CB, in situ (after
clearing it of red cells) with artificial media. Typical results
from a superfused preparation are shown in Figure 4 (Whalen[9]). The
results led us to conclude that the isolated, superfused preparations used by others., e.g. Eyzaguirre[10], were probably adequately
oxygenated (Whalen[9]).

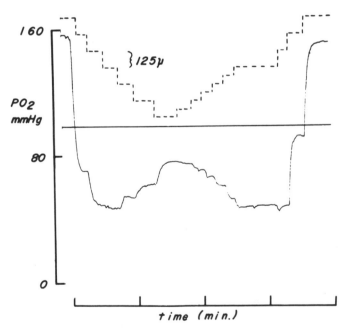

Figure 4: O_2 profile in a cat carotid body superfused in situ. Saline equilibrated with air flowed over the upper surface and saline
equilibrated with 50% O_2 flowed underneath. The electrode was, as
usual, calibrated in the solution flowing over the CB then inserted
into (and out of) the CB in steps as indicated by the dashed lines.

Modifications of the preparation have allowed us to stop the blood flow (or perfusion solution) at will, and to record sinus nerve discharge. Blood flow is stopped by occluding the common carotid artery and opening a cannula in the external carotid artery to allow a low resistance outflow path for any blood coming through collaterals. Total sinus nerve activity is measured via a suction electrode connected to a filter-square-averager (Biro[11]) of our own design. Figure 5 illustrates the rapid fall in TPO₂ following an occlusion and the slightly delayed rise in sinus nerve activity. Release of the occlusion results in a characteristic overshoot of TPO₂ and rapid cessation of sinus nerve discharge. In this experiment discharge began at a TPO₂ of about 25 mmHg which was the lowest "threshold" we found. In 19 trials discharge began when TPO₂ averaged 52 mmHg (Whalen[12]). We interpret these and our earlier results to indicate that chemoreceptor discharge does not result from hypoxia of the sensors in the classical sense wherein PO₂ would have to fall below 5 mmHg (Jobsis[13]). However, the interpretation of the results from the disappearance curves of O₂ is open to some question since CO₂ must be accumulating during this period and could be responsible for the early response (Whalen[14]).

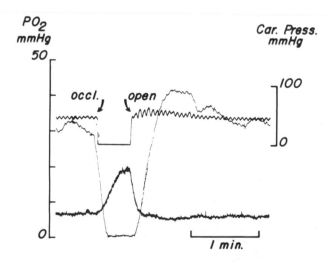

Figure 5: O₂ disappearance curve (thin trace) and chemoreceptor discharge (broad trace) during stoppage of the blood flow to the carotid body.

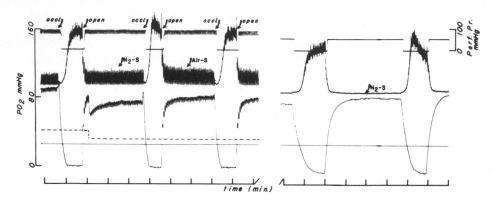

Figure 6:   Disappearance curves (DCs) of O_2 (lower trace) and chemoreceptor discharge (middle trace) during stoppage of the blood flow
(left segment) or the cell-free perfusion solution (right segment).
The O_2 micro electrode was in the same location during the last
four DCs.   About 3 minutes intervened between the two segments during which time the CB was cleared of red cells.   The saline flowing
over the CB was equilibrated with N_2 (N_2-s) or air (air-s).

        The O_2 consumption ($\dot{V}O_2$) of the CB is a matter of some contro-
versy.   In the blood-perfused, normal preparation very high values
of about 7-9 ml/100g/min have been reported (Daly[15], Purves[16]).
Fay[17] however found much lower values in the CB perfused with artificial, cell-free (c-f) solutions (see also Leitner[18]).   We have
perfused the CB in situ (through the cannula in the external carotid) with solutions similar to Fay's and find TPO_2 to be very close
to the PO_2 in the perfusing solutions (Whalen[9]).   Thus, Fay's low
value for $\dot{V}O_2$ cannot be due to tissue hypoxia.

        One can obtain some information regarding the $\dot{V}O_2$ from the O_2
disappearance curves (DCs) especially when not complicated by the
presence of red cells.   Figure 6 shows some rather typical, but still
preliminary, results.   Surprisingly, the DCs during c-f perfusion
are often slower than during perfusion with blood when "stored"
blood should retard the rate.   This appears to be partly due to the
reduced chemoreceptor discharge (and reduced energy demand?) almost
invariably seen during c-f perfusion.   In support of this suggestion
DCs taken during maximum discharge, induced by nicotine injections,
are significantly faster (Whalen[14]).   There is also the possibility
that the "resting" $\dot{V}O_2$ is depressed in the absence of blood.   These
possibilities are currently being explored.

References

1. Biscoe, TJ: Carotid body: structure and function. Physiol.
    Rev. 51: 437-495, 1971.

2. Butler, PJ, and Osborne, MP: A new theory for the receptor
    mechanism of the carotid body. J. Physiol. (London) 248:
    22P-23P, 1975.

3. Howe, A, and Neil E: Arterial chemoreceptors. In Neil, E
    (Editor): Enteroceptors. New York, Springer-Verlag, 1972,
    pp 47-80.

4. Whalen, WJ, Savoca, J, and Nair, P: Oxygen tension measurements
    in carotid body of the cat. Am. J. Physiol. 225: 986-991,
    1967.

5. Whalen, WJ, Riley, J, and Nair, P: A microelectrode for meas-
    uring intracellular PO$_2$. J. Appl. Physiol. 23: 798-801,
    1967.

6. Ganfield, RA, Nair, P, and Whalen, WJ: Mass transfer, storage,
    and utilization of O$_2$ in cat cerebral cortex. Am. J. Physiol.
    219: 814-821, 1970.

7. Whalen, WJ, and Nair, P: Some factors affecting tissue PO$_2$ in
    the carotid body. J. Appl. Physiol. 39: 562-566, 1975.

8. Acker, H, Lubbers, DW, and Purves, MJ: Local oxygen tension
    field in the glomus caroticum of the cat and its change at
    changing arterial PO$_2$. Arch. Ges. Physiol. 329: 136-155,
    1971.

9. Whalen, WJ and Nair, P: PO$_2$ in the carotid body perfused and/or
    superfused with cell-free media. J. Appl. Physiol. 41: 180-
    184, 1976.

10. Eyzaguirre, C, and Lewin, J: Effect of different oxygen ten-
    sions on the carotid body in vitro. J. Physiol. (London)
    159: 238-250, 1961.

11. Biro, G, and Partridge, LD: Analysis of multiunit spike records.
    J. Appl. Physiol. 30: 521-526, 1971.

12. Whalen, WJ, and Nair, P: "Hypoxic" discharge of chemoreceptors
    in the carotid body. Presented at Symposium: Tissue Re-
    sponses to Anoxia and Ischemia. I.S.O.T.T. meetings, Anaheim,
    1976.

13. Jobsis, FF: Basic processes in cellular respiration. In Fenn, WO, Rahn, H (Editors): Handbook of Physiology, Washington, D.C., American Physiological Society, 1964, vol. I., Sec. III, pp 111.

14. Whalen, WJ and Nair, P: Functional correlates with tissue PO_2 in the carotid body. Presented at Oxygen Electrode Colloquium: Oxygen and Physiological Function. FASEB meetings, Anaheim, 1976.

15. Daly, MdeB, Lambertsen, CJ, and Schweitzer, A: Observations on the volume of blood flow and oxygen utilization of the carotid body in the cat. J. Physiol. (London) 125: 67-89, 1954.

16. Purves, MJ: The effect of hypoxia, hypercapnia and hypotension upon carotid body blood flow and oxygen consumption in the cat. J. Physiol. (London) 209: 395-416, 1970.

17. Fay, FS: Oxygen consumption of the carotid body. Am. J. Physiol. 218: 518-526, 1970.

18. Leitner, LM and Liaubet, MJ: Carotid body oxygen consumption of the cat in vitro. Pflugers Arch: 323: 315-322, 1971.

SOME ASPECTS OF LOCALIZATION, DEPLETION, UPTAKE AND TURNOVER OF CATECHOLAMINES BY GLOMUS CELLS OF THE RAT CAROTID BODY

Arthur Hess

Department of Anatomy, Rutgers Medical School-CMDNJ

Piscataway, New Jersey 08854

The carotid body has been shown biochemically to contain catecholamines, predominantly dopamine[1]. Further evidence for the presence of catecholamines in glomus cells is provided by studies of histofluorescence, and glomus cells fluoresce intently after exposure to hot paraformaldehyde vapor[2, 3, 4], a histochemical test specific for catecholamines[5]. The glomus cells of the rat carotid body contain numerous dense-core or granulated vesicles[6, 7], resembling somewhat the vesicles seen in other catecholaminergic cells and nerve fibers. Presumably these vesicles are the site of location, wholly or in part, of the neurotransmitter substances. The biochemical tests show that the catecholamines are in the carotid body, and the histofluorescence studies demonstrate that the catecholamines are in the glomus cells. However, definitive proof has still not yet been presented that the dense-core vesicles are indeed the site of storage of catecholamines in glomus cells.

One method of localizing catecholamines with a resolution sufficient to detect these substances in cell organelles is by cytochemical stains which are supposed to reveal catecholamines specifically. The core and the matrix (or space between core and outer membrane) of granulated vesicles in noradrenergic nerves show a differential affinity to the zinc iodide-osmium tetroxide (Z10) method according to the temperature and time of impregnation[8]. The dense core is usually stained. At 20°C., the matrices of granulated vesicles in noradrenergic nerves also react intensely with Z10. The Z10 method, when applied at room temperature or 4oC. or for 2 or 24 hours to the carotid body, reveals the dense cores of the granulated vesicles (Fig. 1); the matrix of these vesicles is never stained densely by Z10. Hence, compared to the

233

vesicles of noradrenergic nerves, the granulated vesicles of the
carotid body react differently to Z10.   The Z10 method stains
synaptic vesicles in both cholinergic and catecholaminergic nerve
terminals[9].   Cholinergic vesicles stain densely throughout their
extent and do not exhibit cores, while only the core of the
vesicles of glomus cells stains densely after Z10.   This is
perhaps indicative of the monoaminergic nature of the dense core.

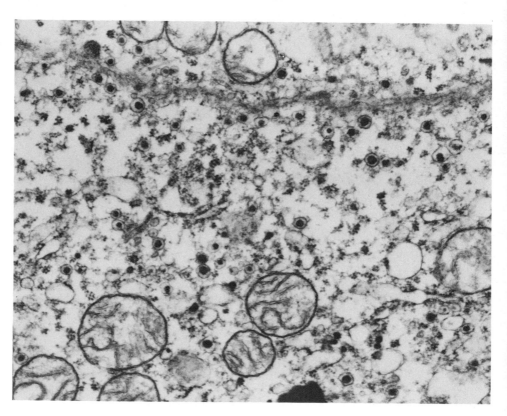

Fig. 1.   Zinc iodide-osmium tetroxide (Z10) method.   The cores of
the vesicles are stained densely, the matrix (between core and
outer membrane) is unstained.   X32,000.

The modified chromaffin reaction of Richards and Tranzer[10] is
said by these authors to be a specific cytochemical technique for
localization of vesicles storing biogenic amines.   With this
procedure (fixation in an aldehyde in a chromate-dichromate buffer),
the dense-core vesicles of the carotid body are similar in
appearance and in apparent number as when other buffers are used
in the fixative.   The dense product seen after the use of the
modified chromaffin reaction in non-osmicated tissues is said to

represent amines. The cores of the vesicles of the glomus cells
are revealed as very dense structures (Fig. 2) after the chromaffin
reaction without osmium tetroxide treatment. Hence, this cytochemical procedure might indicate that the dense core of the
granulated vesicles of the glomus cell is the catecholamine itself.

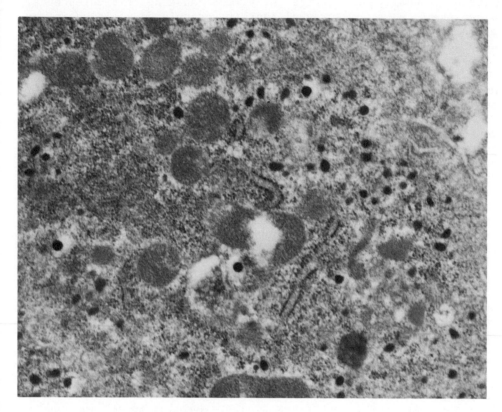

Fig. 2. Modified chromaffin reaction, no treatment with osmium
tetroxide, specific cytochemical stain for catecholamines. The
cores of the vesicles are revealed as densely stained structures.
X32,000.

    Thus, both cytochemical tests employed are consistent with
the view that the dense core in the vesicle of glomus cells
represents the catecholamine itself. However, experiments with
reserpine force a modification of this view. Reserpine depletes
catecholamines from cells by preventing reuptake of these substances
from cytoplasm into vesicle, thus preventing sequestration and
protection of the catecholamines within the vesicle and allowing
monoamine oxidases in the cytoplasm to deaminate and metabolize
the neurotransmitters, resulting in depletion of catecholamines

from the vesicles and from the cells. Reserpine does indeed
deplete the catecholamines from the glomus cells as seen by histofluorescence[2], [4]. The fluorescence of the glomus cells is
virtually absent 3 hours after administration of 15mg/kg intraperitoneally or 1mg/kg subcutaneously or overnight after 5mg/kg
intraperitoneally[11]. Despite the virtual absence of fluorescence,
ultrastructural studies reveal that the granulated vesicles in the
glomus cells are still very numerous and the dense cores are about
as electron dense as normally or before reserpine administration.

To attempt to determine if any changes occur at all in the
number or size of vesicles after reserpine administration, morphometric studies[12] were applied to the carotid body before and after
reserpine administration to ascertain the numerical and volume
densities of dense-core vesicles per volume of cytoplasm[13].
Carotid bodies were fixed in glutaraldehyde in Millonig's phosphate buffer. Sections of 10 levels, spaced 5μ apart, were
photographed. Ten photographs, each in a random location of the
same carotid body, were taken. At least 100 photographs were
taken of each of 4 normal and 4 reserpinized carotid bodies.
Volume and numerical densities of dense-core vesicles expressed
as percentages of glomus cell cytoplasm were determined by a point
counting method; diameters of 800 dense-core vesicles from each
group, normal and reserpinized, were measured. All measurements
and counts were made from photographic prints at a magnification
of X32,000. The numerical density of dense-core vesicles in glomus
cells is not significantly changed after reserpine treatment;
however, the volume density is slightly reduced, indicating that
the vesicles after reserpine are in general smaller. This is
borne out by the diameter measurements. Most vesicles vary from
75-135nm in diameter. Vesicles of 60-90nm are increased in
frequency of occurrence in reserpinized over normal rats by 43%.
Since increase in number of vesicles does not occur after reserpine
(and hence the formation of new smaller vesicles is not induced),
the vesicles have apparently undergone shrinkage in diameter,
perhaps because they have been depleted of some or all of their
content of catecholamines. And yet, as mentioned above, dense
cores are still present.

Reserpine depletes adrenergic substances from dense-core
vesicles of pineal nerves reacting with Z10 at 20°C.[8] Reserpine
administration fails to cause any obvious alterations in appearance
or apparent number of dense-core vesicles of glomus cells revealed
by the Z10 method (Fig. 3).

The organelles which stain selectively by the modified chromaffin reaction could not be observed in sympathetic ganglion cells
from reserpine treated animals[10]. On the contrary, reserpine
does not affect occurrence or apparent number of dense-core

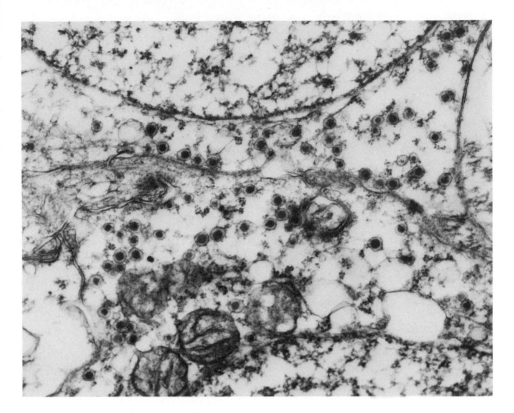

Fig. 3. Reserpine (15mg/kg for 3 hours) followed by the Z10 method. The dense cores of the vesicles are still present and densely stained. Compare with figure 1. X32,000.

vesicles in glomus cells as seen after the chromaffin reaction with or without osmium tetroxide (Fig. 4). The cores are perhaps slightly less dense after reserpine treatment than in normal animals.

The cytochemical tests and the morphometric studies indicate that catecholamines are present in the vesicles of the carotid body. However, both cytochemical tests and ultrastructural studies after reserpine administration, while not contradicting the conclusion that catecholamines are in the vesicles, nevertheless do seem to indicate that the dense core is not composed solely of the catecholamine itself. Perhaps the dense core represents carrier substance to which the catecholamines within the vesicles are bound[2, 14].

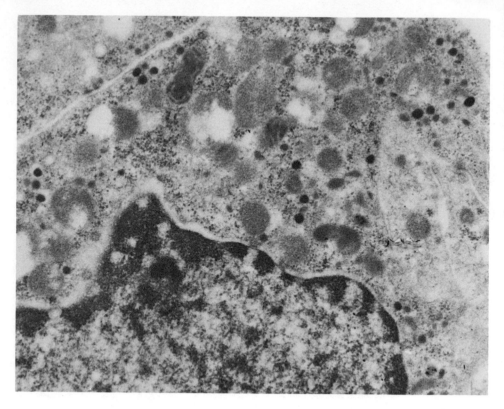

Fig. 4. Reserpine (15mg/kg for 3 hours) followed by the chromaffin
reaction without osmium tetroxide treatment. The dense-core
vesicles are present. Compare with figure 2. X32,000.

Further evidence that catecholamines are within the vesicles
is provided by uptake studies employing 6-hydroxydopamine[15]. This
dopamine analogue is accumulated specifically by the neuronal
membrane pump of catecholaminergic nerve cells and fibers. The
histofluorescence of the carotid body is reduced after 6-hydroxy-
dopamine administration[3]; however, the glomus cells after glutaraldehyde fixation appear unaffected and the dense-core vesicles are
present and normal in appearance. Initial fixation in osmium
tetroxide results in lightly stained or empty vesicles in the
glomus cells[16]. After 6-hydroxydopamine and initial fixation in
osmium tetroxide, the vesicles appear full of dense material[15].
The glomus cells are apparently able to take up 6-hydroxydopamine
and to sequester this substance within the vesicles. The 6-hydroxy-
dopamine does not fluoresce, hence histofluorescence is reduced in

amount and intensity. The 6-hydroxydopamine within the vesicle is
apparently not soluble in osmium tetroxide and hence appears as a
dense reaction product. After 6-hydroxydopamine and reserpine
administration (followed by initial fixation in osmium tetroxide),
the vesicles appear again as they do after initial fixation in
osmium tetroxide alone without any drug treatment[15]. Reserpine is
therefore able to cause depletion of the 6-hydroxydopamine from the
vesicles, and the 6-hydroxydopamine is either metabolized by
monamine oxidases in the cytoplasm like catecholamines or, after
release from protection within the vesicle, is now subject to
being washed out of the cell by fixatives. The uptake of 6-hydroxy-
dopamine by the glomus cell, its incorporation within the vesicle,
and its depletion by reserpine indicate that the catecholamines in
the glomus cell are localized within the vesicle.

Preliminary morphometric studies[13] indicate that the numerical
density of dense-core vesicles is higher in animals treated with
6-hydroxydopamine than in normals, but that the volume density of
normal animals is greater than in those after drug treatment.
Hence, there are more small dense-core vesicles in the glomus cells
after 6-hydroxydopamine treatment, either because 6-hydroxydopamine
causes vesicles to shrink in size or perhaps because the drug
stimulates the biogenesis of new smaller vesicles. This problem
is still under active investigation.

Prolonged administration of the adrenergic neuron blocking
agent guanethidine to adult rats produces a marked and permanent
destruction of the cell bodies of sympathetic neurons and fibers
of the peripheral sympathetic nervous system[17, 18]. In the hopes
of achieving a "glomectomy", guanethidine sulfate was administered
intraperitoneally at 20mg/kg daily for 30 days to adult rats and
the animals studied at 5, 10, 15, 22, 27, and 30 days[19]. Despite
severe degeneration and disappearance of almost the total cell
population of the superior cervical ganglion and the nerves
emanating from it, the glomus cells of the carotid body are intact
and appear unaffected (Fig. 5).

It has been suggested that the damaging effect of guanethidine
will be more marked in those neurons which have a low transmitter
turnover, such as those supplying the vas deferens[20, 21].

To determine the turnover rate of catecholamines in glomus
cells, 400mg/kg of alpha-methyl-para-tyrosine were administered
intraperitoneally in one dose or in each of 3 separate doses to
rats, and the carotid bodies examined for histofluorescence
intensity 2 to 24 hours after injection. Turnover rate is defined
as the rate at which tissue stores of catecholamines are used and
replaced by newly synthesized amines. Administration of alpha-
methyl-para-tyrosine inhibits tyrosine hydroxylase, the rate-

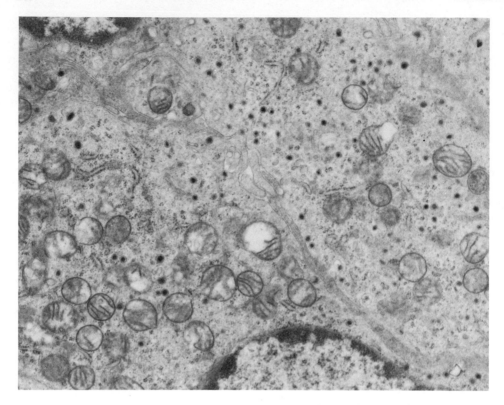

Fig. 5. Guanethidine (20mg/kg for 15 days). The carotid body
appears normal. Sympathetic ganglion cells (not shown) are
severely degenerated and depleted in number in this animal.
X16,000.

limiting enzyme in catecholamine synthesis, and results in depletion of catecholamines from cells. Thus, the rate of decline of
catecholamines in cells that have been treated with this tyrosine
analogue provides a reflection of the turnover rate of catecholamines. After the times and dose of the present schedule, sufficient
to result in marked depletion of catecholamines in peripheral and
central nervous structures, the carotid body still fluoresces
intently. Quantitative studies are in progress to determine the
exact change in intensity of histofluorescence induced by alpha-
methyl-para-tyrosine. However, the alterations in fluorescence
intensity from normal animals are minimal, and it thus appears that
the glomus cells have a low transmitter turnover and are probably
firing off or releasing catecholamines at a very low rate, so that

inhibition of synthesis of catecholamines results in a minimal depletion of catecholamines from glomus cells. It is probably true that, during normoxia, the carotid body is hardly being stimulated. Despite this low turnover rate, the glomus cells appear unaffected morphologically by guanethidine.

The cells of the adrenal medulla[18] and the small intensely fluorescent (SIF) cells in sympathetic ganglia are similarly not affected[22] or only minimally affected[23] by guanethidine. It is perhaps significant that all 3 cell types not affected by guanethidine have large numbers of dense-core vesicles in their cytoplasm, while sympathetic ganglion neurons, markedly degenerated after guanethidine, are almost devoid of such vesicles. Exogenous guanethidine is accumulated in the cell cytoplasm and sequestered in catecholamine storage granules[24] like a "false transmitter". It may be that cells with large numbers of dense-core vesicles are able to sequester large amounts of guanethidine in these vesicles, leaving guanethidine in the cytoplasm insufficient in amount to exert a destructive effect[18].

Further information about the localization, depletion, uptake, and turnover of catecholamines in glomus cells should contribute greatly to knowledge about the neurotransmitter functions of these substances in carotid body physiology and provide evidence for ascertaining the definitive role of glomus cells in the working of the carotid body.

The author's investigations were supported by NIH research grant NS-07662. Thanks to Dr. Elaine S. Hearney and Dr. Gordon J. Macdonald, collaborators in some of the above investigations, for permission to present the unpublished results. Mr. P. J. Adamo, Ms. I. Cassady, and Ms. H. Ferguson provided technical assistance. Ciba-Geigy Corporation gave the guanethidine.

REFERENCES

1. Zapata P, Hess A, Bliss EL, Eyzaguirre C: Chemical, electron microscopic and physiological observations on the role of catecholamines in the carotid body. Brain Res. 14:473-496, 1969.

2. Niedorf HR, Rode J, Blümcke S: Feinstruktur und Catecholamingehalt des Glomus caroticum der Ratte nach einmaliger Reserpin-Injektion. Virchows Arch. Abt. B Zellpath. 5:113-123, 1970.

3. Lassman H, Böck P: Die Wirkung von 6-Hydroxydopamin auf den Katecholamingehalt des Glomus caroticum der Ratte. Z Zellforsch. 127:220-229, 1972.

4. Hess A: Hyposensitivity of deafferented receptor cells in the rat carotid body. Brain Res. 98:348-353, 1975.

5. Fuxe K, Hökfelt T, Jonsson G, Ungerstedt U: Fluorescence microscopy in neuroanatomy. In Nauta WJH, Ebbesson SOE (Editors): Contemporary Research Methods in Neuroanatomy. New York, Springer, 1970, pp 275-314.

6. McDonald DM, Mitchell RA: The innervation of glomus cells, ganglion cells and blood vessels in the rat carotid body: a quantitative ultrastructural analysis. J. Neurocytol. 4:177-230, 1975.

7. Hess A: The significance of the ultrastructure of the carotid body in structure and function of chemoreceptors. In Purves MJ (Editor): The Peripheral Arterial Chemoreceptors. Cambridge University Press, 1975, pp 51-73.

8. Pellegrino de Iraldi A: Z10 staining of monoaminergic granulated vesicles. Brain Res. 66:227-233, 1974.

9. Akert K, Sandri C: Significance of the Maillet method for cytochemical studies of synapses. In Santini M (Editor): Golgi Centennial Symposium: Perspectives in Neurobiology. New York, Raven Press, 1975, pp 387-399.

10. Richards JG, Tranzer JP: Localization of amine storage sites in the adrenergic cell body. J. Ultrastruc. Res. 53:204-216, 1975.

11. Hess A: Calcium inhibits catecholamine depletion by reserpine from carotid body glomus cells. Brain Res. Bull. In Press, 1976.

12. Weibel ER: Stereological principles for morphometry in electron microscopic cytology. Int. Rev. Cytol. 26:235-302, 1969.

13. Hess A, Hearney ES: In preparation.

14. Duncan D, Yates R: Ultrastructure of the carotid body of the cat as revealed by various fixatives and the use of reserpine. Anat. Rec. 157:667-682, 1967.

15. Hess A: The effects of 6-hydroxydopamine on the appearance of granulated vesicles in glomus cells of the rat carotid body. Tiss. Cell 8:379-385, 1976.

16. Knoche H, Kienecker E-W, Schmitt G: Elektronen mikroskopischer Beitrag zur Kenntnis des Glomus caroticum (Katze). Z. Zellforsch. 112:494-515, 1971.

17. Burnstock G, Evans B, Gannon BJ, Heath JW, James V: A new method of destroying adrenergic nerves in adult animals using guanethidine. Brit. J. Pharmacol. 43:295-301, 1971.

18. Johnson EM, O'Brien F: Evaluation of the permanent sympathectomy produced by the administration of guanethidine to adult rats. J. Pharmacol. Exp. Ther. 196:53-61, 1976.

19. Hess, A, Macdonald GJ: In preparation.

20. Burnstock G, Costa M: Adrenergic Neurons. London, Chapman and Hall, 1975, pp 225.

21. Laverty R, Robertson A: Effects of alpha-methyl tyrosine in normotensive and hypertensive rats. In Catecholamines in Cardiovascular Physiology and Disease. Am. Heart Assn. Monograph 17:127-133.

22. Eränkö O, Eränkö L: Effect of guanethidine on nerve cells and small intensely fluorescent cells in sympathetic ganglia of newborn and adult rats. Acta pharmacol. toxicol. 30:403-416, 1971.

23. Heym C, Grube D: Effects of guanethidine on para-ganglionic cells in the superior cervical ganglion of the rat. Anat. Embryol. 148:89-97, 1975.

24. Maitre L, Staehelin M: Guanethidine uptake and noradrenaline depletion in noradrenaline storage particles of the rat heart. Biochem. Pharmacol. 20:1233-1242, 1971.

CATECHOLAMINES AND 3',5' CYCLIC AMP IN CAROTID BODY CHEMORECEPTION IN THE CAT

Robert S. Fitzgerald, Ellen M. Rogus, Abbas Dehghani

The Department of Environmental Medicine and The Department of Physiology, The Johns Hopkins University Baltimore, Maryland   21205

INTRODUCTION

Almost fifty years have passed since the discovery of the carotid body. Its proper functioning seems essential to the organism's normal respiratory (1), circulatory (2), endocrine (3) responses to hypoxia. It is common knowledge that the carotid body normally responds to changes in carbon dioxide and hydrogen ion as well. But exactly which structure or structures in the carotid body act as the receptor for these stimuli, and what processes or mechanisms are operating to transduce changes in oxygen, carbon dioxide, and hydrogen ion into changes in neural output are not known.

Recently attention has been focused on the possibility of a role in chemoreception for catecholamines. Among the many investigators experimenting with the catecholamines Sampson (4), Mitchell and McDonald (5) and we ourselves (Fig. 1) have shown that an injection of dopamine (DA), norepinephrine (NE), or epinephrine (E) close to the carotid body transiently decreases neural output (imp/sec) from the carotid body.

Further, considerable progress has been made recently in providing a more detailed description of the elements of the carotid body and their interrelationships. The Bristol Symposium of 1973 (6) presents an extensive account and bibliography of these advances. Among them has been the frequent observation of high concentrations of catecholamines in the glomus (or Type I) cells of the carotid body. Fillenz concluded that the rate of release of DA seemed too high for DA merely to mediate chemoreceptor

245

impulses and there seemed little correlation between storage and release of catecholamines and chemoreceptor function (7). However, other investigators seem more disposed to find a primary role for the catecholamines as a modulator of chemoreception (8,9,10). The observation of McDonald and Mitchell (8) of reciprocal synapses between glomus cells and afferent nerves reinforces the possibility that the catecholamines modulate chemoreception.

If one assumes that the endogenous catecholamines of the glomus cell inhibit carotid body neural output as does exogenously administered catecholamines, a next question to be asked is--how? How does DA or the other catecholamines inhibit neural activity?

Comparisons have been made between the small intensely florescent (SIF) cells of the superior cervical ganglion (SCG) and the glomus cells of the carotid body (5,7,8). Greengard and Kebabian have presented considerable evidence that the DA of the SIF cells in the bovine SCG is responsible for the inhibitory post synaptic potential (11). It achieves this by activating an adenylate cyclase-cyclic AMP system which phosphorylates a membrane protein and so provokes a hyperpolarization (Fig. 2). The present experiments were performed to see if in the cat carotid body: (1) there was an adenylate cyclase-cAMP system; and

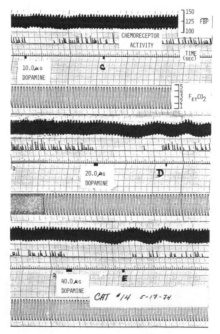

Fig. 1. Single fiber response to increasing doses of dopamine. Drug injected into the thyroid artery. C, D, E mark the end of injection of 1 ml of solution.

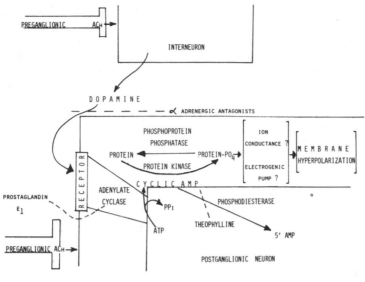

Figure 2

(2) if present, was it activated by DA. Up to the present we
have performed four sets of experiments, one to test for the
presence of adenylate cyclase and its susceptibility to DA
stimulation, and three to see the effect of DA on levels of cAMP
in carotid body homogenates.

METHODS

1. General Methods

Mature cats of both sexes ranging in weight from 2.5 to 5 kg
were anesthetized with sodium pentobarbital 30 mg/kg. Catheters
were placed in the femoral artery and vein. After inserting a
tracheal cannula 1 cm rostral to the sternum the rostral section
of the transected trachea and esophagus were drawn forward to
expose both carotid bifurcations. Small cannulae were inserted
into either the superior thyroid or lingual artery depending upon
the procedure which followed. Carotid bodies were exposed by
carefully dissecting away connective tissue and fat. Arterial
circulation to the carotid body was left intact, the ascending
pharyngeal and occipital arteries being tied off central to the
carotid body. Venous circulation from the carotid body was left
untouched until the carotid body was removed. All sympathetic
input was removed and the carotid nerve itself was sectioned where
it entered the connective tissue surrounding the carotid body.

Ligatures were then loosely placed around the arterial and venous supply of the carotid body. There followed a period of recovery of 0.5-2.0 hours. The area of dissection was continually moistened with saline and maintained at a temperature not less than 1° below rectal temperature. When carotid bodies were removed, the arterial ligature was tightened first, then the venous. The whole removal generally took less than 30 seconds. It was then placed on a piece of saline-moistened cotton and the excess fat, connective tissue and superficial vessels trimmed away. Finally, it was then put into the appropriate solution for homogenization or incubation.

2. Assay for Adenylate Cyclase Activity

In three experiments both carotid bodies were homogenized in 0.4 ml of isotonic sucrose (0.25 M in 1 mM Tris buffer, pH 7.4). These contents were transferred to centrifuge tubes and initially centrifuged at 10,000 g for 10 minutes to obtain nuclei and mitochondria. Supernatant was transferred to new tubes and centrifuged at $\geq$ 100,000 g for 30 minutes to obtain the microsomal fraction. Each pellet was suspended in 0.2-0.4 ml of sucrose. The final volume of each assay tube contained 0.1 ml (Tris buffer pH 6, 25 mM; $MgCl_2$, 5 mM; phosphocreatine, 10 mM; creatine phosphokinase, 0.05 mg/ml; EDTA, 1.4 mM; cAMP, 1 mM; ATP, 0.4 mM; ^{32}P-ATP, $5x10^6$ cpm/tube; protein, 30 μl of enzyme suspension containing 1-30 μg; GTP, 10^{-6} M; when used, NaF, 8 mM; DA, $2x10^{-4}$ M). This was incubated for 20 minutes at 37^oC, returned to the ice bath and 20 μl of "stopping solution" (40 mM ATP in 0.5 NHCl + trace of ^{14}C-cAMP to give about 10^3 CPM/20 μl) was added. This mixture was then boiled for 2 minutes. The separation of the ^{32}P-cAMP was done by alumina column chromatography according to the method of White (12).

In three other experiments both carotid bodies were homogenized and compared with an homogenate of the carotid sinus nerve including 1-2 mm of the glossopharyngeal nerve central to the junction of the former nerve with the latter. The above procedures were followed for the determination of adenylate cyclase activity. Protein was determined according to the method of Lowry (13).

3. Perfusion of the Carotid Body In Situ and Assay for cAMP

After preparation of the carotid bodies the animal was ventilated with 8-10% O_2 (PaO_2 = 27 $\pm$ 4.6; $PaCO_2$ = 20.2 $\pm$ 3.3; pH_a = 7.437 $\pm$ 0.080) for about 4-6 minutes. At the end of this exposure the left carotid bodies were quickly removed to 600 μl of ice cold 6% TCA. They were homogenized in ice for two minutes. The homogenate was immediately transferred to centrifuge tubes, capped and frozen at -15^oC. After a period of recovery the animal was ventilated with oxygen (PaO_2 = 409 $\pm$ 94.5; $PaCO_2$ = 30.6 $\pm$ 7.3;

pH_a = 7.321 $\pm$ 0.062).   Immediately before removal of the carotid body DA (110 $\pm$ 27 μg) was injected into the superior thyroid artery.   Subsequent homogenization and freezing was identical to the procedures followed above.

The homogenates were subsequently analyzed for cAMP according to a modification of the technique of Brown et al. (14).

4.   Incubation of the Carotid Body and Assay for cAMP

After preparation as above, carotid bodies were removed and incubated for 15 minutes at 37°C in one of two Krebs-Ringer solutions. Solution 1 was 10 mM theophylline (P_{O_2} = 355; P_{CO_2} = 40.7; pH = 7.373).   Solution 2 was 10 mM theophylline and 200 μM DA (P_{O_2} = 365; P_{CO_2} = 40.7; pH = 7.397).   After incubation these carotid bodies were placed in 600 μl of ice-cold 6% TCA and homogenized for two minutes in ice.   The homogenates were immediately transferred to centrifuge tubes and frozen at -15°C.

The homogenates were subsequently analyzed for cAMP as above.

5.   Perfusion of the Carotid Body In Situ, Removal to Incubation Medium and Assay for cAMP

Carotid bodies were prepared as above except that ligatures were placed around the common carotid artery and external carotid costral to the lingual artery.   Immediately before removal the common carotid and external carotid arteries were tied and 3-8 ml of solution 1 or 2 (above) were infused (1.5-3.0 minutes).   Toward the end of the infusion the carotid body circulation was tied off as above.   The carotid bodies were quickly excised as above, incubated for 15 minutes as above, homogenized in ice-cold 6% TCA, frozen, and later analyzed for cAMP.

RESULTS

1.   Assay of Carotid Bodies for Adenylate Cyclase Activity

In the first set of experiments we attempted to see if an adenylate cyclase system was present, was stimulated by DA, and was located preferentially in any fraction of cellular components. Figure 3 presents the results of three experiments using a homogenate of 2 carotid bodies per experiment.   There was barely detectable activity in the basal or DA tubes.   Fluoride stimulated adenylate cyclase activity in both the carotid body and nerve. But this is a small amount in comparison to other tissues, being only about 1% of what is found in muscle.   Kebabian and Greengard (15) report an adenylate cyclase activity in the DA-stimulated (7 μM) SCG of 0.059 n moles/mg protein/min.

Figure 4 shows the results of three experiments in which NaF was used to provoke adenylate cyclase activity in the mitochondrial-nuclear and microsomal fractions. Though the variation of activity in the microsomal fraction is large, there is the suggestion that the microsomal fraction has more activity than the mitochondria and heavier particles. In the three experiments there was 1.7, 2.2, and 6.4 times as much activity in the microsomal fraction as in the mitochondrial fraction.

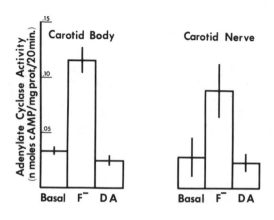

Figure 3

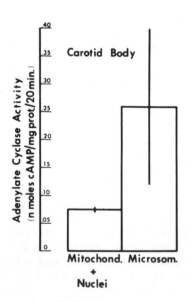

Figure 4

2. Perfusion with DA

The purpose of these experiments was to see if a given amount of DA, known to reduce transiently the neural activity from the carotid body, increases the cAMP in the carotid body. In six out of seven experiments we observed that the DA-injected carotid body had a higher cAMP content that the hypoxia-exposed carotid body (Table 1). But the magnitude of the difference was not great. We felt that perhaps magnitude of the difference might be increased and the variability decreased if exposure of the carotid body to DA were prolonged.

TABLE 1

TRANSIENT PERFUSION OF THE CAROTID BODY WITH DA DURING

HYPEROXIA VS. NO PERFUSION DURING HYPOXIA

| EXPT. NO. | TREATMENT | | % CHANGE |
| | Low O_2 | DA/high O_2 | |
	(p moles cAMP/carotid body)		
1	2.87	3.32	15.7
5	2.90	3.75	29.3
7	5.60	6.40	14.3
8	11.40	7.56	- 33.7
10	4.85	6.30	29.9
11	4.35	10.00	129.9
12	4.80	14.30	197.9
$\overline{X}$	5.25	7.38	54.8
$\pm$ S.E.	1.18	1.55	32.6

3. Incubation with DA

In three successful experiments we incubated for 15 minutes whole carotid bodies either in a Krebs-Ringer solution which was 10 mM theophylline equilibrated with 95% O_2 and 5% CO_2 at 37°C, or in the same solution made also 200 μM DA. In some experiments the DA became oxidized. These were discarded. Once again, the DA-treated carotid bodies have the greater content of cAMP; but

TABLE 2

FIFTEEN MINUTE INCUBATION IN KREBS-RINGER SOLUTION WITH:

| EXPT. NO. | TREATMENT | | % CHANGE |
| | 10 mM Theophylline | 10 mM Theophylline + 200 μM DA | |
	(p moles cAMP/carotid body)		
15	6.60	6.95	5.3
17	5.45	6.55	20.2
19	22.50	37.90	68.4

TABLE 3

PERFUSION AND INCUBATION IN KREBS-RINGER SOLUTION WITH:

| EXPT. NO. | TREATMENT | | % CHANGE |
| | 10 mM Theophylline | 10 mM Theophylline + 200 μM DA | |
	(p moles cAMP/carotid body)		
20	21.00	12.00	-42.9
21	14.62	13.88	- 5.1
22	34.88	21.75	-37.6
23	20.25	15.38	-24.0
25	15.75	16.50	+ 4.7
$\overline{X}$	21.30	15.90	-21.0
± S.E.	4.04	1.84	10.2

there is again a good deal of variation in the three results
(Table 2).   Inasmuch as these carotid bodies were not minced, we
felt that differences in cAMP may be due to different distances
through which the medium had to diffuse.

4.   Perfusion and Incubation

This last series of five experiments was performed to try
once again to give maximum exposure of the carotid body to DA in
hopes of maximizing cAMP production and reducing interexperiment
variability.   Hence, immediately before excising the carotid
bodies their arterial circulation was tied off and they were
perfused in situ with the solution in which they were about to be
incubated.   Table 3 presents the results.   It is apparent this
procedure provoked more consistent and higher levels of cAMP for
both treatments.   However, in the three of the five experiments
there is a significantly smaller amount of cAMP in the DA-treated
carotid body (Expts. 20,22,23).   On the basis of the previous
experiments this is the opposite of what we expected.

DISCUSSION

Cyclic AMP regulates key functions in many tissues: lipolysis
in fat, secretion in endocrine glands, gluconeogenesis in liver.
Presently a variety of evidence also supports the hypothesis that
cAMP and cGMP exercise regulatory roles in neuronal function.   The
phenomenon has been studied in a number of different preparations
including incubated brain slices, cells of neuronal or glial
origin, functional ganglia or discrete central neurons.   Initially,
high levels of adenylate cyclase were detected in the brain.
Indeed the levels of adenylate cyclase activity and the concentration of cAMP are higher in the brain than in any other tissue.
Equally impressive levels of phosphodiesterases were found in the
brain.   Both enzymes along with cAMP-dependent protein kinases
were later found to be associated with synaptic elements.   Later
still, presumed neurotransmitters like norepinephrine, DA,
serotonin, histamine were shown to provoke increases in intracellular cAMP in brain slices.   And the currently accepted
mechanism has the neurotransmitter activating adenylate cyclase
which promotes the formation of cAMP from ATP.   Cyclic AMP
activates a protein kinase which phosphorylates enzymes and other
functional proteins altering their properties; it is deactivated
by degradation to a 5' phosphate by phosphodiesterases.   The
phosphorylated protein is dephosphorylated by a phosphoprotein
phosphatase (Fig. 2).

During the past decade considerable evidence has appeared pointing to the cAMP-dependent mechanisms operating post-synaptically in the CNS. This means that the five proteins involved would be located in the post-synaptic neuron and the effect of the nucleotide would depend not only on the intracellular site of its generation, but also on the substrate specificity of the activated kinase, the availability of the protein substrate and effect-releasing proteins. A priori one would expect from the complexity of such a system that identical treatment of sensitive synapses might produce some degree of variability in the results. The possibility for inter-species differences would also seem high. Such indeed is the case.

In a recent review Daly (16) remarks that in the brain, for example, there are profound differences in the amount of cAMP elicited by stimulatory agents depending on the region of the brain and/or the species of animal. And even for the same brain region from the same species results are often quantitatively different. This is due to variability in individual animals, groups of animals, inadequate experimentation and variations in experimental technique. This variability is also found in peripheral systems. For example, in bovine SCG DA and higher concentrations of NE will elicit about a ten-fold increase in endogenous cAMP. This response to DA is blocked by alpha-antagonists, not by beta-antagonists. But beta-antagonists do reduce the effects of NE. In contrast to this NE and isoproterenol increase the level of cAMP in the cultured rat SCG transiently 8-20-fold. But even higher concentrations of DA have only a marginal effect.

Inasmuch as our study is, as far as we know, the first effort to determine the possible presence and characteristics of an adenylate cyclase-cAMP system in the carotid body we have no criterion for what constitutes a significant change in cAMP consequent to DA activity. One would ordinarily compare the changes in cAMP with those found for other tissues. But the problems inherent in this are clear from the above.

We presently have no explanation as to why the NaF stimulated increase in adenylate cyclase activity is so low even though it does show a 3-4-fold increase over basal levels. The fact that DA does not stimulate any increase in activity may be due to some disruption of the hormone receptor element during homogenization. The similarity in the response profile between the carotid body and the carotid nerve is compatible with the possibility that the adenylate cyclase-cAMP system is located post-synaptically to the Type I cell, namely in the afferent nerve.

The results shown in Tables 1 and 2 taken together, though not conclusive, do suggest that transient or prolonged but limited exposure to DA does provoke an increase in cAMP somewhere in the carotid body. The fact that these differences are small may be due in the first case to the DA being too transitory and in the second case to the problems of diffusion from the incubation medium into the carotid body.

Table 3 presents the most perplexing results. However, several investigations of the effect of hormones on cAMP in other tissues present a possible explanation (17-22). Ho and Sutherland (17) reported that fat cells responded to epinephrine with a 35-fold increase in cAMP levels by 3 minutes. This was followed by a rapid decrease so that at 9 minutes the level was only 4-fold greater than control. Additional hormone produced little or no increase in cAMP. They interpreted this as a resistance of the

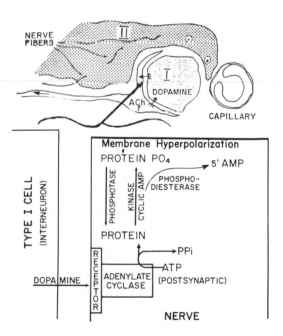

Figure 5

cell to epinephrine. Similar results are reported for the perfused rat heart (18), rat cerebral slices (19), rat epididymal fat pad (20), and perfused rat livers (21). Ho et al. (23) later obtained direct evidence showing the cellular formation and subsequent release of a potent inhibitor of adenylate cyclase by adipocytes stimulated with epinephrine. Hence, it is not impossible that treatment with both the theophylline and DA via perfusion and incubation overly exposed the carotid body to the hormone, and some inhibitor was generated. It is interesting to note that a biphasic response of the carotid body to some catecholamine injections has been observed (3,24,25), an initial decrease in neural activity followed by an increase in activity.

In summary, we have presented evidence which does not contradict the hypothesis that the modulation of chemoreceptor activity seen with injections of catecholamines near the carotid body is accomplished by the activation of an adenylate cyclase-cAMP system such as that depicted in Figure 5. Endogenous catecholamines of the carotid body may act in the same way to modulate chemoreception.

ACKNOWLEDGEMENTS

The authors gratefully acknowledge Drs. Robert A. Mitchell and Alan Berger of CVRI, University of California, San Francisco. It was their suggestion that initiated these investigations. The authors also acknowledge the generous assistance of Dr. Elizabeth Gillespie and Miss Jane Benson in the analysis of cAMP, and Miss Judy Wagner in the preparation of the manuscript.

REFERENCES

1. Heymans, C., Neil, E. Reflexogenic Areas of the Cardiovascular System. London, Churchill, 1958.

2. Korner, P.I. Integrative neural cardiovascular control. Physiol. Rev. 51:312-367, 1971.

3. Lau, C. Role of respiratory chemoreceptors in adrenocortical activation. Am. J. Physiol. 221:602-606, 1971.

4. Sampson, S.R. Pharmacology of feedback inhibition of carotid body chemoreceptors in the cat. In: The Peripheral Arterial Chemoreceptors, M.J. Purves (Editor). London, Cambridge University Press, 1975, pp. 207-220.

5. Mitchell, R.A., McDonald, D.M. Adjustment of chemoreceptor
    sensitivity in the cat carotid body by reciprocal synapses.
    In: The Peripheral Arterial Chemoreceptors, M.J. Purves
    (Editor). London, Cambridge University Press, 1975, pp. 269-292.

6. Purves, M.J. (Editor). The Peripheral Arterial Chemoreceptors.
    London, Cambridge University Press, 1975.

7. Fillenz, M. The function of the Type I cell of the carotid
    body. In: The Peripheral Arterial Chemoreceptors, M.J.
    Purves (Editor). London, Cambridge University Press, 1975,
    pp. 133-142.

8. McDonald, D.M., Mitchell, R.A. A quantitative analysis of
    synaptic connections in the rat carotid body. In: The
    Peripheral Arterial Chemoreceptors, M.J. Purves (Editor).
    London, Cambridge University Press, 1975, pp. 101-132.

9. Sampson, S.R., Nicolaysen, G., Jaffe, R. Influence of
    centrifugal sinus nerve activity on carotid body catecholamines:
    microphotometric analysis of formaldehyde-induced fluorescence.
    Brain Res. 85:437-446, 1975.

10. Mills, E., Slotkin, T.A. Catecholamine content of the carotid
    body in cats ventilated with 8-40% oxygen. Life Science 16:
    1555-1562, 1975.

11. Greengard, P., Kebabian, J.W. Role of cyclic AMP in synaptic
    transmission in the mammalian peripheral nervous system. Fed.
    Proc. 33:1059-1067, 1974.

12. White, A.A. Separation and purification of cyclic nucleotides
    by alumina column chromatography. In: Methods in Enzymology,
    J.G. Hardman and B.W. O'Malley (Editors). New York, Academic
    Press, 1974, Vol. 38, pp. 41-46.

13. Lowry, O.H., Rosebrough, N.J., Farr, A.L., Randall, R.J.
    Protein measurement with the folin phenol reagent. J. Biol.
    Chem. 193:265-275, 1951.

14. Brown, B.L., Albano, J.D.M., Ekins, R.P., Sgherzi, A.M. A
    simple and sensitive saturation assay method for the measure-
    ment of adenosine 3':5'-cyclic monophosphate. Biochem. J.
    121:561-562, 1971.

15. Kebabian, J.W., Greengard, P. Dopamine-sensitive adenyl

cyclase: possible role in synaptic transmission. Science 174:1346-1349, 1971.

16. Daly, J. Role of cyclic nucleotides in the nervous system. In: Handbook of Psychopharmacology, L.L. Iversen, S.D. Iversen, S.H. Snyder (Editors). New York, Plenum Press, 1975, Vol. 5, pp. 47-130.

17. Ho, R.J., Sutherland, E.W. Formation and release of a hormone antagonist by rat adipocytes. J. Biol. Chem. 246:6822-6827, 1971.

18. Robison, G.A., Bukher, R.W., Øye, I., Morgan, H.E., Sutherland, E.W. The effect of epinephrine on adenosine 3',5'-phosphate levels in the isolated perfused rat heart. Molec. Pharmacol. 1:168-177, 1965.

19. Kakiuchi, S., Rall, T.W., McIlwain, H. The effect of electrical stimulation upon the accumulation of adenosine 3',5'-phosphate in isolated cerebral tissue. J. Neurochem. 16:485-491, 1969.

20. Butcher, R.W., Ho, R.J., Meng, H.C., Sutherland, E.W. Adenosine 3',5' monophosphate in biological materials. J. Biol. Chem. 240:4515-4523, 1965.

21. Exton, J.H., Robison, G.A., Sutherland, E.W., Park, C.R. Studies on the role of adenosine 3',5'-monophosphate in the hepatic action of glucogon and catecholamines. J. Biol. Chem. 246:6166-6177, 1971.

22. Kuo, J.F., DeRenzo, E.C. A comparison of the effects of lipolytic and antilipolytic agents on adenosine 3',5'-monophosphate levels in adipose cells as determined by prior labeling with adenine-8-[14]C. J. Biol. Chem. 244:2252-2260, 1969.

23. Ho, R.J., Russell, T.R., Asakawa, T., Sutherland, E.W. Cellular levels of feedback regulator of adenylate cyclase and the effect of epinephrine and insulin. PNAS (USA) 72:4739-4743, 1975.

24. Sampson, S.R. Catecholamines as mediators of efferent inhibition of carotid body chemoreceptors in the cat. Fed. Proc. 30:551, 1971.

25. Fitzgerald, R.S. Unpublished observations, 1973.

Circulatory and Metabolic Aspects
of Cerebral Hypoxia-Ischemia

Chairman: M. Reivich

METABOLIC ASPECTS OF CEREBRAL HYPOXIA-ISCHEMIA

B.K. Siesjö, C.-H. Nordström and S. Rehncrona

Brain Research Laboratory, E-Blocket, the University Hospital, and Department of Neurosurgery, University of Lund, Lund, Sweden

This communication, which is focused on changes in brain metabolism in hypoxia and ischemia, briefly summarizes results obtained in this and other laboratories during the last 4-5 years. An attempt will be made to describe the characteristic features of hypoxic hypoxia, both at normal and at reduced perfusion pressures, as well as of incomplete and complete ischemia, and to discuss how the metabolic changes relate to irreversible neuronal damage. The references quoted are highly selective. For further references, and for a somewhat more detailed account of the topics discussed, the reader is referred to original papers quoted in the text and to some recent review articles (Nilsson et al. 1974, Siesjö et al. 1974, 1975, 1976, Siesjö 1977).

1. Uncomplicated Hypoxia

Arterial hypoxia occurs when there is either a decrease in arterial pO_2 (hypoxic hypoxia) or in hemoglobin concentration (anemic hypoxia). We will use the expression "uncomplicated hypoxia" to denote conditions in which the cerebral perfusion pressure is either normal or increased, and in which there is no occlusion of inflow vessels. Typical of uncomplicated hypoxia is a reduction in oxygen delivery with unlimited supply of substrate. There is invariably an increase in CBF.

When arterial pO_2 is reduced in steps from the normal values of about 90 mm Hg, the first detectable metabolic signs occur at a pO_2 of about 50 mm Hg and consist of an accumulation of lactic acid (Siesjö and Nilsson 1971), reduction of cytoplasmic and mitochondrial redox couples (Siesjö et al. 1975, Rosenthal et al. 1976), and a

261

reduced rate of synthesis of catechole- and indolamines (Davis and
Carlsson 1973, Davis et al. 1973). At these levels of hypoxia, there
is also a steep increase in CBF (Kogure et al. 1970, Jóhannsson and
Siesjö 1975, Borgström et al. 1975). Although this CBF response indicates a coupling to the metabolic events, CBF varies inversely with
arterial pO_2 even within the physiological pressure range (Borgström
et al. 1975).

The initial activation of glycolysis occurs at the phosphofructokinase step (Norberg and Siesjö 1975 a, Norberg et al. 1975),
but, probably due to secondary acceleration of hexokinase activity
and to breakdown of glycogen, the concentrations of all glycolytic
intermediates (and end products) are subsequently increased (Duffy
et al. 1972, Bachelard et al. 1974). Citric acid cycle changes are
initially dominated by decreases in the concentrations of α-ketoglu-
tarate (α-KG) and oxaloacetate (OAA) (Duffy et al. 1972, Norberg
and Siesjö 1975 b). Later, there is an increase in the size of the
citric acid cycle pool (Norberg and Siesjö 1975 b), an increase in
alanine and a decrease in aspartate concentration (Duffy et al.
1972, Norberg and Siesjö 1975 b, Siesjö et al. 1975). All these
changes can be satisfactorily explained as being caused by the accumulation of pyruvate, and by the redox change (see Duffy et al. 1972,
Norberg and Siesjö 1975 b). Thus, accumulation of pyruvate may explain the increase in alanine concentration (via its effect on the
alanine aminotransferase reaction) and the increase in the size of
the citric acid cycle pool (via its effect on the pyruvate carboxylase and the alanine aminotransferase reactions), while a redox-de-
pendent increase in malate/OAA ratio (and relative decrease in OAA
concentrations), by its effect on the aspartate-aminotransferase
reaction, may explain the initial fall in α-KG concentration, and
the decrease in aspartate concentration. Previously, it has been
well documented that hypoxia leads to an increase in GABA concentration (Wood et al. 1968, see also Duffy et al. 1972). Presumably, this
is due to lack of NAD^+ for the succinic semialdehyde dehydrogenase
reaction.

The changes described are observed in the approximate pO_2 range
50 to 20 mm Hg. At these levels of hypoxia, cerebral oxygen utilization (CMR_{O_2}) is not measurably reduced (Kety and Schmidt 1948, Cohen
et al. 1967, Jóhannsson and Siesjö 1975), and the tissue concentrations of ATP, ADP and AMP are close to normal (Schmahl et al. 1966,
Siesjö and Nilsson 1971, Duffy et al. 1972, MacMillan and Siesjö
1972, Bachelard et al. 1974). Presumably, energy homeostasis is due
solely to the increase in CBF. Despite considerable experimentation
and speculation, the mechanisms triggering the hyperemia have never
been clarified. It has been customary to ascribe the increase in CBF
to extracellular acidosis, secondary to lactic acid production (Lasse
1968, Kogure et al. 1970, Betz 1972), but recent results have failed
to corroborate this hypothesis (Siesjö et al. 1975, Nilsson et al.

1975, Astrup et al. 1976). Histopathological evidence supports the view that these degrees of tissue hypoxia do not critically encroach upon neuronal energy production. Thus, when rats are subjected to unilateral carotid artery clamping and the arterial pO_2 is reduced to below 25 mm Hg for 30 min, the unclamped side is devoid of neuronal damage (Salford et al. 1973 b).

2. Hypoxia with Relative Ischemia

At arterial pO_2 values of 20-25 mm Hg (about 5% O_2) there is a gradual failure of the heart, with a fall in blood pressure. The resulting reduction in perfusion pressure curtails the increase in CBF and creates a condition of relative ischemia (see Siesjö et al. 1974). Experimentally, this occurs as a complication to studies of hypoxic hypoxia (Siesjö and Nilsson 1971), or has been studied by combining hypoxia with unilateral carotid artery ligation (Salford et al. 1973 a and b, Salford and Siesjö 1974, Levy et al. 1975). Even though CBF may not fall below normal there is energy failure with reduced ATP and increased ADP and AMP concentrations. Since substrate supply is maintained, there is a progressive lactic acidosis with individual values sometimes exceeding 40 μmol·g^{-1}. In the citric acid cycle, both α-KG and OAA fall, probably due to ammonia accumulation and reduction of cellular redox systems. When this degree of cellular hypoxia is maintained for 15-30 min there are ischemic cell changes affecting neurons in selectively vulnerable areas (Salford et al. 1973 b, Levy et al. 1975).

3. Incomplete Ischemia

When CBF is reduced below about 50% of control there are changes in cerebral metabolism, similar to those observed in hypoxia with relative ischemia. Thus, there is accumulation of lactic acid and deterioration of the phosphorylation state (Siesjö and Zwetnow 1970, Eklöf and Siesjö 1972, Eklöf et al. 1972). Results on cerebral energy state and cerebral venous pO_2 indicate that cerebral ischemia develops in an inhomogenous fashion, and that relatively well perfused areas may coexist with others in which flow has ceased (Eklöf et al. 1973). Even if CBF is reduced to very low values (5-10% of control), continued substrate supply leads to a gradually progressive lactic acidosis that may become excessive. If CBF is reduced to such low values for 30 min, the tissue does not recover its phosphorylation state upon recirculation, and there is a pronounced, lingering lactic acidosis (Nordström et al. 1976, Nordström et al., in preparation). These findings are in line with previous histopathological results which have shown that incomplete ischemia, lasting 15 min or longer, gives rise to permanent neuronal damage, localized to arterial boundary zones (Brierley et al. 1969, Brierley 1973).

4. Complete Ischemia

This condition differs from incomplete ischemia (and hypoxia with relative ischemia) in that the supply of oxygen and glucose is nil. Since no exogenous substrate is provided the lactic acidosis is limited by the preischemic stores of glucose and glycogen (see Ljunggren et al. 1974 c). Complete ischemia leads to rapid depletion of glucose, glycogen, pyruvate, α-KG and OAA, and to accumulation of lactate, succinate, alanine, GABA and ammonia (Lowry et al. 1964, Goldberg et al. 1966, Ljunggren et al. 1974 a, Folbergrová et al. 1974). There is an increase in the size of the citric acid cycle pool, presumably due to CO_2 fixation and reversal of the terminal reactions of the cycle (Folbergrová et al. 1974). In all probability, depletion of OAA is caused by the rapid reduction of NAD^+ in both cytoplasm and mitochondria, while depletion of α-KG can be ascribed to ammonia fixation via the glutamate dehydrogenase reaction. Since there is no accumulation of pyruvate at any time (Nordström and Siesjö, in preparation) CO_2 fixation must occur by other reactions than the pyruvate carboxylase reaction, and the shift in the alanine aminotransferase reaction may be caused by a fall in α-KG concentration (relative to that of pyruvate).

In spite of these dramatic changes, and despite the fact that energy depletion occurs within the first 5 min, recirculation of the brain after ischemic periods of 15 or 30 min leads to the subsequent restoration of adenylate energy change to within 1% of control and to reoxidation of the lactate accumulated (Ljunggren et al. 1974 b, Nordström et al. 1976). In cats under barbiturate anaesthesia, a certain proportion of animals regain some electrophysiological functions, such as the EEG and evoked cortical responses, and show a fair restoration of cerebral energy state (Hossmann and Kleihues 1973, Kleihues et al. 1974). These findings argue against any extensive mitochondrial damage. In support, studies of mitochondria isolated from brains following 30 min of ischemia have failed to give evidence of damage to mitochondrial function (Schutz et al. 1973). There is, though, a lingering perturbation of amino acid levels and of mono-amine metabolism (Ljunggren et al. 1974 b, Folbergrová et al. 1974, Brown et al. 1974), possibly contributing to lack of restoration of function.

5. Biochemical Basis of Irreversible Neuronal Damage

In general, little is known about the biochemical mechanisms underlying cell death. In considering the metabolic basis of neuronal damage, two recent findings should be stressed. First, although both hypoxia with relative ischemia and incomplete ischemia of 30 min duration may give rise to a permanent metabolic lesion (and to irreversib. histopathologic changes), animals tolerate 30 min of complete ischemia without showing signs of such a lesion (see above, and Hossmann and Kleihues 1973). Second, when animals are pretreated with phenobarbital before being subjected to incomplete ischemia, most of the brains show energy depletion within 5 min but none fails to recover their energy state after 30 min of ischemia (Nordström et al. 1976). There are three possible explanations.

(1) There is deficient recirculation of the tissue following hypoxia with relative ischemia and following incomplete ischemia, but not following complete ischemia. Although this possibility cannot yet be excluded, CBF measurments indicate that recirculation occurs upon termination of the hypoxia-ischemia, and that any deterioration occurs later (see Hossmann et al. 1973, Snyder et al. 1975). Possibly, failure of mitochondrial metabolism causes gradual cell swelling which secondarily compromises capillary circulation (see Leaf 1973).

(2) The excessive acidosis occurring in hypoxia with relative ischemia, and in incomplete ischemia, adversely affects cellular metabolism and/or cell structure. So far, attempts to demonstrate an effect of acidosis have failed (Ljunggren et al. 1974 c). Furthermore, phenobarbital does not prevent the development of pronounced acidosis in incomplete ischemia. Thus, if acidosis is detrimental, its effect should be blocked by the barbiturate.

(3) A continued supply of oxygen allows oxygen-dependent autolytic degradation of cell structures. There are several possible mechanisms, including peroxidation of membrane lipids by release of free radicals (Demoupoulus et al. 1976). This hypothetical mechanism may explain why there is damage following both hypoxia with relative ischemia, and incomplete ischemia, but not following complete ischemia. It would also explain the effect of barbiturates which are considered to be efficient free radical scavengers.

At the present time, there is insufficient information to distinguish between these three possibilities. However, the mere fact that the final outcome of a period of hypoxia-ischemia does not correlate to the degree (or duration) of cellular oxygen lack suggests that an intense study of the biochemical mechanisms leading to cellular damage is warranted.

Acknowledgements

This study was supported by grants from the Swedish Medical Research Council (Project No. 14X-00263), and from U.S. PHS No. 2 R01 NS07838-07 from N.I.H.

References

Astrup, J., D. Heuser, N.A. Lassen, B. Nilsson, K. Norberg and
B.K. Siesjö: Evidence against H^+ and K^+ as the main factors in
the regulation of cerebral blood flow during epileptic discharges,
acute hypoxemia, amphetamine intoxication and hypoglycemia. A
microelectrode study. Workshop on Vascular Smooth Muscle, Tübingen
1976. Springer Verlag, Berlin–Heidelberg–New York.

Bachelard, H.S., L.D. Lewis, U. Pontén and B.K. Siesjö: Mechanisms
activating glycolysis in the brain in arterial hypoxia. J. Neurochem. 22. 395–401. 1974.

Betz, E.: Cerebral blood flow: its measurements and regulation.
Physiol. Rev. 52. 595–630. 1972.

Borgström, L., H. Jóhannsson and B.K. Siesjö: The relationship between arterial pO_2 and cerebral blood flow in hypoxic hypoxia.
Acta physiol. scand. 93. 423–432. 1975.

Brierley, J.B., A.W. Brown, B.J. Excell and B.S. Meldrum: Brain
damage in rhesus monkey resulting from profound arterial hypotension. I. Its nature, distribution and general physiological
correlates. Brain Res. 13. 68–100. 1969.

Brierley, J.B.: Pathology of cerebral ischemia. In: Cerebral Vascular
Diseases. (eds. F.H. McDowell and R.W. Brennan) pp. 59–75. Grune
and Straton, New York–London 1973.

Brown, R.M., A. Carlsson, B. Ljunggren, B.K. Siesjö and S.R. Snider:
Effect of ischemia on monoamine metabolism in the brain. Acta
physiol. scand. 90. 789–791. 1974.

Cohen, P.J., S.C. Alexander, T.C. Smith, M. Reivich and H. Wollman:
Effects of hypoxia and normocarbia on cerebral blood flow and
metabolism in conscious man. J. appl. Physiol. 23. 183–189. 1967.

Davis, J.N. and A. Carlsson: Effect of hypoxia on tyrosine and tryp-
tophan hydroxylation in unanaesthetized rat brain. J. Neurochem.
20. 913–915. 1973.

Davis, J.N., A. Carlsson, V. MacMillan and B.K. Siesjö: Brain trypto-
phan hydroxylation: Dependence on arterial oxygen tension. Science
182. 72–74. 1973.

Demopoulus, H., F. Flamm and J. Ransohoff: Molecular pathology of
lipids and CNS membrane. 60th FASEB Annual Meeting, Anaheim,
April 1976.

Duffy, T.E., S.R. Nelson and O.H. Lowry: Cerebral carbohydrate metabolism during acute hypoxia and recovery. J. Neurochem. 19.
959–977. 1972.

Eklöf, B. and B.K. Siesjö: The effect of bilateral carotid artery
ligation upon the blood flow and the energy state of the rat brain
Acta physiol. scand. 86. 155–165. 1972.

Eklöf, B., V. MacMillan and B.K. Siesjö: The effect of hypercapnic acidosis upon the energy metabolism of the brain in arterial hypotension caused by bleeding. Acta physiol. scand. 87. 1-14. 1973.

Folbergrová, J., B. Ljunggren, K. Norberg and B.K. Siesjö: Influence of complete ischemia on glycolytic metabolites, citric acid cycle intermediates, and associated amino acids in the rat cerebral cortex. Brain Res. 80. 265-279. 1974.

Goldberg, N.D., J.V. Passonneau and O.H. Lowry: Effects of changes in brain metabolism on the levels of citric acid cycle intermediates. J. biol. Chem. 241. 3997-4003. 1966.

Hossmann, K.-A. and P. Kleihues: Reversibility of ischemic brain damage. Arch. Neurol. 29. 375-384. 1973.

Jóhannsson, H. and B.K. Siesjö: Cerebral blood flow and oxygen consumption in the rat in hypoxic hypoxia. Acta physiol. scand. 93. 269-276. 1975.

Kety, S.S. and C.F. Schmidt: The effects of altered arterial tensions of carbon dioxide and oxygen on cerebral oxygen consumption of normal young men. J. clin. Invest. 27. 484-492. 1948.

Kleihues, P., Kobayashi, K. and Hossmann, K.-A.: Purine nucleotide metabolism in the cat brain after one hour of complete ischemia. J. Neurochem. 23. 417-425. 1974.

Kogure, K.P., O.M. Scheinberg, M. Reinmuth and R. Busto: Mechanisms of cerebral vasodilatation in hypoxia. J. appl. Physiol. 29. 223-229. 1970.

Lassen, N.A. : Brain extracellular pH: The main factor controlling cerebral blood flow. Scand. J. clin. Lab. Invest. 22. 247-251. 1968.

Leaf, A.: Cell swelling a factor in ischemic tissue injury. Circulation. 48. 455-458. 1973.

Levy, D.E., J.B. Brierley, D.G. Silverman and F. Plum: Brief hypoxia-ischemia initially damages cerebral neurons. Arch. Neurol. 32. 450-456. 1975.

Ljunggren, B., H. Schutz and B.K. Siesjö: Changes in energy state and acid-base parameters of the rat brain during complete compression ischemia, Brain Res. 73. 277-289. 1974 a.

Ljunggren, B., R.A. Ratcheson and B.K. Siesjö: Cerebral metabolic state following complete compression ischemia. Brain Res. 73. 291-307. 1974 b.

Ljunggren, B., K. Norberg and B.K. Siesjö: Influence of tissue acidosis upon restitution of brain energy metabolism following total ischemia. Brain Res. 77. 173-186. 1974 c.

Lowry, O.H., Passonneau, J.V., F.X. Hasselberger and D.W. Schulz: Effect of ischemia on known substrates and cofactors of the glycolytic pathway in brain. J. biol. chem. 239. 18-30. 1964.

MacMillan, V. and B.K. Siesjö: Brain energy metabolism in hypoxemia. Scand. J. Clin. Lab. Invest. 30. 127-136. 1972.

Nilsson, B., K. Norberg, C.-H. Nordström and B.K. Siesjö: Influence of hypoxia and hypercapnia on CBF in rats. In: Blood Flow and Metabolism in the Brain (eds. M. Harper, B. Jennet, D. Miller, J. Rowan) pp. 9.19-9.23. Churchill Livingstone, Edinburgh-London-New York 1975.

Nilsson, B., K. Norberg and B.K. Siesjö: Biochemical events in cerebral ischemia. Brittish J. Anaesth. 47. 751-760. 1975.

Norberg, K. and B.K. Siesjö: Cerebral metabolism in hypoxic hypoxia. I. Pattern of activation of glycolysis; a re-evaluation. Brain Res. 86. 31-44. 1975 a.

Norberg, K. and B.K. Siesjö: Cerebral metabolism in hypoxic hypoxia. II. Citric acid cycle intermediates and associated amino acids. Brain Res. 86. 45-54. 1975 b.

Norberg, K., B. Quistorff and B.K. Siesjö: Effects of hypoxia of 10-45 seconds duration on energy metabolism in the cerebral cortex of unanaesthetized and anaesthetized rats. Acta physiol. scand. 95. 301-310. 1975.

Nordström, C.-H., S. Rehncrona and B.K. Siesjö: Restitution of cerebral energy state after complete and incomplete ischemia of 30 min duration. Acta physiol. scand. In press.

Rosenthal, M., J.C. LaManna, F.F. Jöbsis, J.E. Levassen, H.A. Kontos and J.L. Patterson: Effects of respiratory gases on cytochrome a in intact cerebral cortex: is there a critical pO$_2$? Brain Res. In press.

Salford, L.G., F. Plum and B.K. Siesjö: Graded hypoxia-oligemia in rat brain. I. Biochemical alterations and their implications. Arch. Neurol. 29. 227-233. 1973 a.

Salford, L.G., F. Plum and J.B. Brierley: Graded hypoxia-oligemia in rat brain. II. Neuropathological alterations and their implications. Arch. Neurol. 29. 234-238. 1973 b.

Salford, L.G. and B.K. Siesjö: The influence of arterial hypoxia and unilateral carotid artery occlusion upon regional blood flow and metabolism in the rat brain. Acta physiol. scand. 92. 130-141.

Schmahl, F.W., E. Betz, E. Dellinger and H.J. Hohorst: Energiestoffwechsel der Grosshirnrinde und Elektroencephalogram bei Sauerstoffmangel. Pflüg. Arch. ges. Physiol. 292. 46-59. 1966.

Siesjö, B.K. and N.N. Zwetnow: Effects of increased cerebrospinal
    fluid pressure upon adenine nucelotides and upon lactate and
    pyruvate in rat brain tissue. Acta neurol. scand. 46. 187-202.
    1970.

Siesjö, B.K. and L. Nilsson: The influence of arterial hypoxemia
    upon labile phosphates and upon extracellular and intracellular
    lactate and pyruvate concentration in the rat brain. Scand. J.
    Clin. Lab. Invest. 27. 83-96. 1971.

Siesjö, B.K., H. Jóhannsson, B. Ljunggren and K. Norberg: Brain dys-
    function in cerebral hypoxia and ischemia. In: Brain Dysfunction
    in Metabolic Disorders (ed. F. Plum) vol. 53. pp. 73-112. Raven
    Press, New York 1974.

Siesjö, B.K., H. Jóhannsson, K. Norberg and L.G. Salford: Brain
    function, metabolism and blood flow in moderate and severe arterial
    hypoxia. Alfred Benzon Symposium VIII. Brain Work. pp. 101-125.
    Munksgaard, Copenhagen 1975.

Siesjö, B.K. and C.-H. Nordström: Brain metabolism in relation to
    oxygen supply. 60th FASEB Annual Meeting, Anaheim, April 1976.

Siesjö, B.K.: Brain Energy Metabolism. To be published by John
    Wiley and Sons Ltd., London.

Snyder, J.V., E.M. Nemoto, R.G. Carroll and P. Safar: Global ischemia
    in dogs: intracranial pressures, brain blood flow and metabolism.
    Stroke. 6. 21-27. 1975.

Wood, J.D., W.J. Watson and A.J. Ducker: The effect of hypoxia on
    brain γ-aminobutyric acid levels. J. Neurochem. 15. 603-608. 1968.

DISCUSSION: METABOLIC ASPECTS OF CEREBRAL HYPOXIA-ISCHEMIA

Thomas E. Duffy
David E. Levy
Departments of Neurology and Biochemistry
Cornell University Medical College
New York, New York

To Dr. Siesjö's list of possible explanations for the relative susceptibility of brain to sub-total ischemia and for the protection afforded by barbiturates, our own studies (1) in the gerbil suggest that an additional factor, i.e., hypermetabolism of variably damaged tissue, may also play a role.

Gerbils lack posterior communicating arteries and are therefore vulnerable to unilateral carotid artery occlusion. Cerebral ischemia was induced in adult male gerbils (50-70 g) by occluding the right common carotid artery with an aneurysm clip under brief (3 min) halothane anesthesia. Clinical status (gait, responsiveness, seizures) was assessed during one hour of occlusion, and the clip was removed. Animals were frozen head-first in liquid nitrogen after 15 or 60 minutes of carotid occlusion and at one, four, and 24 hours after release of the clip. One day prior to the experiment, the skin overlying the calvarium had been removed under local anesthesia to facilitate freezing of the brain.

Frozen slices (1-1.5 mm thick) of parietal cortex from each hemisphere (right, ipsilateral to the occluded artery; left, contralateral) were separately weighed, extracted with perchloric acid, and analyzed according to the fluorometric, enzymatic methods of Lowry and Passonneau (2).

Of 170 gerbils subjected to unilateral carotid artery occlusion, 68 (40%) had motor abnormalities consistent with stroke during the period of occlusion; this incidence of stroke is consistent with data of others (3,4). Biochemical changes were most marked in the ipsilateral cortex of animals with clinical evidence of stroke. Thus, phosphocreatine and ATP both fell to 15% of control by 15 minutes

271

Table 1

Metabolite levels (mmol/kg) in ipsilateral cerebral cortex during
and following 1 hour of right carotid artery occlusion in gerbils.

Treatment	Phosphocreatine	ATP	ADP	AMP
Sham-operated (9)	4.19	2.76	0.50	0.014
Occlusion 15 min (6)	0.65*	0.42*	0.35§	1.41*
Occlusion 60 min (5)	0.39*	0.32*	0.32*	0.82*
Occlusion 60 min and recovery 1 hr (5)	4.60§	1.78*	0.31*	0.012
and recovery 4 hr (7)	4.79§	2.26*	0.40§	0.020
and recovery 24 hr (6)	3.50	2.13§	0.37§	0.031

* Different from sham-operated with $P<0.01$; § $P<0.05$.

of occlusion and were even further reduced after 60 minutes (Table
1). The changes in ATP were partly realized as increased AMP; ADP
was also substantially decreased. The sum of the adenine nucleotides (ATP + ADP + AMP) fell from 3.3 mmol/kg to 1.6 mmol/kg after
60 minutes of occlusion.

There were changes in the contralateral cortex of gerbils with
stroke (ATP and ADP fell, whereas AMP rose) but these differences,
though significant, were small.

Following ischemia, concentrations of the adenine nucleotides
tended to return toward control. However, normal values of ATP and
ADP were never fully achieved, and the total adenylate pool remained
depressed (77% of control) even after 24 hours, despite the fact
that the energy charge potential (5) had returned to within 1% of
control. Because enzymes respond to substrates and effectors rather
than to ratios per se (6), the persistent decline in ATP at 24 hours
must be expected to alter ATP-dependent reactions and energy metabolism would therefore still be abnormal even though the energy charge
potential returned to normal.

In order to assess the dynamics of cerebral energy metabolism
in gerbils recovering from stroke, we adopted Lowry's technique (7)
for estimating energy utilization rates. Normal gerbils and animals
that were subjected to 1 hour of unilateral carotid occlusion and
allowed to recover for one, four, or 24 hours, were decapitated
and the heads frozen after 10 seconds of total ischemia. Energy
use was calculated from differences in concentrations of ATP, ADP,

Table 2

High-energy phosphate utilization (~P use) following one hour of
right common carotid artery occlusion in gerbils with stroke.

Treatment	~P Use (mmol/kg/min)	
	Right Cortex	Left Cortex
Sham-operated (11)	9.65 ± 0.46	
Occlusion 60 min		
and recovery 1 hr (5)	10.05	8.90
and recovery 4 hr (10)	15.76*	10.20
and recovery 24 hr (6)	4.86§	7.57§

The sham-operated value represents the mean ± SEM for pooled samples from right and left cortices.
* Different from sham-operated with P<0.01; § P<0.05.

and phosphocreatine in the decapitated versus intact animals according to the formula: Δ~P = Δ(2ATP + ADP + Phosphocreatine). At one
hour of recovery, there were no significant differences from sham
(Table 2); at 24 hours, energy use was below normal in both cerebral
cortices of animals with stroke. After four hours of recovery, however, energy consumption was 50% higher on the occluded side of animals with stroke.

Generalized convulsions are a frequent manifestation of cerebral
ischemia in gerbils, and sometimes occur in human stroke (8). Because seizures increase cerebral energy metabolism, one might sus-
pect that seizures were responsible for the abnormally increased
metabolic activity observed at four hours. This does not appear to
be the case. When the data were computed for seizure-free animals
alone, cortical energy consumption was still significantly elevated
on the occluded side after four hours of recovery. Moreover, cerebral glucose consumption, as assessed autoradiographically after the
administration of [1-^{14}C]2-deoxyglucose, was also increased four
hours after ischemia, despite pretreatment of the animals with
Dilantin (25 mg/kg) to control seizure activity. Gerbils that had
evidence of stroke during one hour of right common carotid artery
occlusion received [1-^{14}C]2-deoxyglucose four hours after release
of the carotid clip. Autoradiographs of coronal brain sections
showed increased glucose utilization in the ipsilateral cortex,
hippocampus, and thalamus, findings consistent with increased energy
demands in the damaged hemisphere.

How is this additional energy being used? Whittam (9) has estimated from in vitro studies that ion pumping accounts for about

40% of the cerebral oxidative energy consumption; the percentage is almost certainly higher for the cerebral cortex in vivo. Increased ion translocation in association with the development of post-ische-mic cerebral edema would further increase energy demands. We believe that the hypermetabolism observed at 4 hours after ischemia reflects the energy requirements for cell repair superimposed upon the energy needed for recovering neurological function. Since anesthetics de-press cerebral energy consumption, the protection of the ischemic brain by barbiturates may be mediated by selective suppression of neuronal excitability, thereby channeling more of the available energy toward repair of cellular damage.

These observations of post-ischemic hypermetabolism may be rele-vant in connection with Dr. Siesjö's comments regarding the adverse effects of excessive acidosis on cellular metabolism and structure. Swanson (10) showed that guinea pig cerebral cortex incubated in vitro under mildly acidic conditions (pH 6.5) responded normally to electrical stimulation by gaining Na^+ and losing K^+, by utilizing high-energy phosphates, and by increasing respiration. However, after termination of the stimulus, the recovery of cations and acid-soluble phosphates was less complete in acidotic slices than in con-trols at pH 7.5. Recent studies by Myers (11) provide indirect evi-dence that acidosis is harmful to the ischemic brain. He found that pretreatment of monkeys with glucose markedly increased their sus-ceptibility to brain damage during 14 minutes of circulatory arrest. Glucose treatment would be expected to lead to a greater accumulation of lactic acid in brain during ischemia and perhaps to prolong brain activity by increasing energy stores.

It thus appears that whereas acidosis is harmful to the ischemic brain, acidosis plus increased metabolic/functional demands may be devastating.

1.   Levy, D.E. and Duffy, T.E. (1977) J. Neurochem., in press.
2.   Lowry, O.H. and Passonneau, J.V. (1972) A Flexible System of Enzymatic Analysis, Academic Press, New York.
3.   Levine, S. and Payan, H. (1966) Exp. Neurol. 45, 503-508.
4.   Levy, D.E., Brierley, J.B., and Plum, F. (1975) J. Neurol. Neurosurg. Psychiat. 38, 1197-1205.
5.   Atkinson, D.E. and Walton, G.M. (1967) J. Biol. Chem. 242, 3239-3241.
6.   Purich, D.E. and Fromm, H.J. (1973) J. Biol. Chem. 248, 461-466.
7.   Lowry, O.H., Passonneau, J.V., Hasselberger, F.X., and Schulz, D.W. (1964) J. Biol. Chem. 239, 18-30.
8.   Louis, S. and McDowell, F. (1967) Arch. Neurol. 17, 414-418.
9.   Whittam, R. (1962) Biochem. J. 7, 260-263.
10. Swanson, P.D. (1969) Arch. Neurol. 20, 653-663.
11. Myers, R.E. (1976) Neurology 26, 345.

REGIONAL CHANGES IN METABOLISM IN HYPOXIA-ISCHEMIA

F.A. Welsh, M.J. O'Connor, W. Rieder, and V.R. Marcy

Division of Neurosurgery, Univ. of Penna.

Philadelphia, Pennsylvania 19104

The purpose of this study is to describe regional metabolic changes following an episode of cerebral ischemia in the cat. Regional characterization of metabolic derangements is imperative because it is unlikely that cerebral blood flow is uniformly reduced in most hypoxic-ischemic episodes.[1, 2, 3] Furthermore, neurons in discrete anatomic regions such as hippocampus or arterial border zones[4] are selectively vulnerable to hypoxia-ischemia. Consequently, we have investigated regional alterations of cerebral metabolites in a model of incomplete ischemia (oligemia).

Three methods of regional metabolic analysis have been used to demonstrate an extremely heterogeneous response to cerebral oligemia. First, dissection of small samples from various brain regions revealed that alterations in high energy phosphates and lactate were greatest in white matter following mild cerebral oligemia. Second, NADH fluorescence from frozen brain slices demonstrated a patchy increase in NADH indicating micro-heterogeneity. These fluorescent patches were most striking in cortex and were characterized by alternating bands of normal and increased NADH. Third, in vivo, continuous measurement on NADH fluorescence from the cortical surface indicated that ischemic metabolic alterations were heterogeneous with respect to time as well as space.

METHODS

Cats of either sex, 2-4 kg, were anesthetized with 20 mg/kg ketamine (Ketalar[R], Parke-Davis), paralyzed with 5 mg/kg/hr gallamine (Flaxedil[R], Davis and Geck), and ventilated with 25% O_2 and 75% N_2O using a Harvard respirator. End-tidal CO_2 was maintained at 4.0% by adjusting respiratory rate and volume.

Cerebral oligemia was induced with bilateral occlusion of the common carotid arteries and reduction of systemic arterial pressure. Mean arterial pressure was reduced by blood withdrawal from a femoral arterial cannula. In 2 groups of animals (n = 3) arterial pressure was held at 50 ± 2 torr and 60 ± 2 torr for 20 minutes. Since the results at the 2 arterial pressures were the same, they have been lumped into one group of 6 animals. After 20 minutes of 50 or 60 torr the brain was frozen in situ by direct application of liquid nitrogen to the skull of the animal. At least 10 minutes freezing was allowed, during which time arterial pressure was held constant and ventilation was continued. A pre-cooled vibrating saw was used to remove 2-3 coronal brain slices 1 cm in thickness for regional metabolic analysis.

The frozen brain slices were first examined for the distribution of NADH fluorescence. To fluoresce tissue NADH, the slices at -196° were illuminated with a 200 watt mercury arc lamp through Corning filter #5840, which transmits 366 nm excitation light. 450nm fluorescence was recorded photographically on Polaroid high contrast film (type 51) through Corning filters #3389 and 5562. In addition, reflected 366 nm light was photographed through a second 5840 filter.

To measure metabolite levels in various brain regions, 5 mg samples were dissected at -30° from the outer 2 mm of the lateral, medial, and cingulate gyri; from subcortical white matter; and from basal ganglia. A total of 10 specimens were taken from each of the 6 animals. The samples were weighed and extracted, the extracts being analyzed for ATP, phosphocreatine (PCr), lactate (Lac), and NADH by fluorometric enzymatic methods.[3, 5]

In one additional animal, in which NADH was monitored in vivo, arterial pressure was lowered to 60 torr 30 minutes after carotid clamping. 450 nm fluorescence and 366 nm reflectance were measured during the 20 minute period of oligemia from the exposed cortical surface with a television fluorometer as described by Schuette et al.[6] The fluorescent and reflectant images were stored on videotape, and the intensity of fluorescence and reflectance from several cortical regions was densitized by replaying the videotape.

CONTROL STUDIES FOR IN SITU FREEZING

Although Pontén et al.[7] have shown that in situ freezing adequately traps metabolite levels in rats and mice, similar control studies have not been carried out for larger animals such as cat. Therefore, a group of 4 control cats were studied to determine the efficacy of in situ freezing.

The upper photograph in Figure 1 shows the low temperature
NADH fluorescence from a coronal slice of a control cat. Also shown
are NADH reference standards (10 μM, 30 μM and 100 μM, right to left) to
which the intensity of tissue fluorescence may be compared. In the
lower photo is shown the same slice from which the reflected excitation light (366 nm) was recorded. The reflectance photograph clearly
delineates white matter from gray and shows some of the larger blood
vessels.

The gray matter 450 nm fluorescence (Figure 1, upper photo) was
much lower than that of white matter in all regions except the depths
of the cortical sulci. The bottom halves of the sulci fluoresced
more intensely than did the surfaces of the gyri. The blood supply
to the cortex within sulci is derived primarily from vessels penetra-
ting from the cortical surface. Since the freezing front begins at
the surface, it appears that the blood supply to the sulci is occluded
before the sulci themselves are frozen. The result is ischemic metabolic changes, reflected by an increase in NADH fluorescence.

Direct chemical analysis for NADH confirmed that the increase
in 450 nm fluorescence is accompanied by a rise in tissue NADH. Figure 2 gives the metabolite levels in samples dissected from the
slice pictured in Figure 1. ATP values ranged from 2.3 to 2.7 m-mole/
kg. Phosphocreatine averaged 6 m-mole/kg in all regions except the
surface cortical sulci, where it was 40% lower. Lactate was found to
be twice as high in the sulci as in other brain regions, and NADH was
4-fold higher. Thus, the metabolic differences seen in the sulci are
best explained by a period of artefactual ischemia during freezing.
Based on the extent of these changes and the rate of metabolic alteration in complete ischemia[8], the period of artefactual ischemia was
only 10 seconds in duration. Other regions such as hippocampus
(Figure 2; D_1, D_2) and midline cortex (Figure 2, C) showed neither
increased NADH fluorescence nor ischemic metabolic changes. Thus it
appears that the in situ freezing technique adequately preserves metabolite levels with a minimum of ischemic artefact in most brain regions.

RESULTS

A group of 6 cats were subjected to 20 minutes of cerebral
oligemia and samples were removed bilaterally from 5 brain regions
for determination of metabolites as described in the methods. Figure
3 illustrates the values found for each metabolite in the various
regions as compared to values from the same region in the control
animals. The greatest changes in lactate, phosphocreatine, and ATP
occured in the subcortical white matter rather than in cortex or basal
ganglia. White matter ATP and PCr were 30% and 90% reduced, and
lactate was 10 times the control values. In gray matter regions, ATP
was altered less than 10%, PCr reduced 20%, and lactate doubled in
cortex and quintupled in basal ganglia when compared to control.

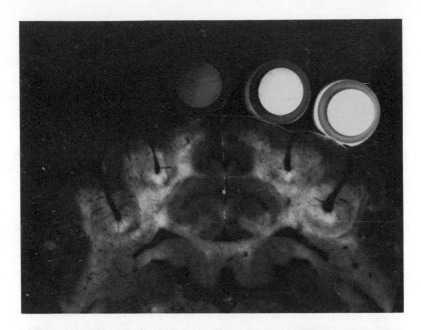

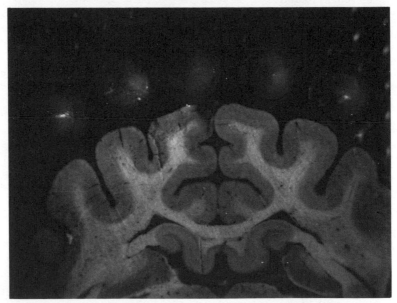

Figure 1

NADH Fluorescence (upper) and 366 nm Reflectance (lower)
from a Frozen Brain Slice of a Control Cat.

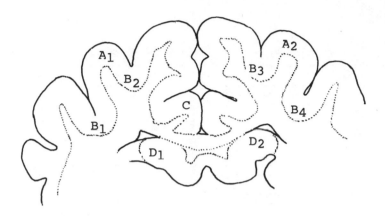

Control Regional Metabolite Values (m—mole/kg)

	ATP	PCr	Lac	NADH
A_1	2.5	6.1	1.4	.008
A_2	2.7	5.8	1.6	.008
B_1	2.3	3.3	3.1	.025
B_2	2.4	3.7	2.3	.030
B_3	2.3	4.4	1.9	.033
B_4	2.3	3.5	2.7	.031
C	2.6	6.0	1.5	.008
D_1	2.6	6.1	1.3	.016
D_2	2.6	5.7	1.5	.016

Figure 2

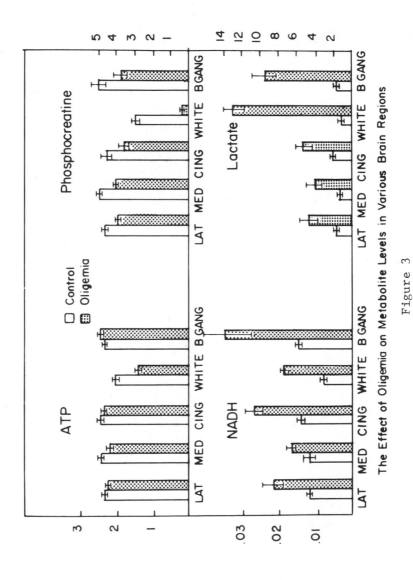

Figure 3

The Effect of Oligemia on Metabolite Levels in Various Brain Regions

NADH was elevated 100% in all but one region. The most important observation is that white matter was the only region to show severe ischemic metabolic changes with this degree and duration of cerebral oligemia.

    In one additional animal, the timecourse of changes of NADH during oligemia was measured from the cortical surface. In Figure 4 is shown the fluorescent traces from 3 adjacent 2 x 3 mm cortical regions. It can be seen that the fluorescence intensity increased steadily in all 3 spots during the 20 minute insult. In the top trace, this increase appeared to plateau at a level 50% above the pre-insult value. In the second trace, there was a steady rise during the first 18 minutes to a level 70% higher than the pre-insult fluor-escence intensity. At the 19th minute, however, there was a sudden further increase in intensity (+60% of the pre-insult level). The third trace exhibits a similar sudden rise, but the rise occurred at an earlier time. These relatively rapid increases in 450 nm fluor-escence occurred with no change in the intensity of 366 nm reflected light. Therefore, the fluorescent increases were not likely due to vascular artefact. In general, the rise in 366 nm reflectance over the 20 minute insult was no more than 10% of the resting level in all of the cortical spots densitized.

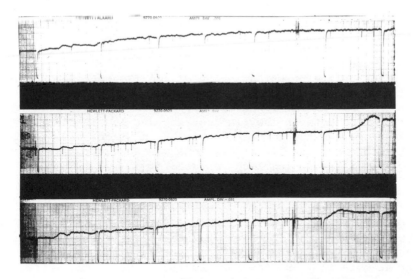

Figure 4

Effect of Oligemia on In Vivo NADH Fluorescence from
3 Cortical Regions

After 20 minutes of oligemia to the animal described above, the brain was frozen and slices prepared for examination of low temperature NADH fluorescence. Figure 5 shows the 450 nm fluorescence and 366 nm reflectance from one of the coronal slices. In this figure, the right hemisphere is on the left side of the pictures. In the right hemisphere a variety of fluorescent patterns can be distinguished. There were 2 regions with low intensity: the tip of the right cingulate gyrus (near the midline), and the tip of the right suprasylvian gyrus. Most of the right surface cortex, however, was characterized by patches or bands of fluorescence which were approximately 0.3 mm in width and appeared to radiate from the stalk of each gyrus. Other cortical regions were more diffusely fluorescent, including much of the left hemisphere.

Figure 6 displays the metabolite values in various regions of the slice pictured in Figure 5. Two cortical regions with the lowest fluorescence contained .015 and .017 m-mole/kg of NADH, which is 50% greater than the values in control animals (Figures 2 and 3). Samples taken from cortical regions with patchy fluorescence contained .023 an .030 m-mole/kg, while samples from uniformly fluorescent regions contained .034 and .036 m-mole/kg of NADH. Higher NADH values were present throughout the left hemisphere.

ATP levels in gray matter were only 10-30% reduced on the right; however, in the left hemisphere the levels were less than 50% of control in all but one sample. PCr values ranged between 20 and 100% of control levels in the right cortex. The 2 samples with highest PCr were from regions of low 450 nm fluorescence, and the lowest PCr level were found in regions where fluorescence was uniformly increased. Lactates were 3-10 fold increased in the right hemisphere and 20-30 fold increased in the left. The lowest lactate value was found in the right cingulate gyrus, a region of low fluorescence. However, the other low-fluorescent area had a value of 10 m-mole/kg, while a lactate of 4 m-mole/kg was found in a region of high fluorescence. Thus, the correlation between low fluorescence and low lactate was not without exception. In the cortex of this brain slice, therefore, a spectrum of ischemic metabolic alterations was seen; from near exhaustion ATP, to only a 3-fold increase in lactate.

DISCUSSION

The results of frozen brain fluorescence and metabolite levels, and the results of in vivo fluorescence, clearly illustrate the heterogeneous response of the brain to oligemia. This heterogeneity was evident at more than one anatomic level. Subcortical white matter was severely affected by an insult which caused rather limited changes in cortex or basal ganglia (Figure 3). When alterations in cortex did occur, they were patchy in appearance, as evidenced from the distribution of NADH fluorescence (Figure 5). Some regions of cortex had a

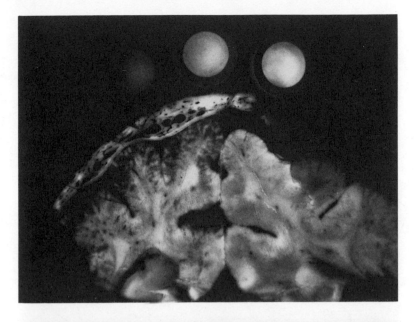

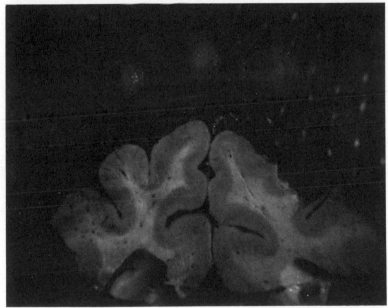

Figure 5

Effect of Oligemia on NADH Fluorescence (upper)
and 366 nm Reflectance (lower)

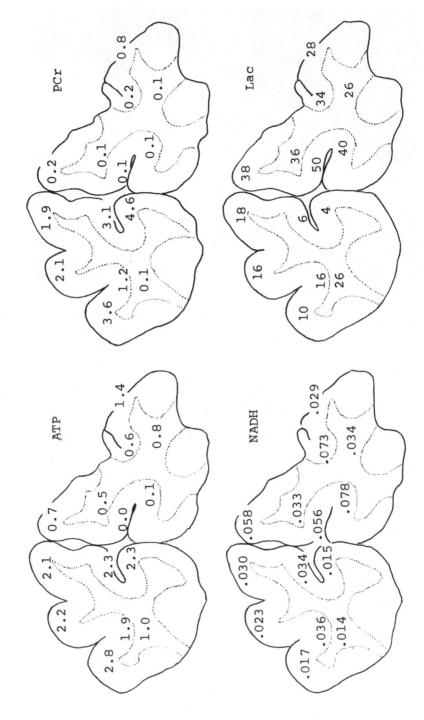

Figure 6. Effect of Oligemia on Regional Metabolite Values (m-mole/kg)

striped appearance, the stripes consisting of alternating bands of normal and increased NADH. The smallest ischemic patches seen on the NADH photographs were less than 100μ in width. Since the inter-capillary distance in cat cortex is 60μ,[9] the observed heterogeneity may extend down to the level of the capillary.

The vulnerability of the white matter was the most suprising finding of this study. Because the metabolic rate of gray matter has been estimated to be twice that of white[10], it has been assumed by many that gray matter suffers first when blood flow is compromised. In the normoxic animal, flow in white matter is much lower than in gray[11], which is consistent with the low metabolic demands. It is possible, however, that when global blood flow is reduced by a decrease in perfusion pressure, blood flow falls proportionally more in white than in gray matter. Thus, in spite of the intrinsically low metabolic rate of white matter, blood flow falls below that required to meet energy demands.

The appearance of ischemic patches in cortex during oligemia has, to our knowledge, not been described before. Micro-heterogeneity of ionic activities[12] has been described, and our data are consistent with those findings. There are 2 possible causes for this heterogeneity. Inhomogeneous flow reduction is the most probable cause. However, homogeneous flow reduction coupled with a heterogeneous metabolic rate would have the same effect and has not yet been ruled out.

REFERENCES

1. Siesjö BK, Johannsson H, Ljunggren B, Norberg K: Brain Dysfunction in Cerebral Hypoxia and Ischemia. Res. Publ. Assoc. Nerve Ment. Dis. 53:75-112, 1974.

2. Eklöf B, Siesjö BK: Cerebral Blood Flow in Ischemia Caused by Carotid Artery Ligation in the Rat. Acta Physiol. Scand. 87:69-77, 2973.

3. Welsh FA, Durity F, Langfitt TW: The Appearance of Regional Variation in Metabolism at a Critical Level of Diffuse Cerebral Oligemia. Submitted to J. Neurochem. 1976.

4. Lindenberg R: Patterns of CNS Vulnerability in Acute Hypoxaemia, including Anaesthesia Accidents. In Schade JP, McMenemey WH (Editors): Selective Vulnerability of the Brain in Hypoxaemia. Philadelphia, FA Davis Pulbishing Company, 1963, pp 189-209.

5. Lowry OH, Passonneau JV: A Flexible System of Enzymatic Analysis. New York, Academic Press, 1972.

6. Schuette WH, Whitehouse, WC, Lewis DV, O'Connor, M, van Buren
    JM: A Television Fluorometer for Monitoring Oxidative Metab-
    olism in Intact Tissue. Med. Instrum. 8:331-333, 1974.

7. Pontén U, Ratcheson RA, Salford LG, Siesjö BK: Optimal Freezing
    Conditions for Cerebral Metabolites in Rats. J. Neurochem. 21:
    1127-1138, 1973.

8. Lowry OH, Passonneau JV, Hasselberger FX, Schulz DW: Effect
    of Ischemia on Known Substrates and Cofactors of the Glycolytic
    Pathway in Brain. J. Biol. Chem. 239:18-30, 1964

9. Lierse W: Die Kapillarastände in verschiedenen Hirnregionen
    der Katze. Z. Zellforsch. 54:199-206, 1961.

10. McIlwain H: Biochemistry and the Central Nervous System.
    Boston; Little, Brown and Company, Third Edition, 1966, p 55.

11. Reivich M: Blood Flow Metabolism Couple in Brain. Res. Publ.
    Assoc. Nerve Ment. Dis. 53:125-139, 1974.

12. Silver IA: Changes in pO_2 and Ion Fluxes in Cerebral Hypoxia-
    ischemia. These Proceedings.

CYCLIC NUCLEOTIDE LEVELS IN THE GERBIL CEREBRAL CORTEX, CEREBELLUM AND SPINAL CORD FOLLOWING BILATERAL ISCHEMIA

W.D. Lust, M. Kobayashi, B. B. Mrsulja, A. Wheaton, and
J.V. Passonneau
Laboratory of Neurochemistry and Laboratory of Neuro-
pathology and Neuroanatomical Sciences, NINCDS, NIH
Bethesda, Maryland   20014,   U.S.A.

It is well established that the levels of cyclic nucleotides
are markedly affected by an ischemic episode. Since the first
demonstration by Breckenridge that cyclic AMP increased in the
decapitated mouse brain[1], a number of laboratories have described
the rapid large accumulation of cyclic AMP in various ischemic
regions of the brain[2-3]. Using the gerbil model of unilateral
ischemia first described by Levine and Payan[4], we have previously
shown that the levels of cyclic AMP increased 10-fold in the ischemic
cerebral cortex, while those of cyclic GMP decreased to 50 percent
of control[5]. The cyclic nucleotides were also determined during
the recovery period following an ischemic episode[6]. The cyclic AMP
levels at 5 min of recirculation after either 1 or 3 hours of
unilateral ischemia exhibited an additional increase to a level
20-fold greater than control. During the recovery period, cyclic
GMP increased from the depressed levels during ischemia to a
concentration more than 2-fold greater than control. Since it is
increasingly evident that the cyclic nucleotides play a role in
neuronal excitability[7-8], these ischemia-induced changes in cyclic
nucleotides may reflect a substantial perturbation in the electrical
excitability of the brain. If such a change in neuronal activity
does occur in ischemic regions of the brain, it would appear likely
that the electrical input through neuronal pathways to non-ischemic
areas of the central nervous system would be affected by these
alterations.

To evaluate the effects of the ischemic cerebral cortex on
other regions of the brain, we measured the cyclic nucleotides in
the cerebellum and the spinal cord, areas whose circulation is
supposedly maintained after carotid artery occlusion. There is a

low incidence of successful unilateral ischemia in gerbils (40%) and
the evaluation of neurological symptoms during short ischemic periods
is difficult. Consequently both common carotid arteries were ligated
to produce bilateral ischemia without ambiguity. All the bilaterally
occluded animals exhibited both the biochemical changes characteristi
of ischemia in the cerebral cortex and the positive neurological
signs of ischemia. The levels of ATP and P-creatine were monitored
and provided evidence that the energy status in both cerebellum and
spinal cord was not severely compromised by either the surgical
procedures or the ischemic episode. While the cyclic nucleotide
changes were much greater in the cerebral cortex, there were
significant alterations in both the spinal cord and cerebellum.

MATERIALS AND METHODS

Mongolian gerbils (Meriones unguiculatus) from Chickline Co.
(Vineland, New Jersey) were deprived of food for 24 hours prior to
experimentation. The gerbils weighing 50-60 g were anesthetized
with 35 mg/kg IP of sodium pentobarbital and the common carotid
arteries were exposed and looped with surgical suture. Approximately
3 hours later when the gerbils had recovered from the anesthesia,
both arteries were occluded with aneurysm clips. The animals were
then frozen in liquid nitrogen at 1,5 and 20 min of occlusion or
after 1, 5 and 30 min of recirculation following the 3 different
periods of ischemia. The tissues were removed in a cryostat maintained at -20°C, extracted with methanol-HCl, followed by precipita-
tion of the protein with 0.3 N perchloric acid containing 1 mM EGTA
and then centrifuged[9]. The supernatant was neutralized with potassiu
bicarbonate and the protein pellet was solubilized in 1 ml of 1 N
NaOH. ATP and P-creatine were analyzed enzymically according to the
fluorometric procedures of Lowry and Passonneau[10]. Cyclic nucleotide
were measured by radioimmunoassay according to the method of Steiner[1]
Proteins were determined by the method of Lowry et al.[12]. Statistics
were performed using the Student t-test.

RESULTS

Neurological Symptoms following Bilateral Ischemia
The gerbils exhibited changes in respiration almost immediately
after bilateral occlusion and within 15 sec assumed a posture
characterized by dorsal flexion of the head and neck with the front
legs extended forward. The behavioral activity of the animals
subsequently increased as reflected by periods of vertical jumping.
These intermittent attacks lasted from 10 to 30 sec and were
interspersed between periods of behavioral quiescence. Other
neurological signs included ptosis of the eyes, positive response to
painful stimuli and an intact righting reflex. Seizures were
frequently observed in the 20 min ischemic gerbils but only rarely
in the 1 and 5 min groups. The occurrence of convulsions in the 20
min ischemic group persisted during the post-ischemic period.

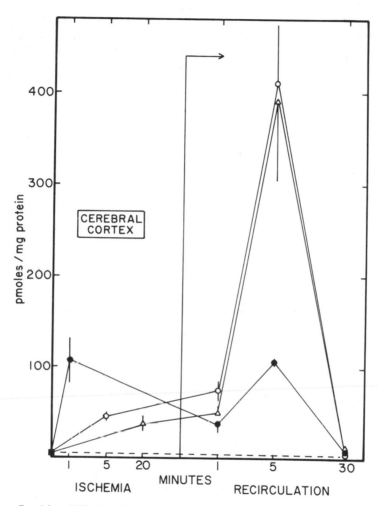

Fig. 1. Cyclic AMP in the cerebral cortex during and after bilateral
ischemia. The experiments were performed as described in the
Materials and Methods. The symbols represent the cortical levels
of cyclic AMP in sham-operated controls, ■ ; 1 min of ischemia, ● ;
5 min of ischemia, O ; and 20 min of ischemia, Δ . The vertical line
with an arrow separates the values during ischemia (left) and during
recirculation (right). The cyclic AMP concentration in sham-operated
controls (designated by dashed line) was 4.68 + 0.37 pmoles/mg protein.
Each point represents the mean of 5 determinations and the vertical
lines the SEM. A total of 65 gerbils were used.

Cyclic Nucleotides in the Ischemic Cerebral Cortex

The levels of ATP (27.7 nmole/mg protein) and P-creatine (42.5 nmole/mg protein) in the cerebral cortex both fell to less than 10 percent of control within 5 min of ischemia, confirming the ischemic insult. During recirculation, the rate of restoration of these metabolites was dependent upon the duration of the ischemia. By 30 min of recirculation, both metabolites were essentially back to control level (data not shown).

The changes in cyclic AMP during and after bilateral ischemia are illustrated in Fig. 1. The levels in cyclic AMP increased 23-, 10- and 8-fold after 1, 5 and 20 min of ischemia, respectively. In the 1 min ischemic group, cyclic AMP then fell to a level 8-fold greater than control at 1 min of recirculation and subsequently returned to 23-fold greater than control at 5 min of recirculation. The changes in cyclic AMP were similar in the 5 and 20 min ischemic groups. At 5 min of recirculation, the cyclic AMP increased by over

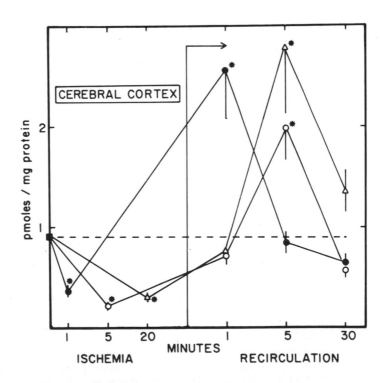

Fig. 2. Cyclic GMP in the cerebral cortex during and after ischemia. For explanation of symbols and procedures, see Fig. 1. The control concentration of cortical cyclic GMP was 0.90 $\pm$ 0.17 pmole/mg protein. * p<0.05.

80-fold in both groups. In all 3 groups, the cyclic AMP was back to control by 30 min of post-ischemia. The changes in cyclic AMP following bilateral ischemia were similar to those previously observed after unilateral ischemia[5-6]. In both cases, the changes in cyclic AMP during recirculation were large, but of relatively short duration.

In contrast, cyclic GMP levels decreased to less than 40 percent of control after 1, 5 and 20 min of bilateral ischemia (Fig. 2). At 1 min of post-ischemia, the cyclic GMP increased to 284 percent of control in the 1 min ischemic group, while those in the other 2 groups were not significantly different from control. At 5 min of recirculation, the cyclic GMP levels in the 1 min group returned to control and those in the 5 and 20 min groups increased more than 2-fold. The changes induced by ischemia in both cyclic AMP and cyclic GMP concentrations indicate that temporally and quantitatively there are marked differences in the effect of 1 min versus 5 or 20 min of ischemia.

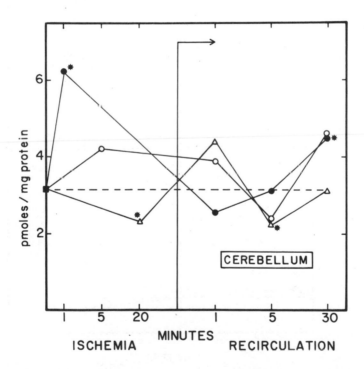

Fig. 3. Cerebellar cyclic AMP during and after bilateral ischemia. For explanation of symbols and procedures, see Fig. 1. The control concentration of cerebellar cyclic AMP was 3.27 ± 0.29 pmole/mg protein. * p<0.05.

Cerebellar Cyclic Nucleotides during and after Carotid Artery Occlusion

ATP (22.2 nmole/mg protein) and P-creatine (42.8 nmole/mg protein) levels were essentially unchanged during and after the ischemic episodes (data not shown). The levels of cerebellar cyclic AMP were not altered as greatly as in the cerebral cortex (Fig. 3). However, significant changes ($p < 0.05$) occurred at 1 and 20 min of ischemia, at 5 min of recirculation after 20 min of ischemia and at min of recirculation after 1 min of ischemia.

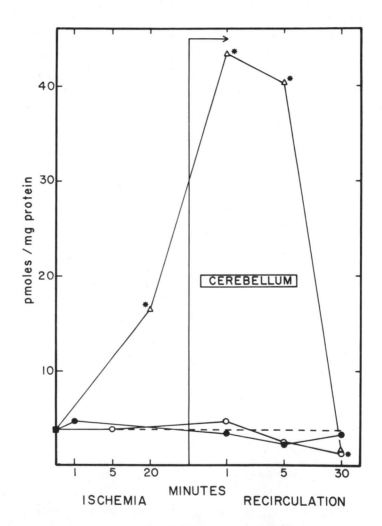

Fig. 4. Cerebellar cyclic GMP during and after bilateral ischemia. For explanation of symbols and procedures, see Fig. 1. The control level of cerebellar cyclic GMP was 3.93 $\pm$ 1.09 pmole/mg protein.

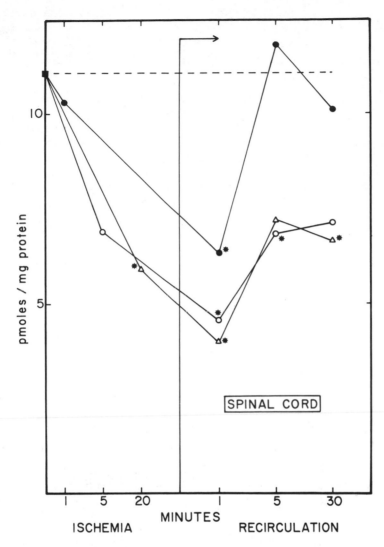

Fig. 5. Cyclic AMP in the spinal cord during and after bilateral
ischemia. For explanation of symbols and procedures, see Fig. 1. The
mean concentration of cyclic AMP in the spinal cord from sham-operated
control was 11.08 ± 1.41 pmole/mg protein. $*$ $p < 0.05$.

     The levels of cyclic GMP in the cerebellum were not changed
during or after ischemia in the 1 and 5 min ischemic groups (Fig. 4).
After 20 min of ischemia, cyclic GMP increased 4-fold and increased
further to 10-fold greater than control after 1 and 5 min of the post-
ischemic period. By 30 min of recovery, the cyclic GMP levels were
less than those of control in all 3 groups. The cyclic GMP response

in the cerebellum also appears to be dependent on the duration of the ischemic insult.

Cyclic Nucleotides in the Spinal Cord during and after Carotid Artery Occlusion

As was observed in the cerebellum, the levels of ATP (17.5 nmole/mg protein) and P-creatine (29.3 nmole/mg protein) were not changed in the spinal cord during and after the occlusion of the common carotid arteries (data not shown). The levels of cyclic AMP decreased during 1, 5 and 20 min of occlusion (Fig. 5). After 1 min of recirculation, the cyclic AMP decreased further in all 3 groups. Cyclic GMP levels were not significantly different from those of control either during or after occlusion (Fig. 6).

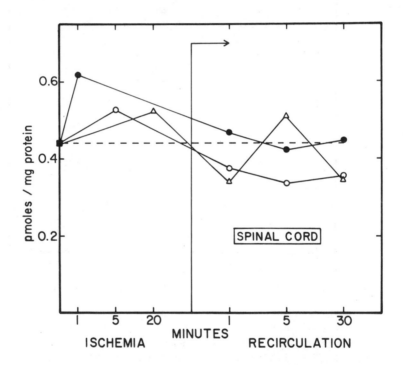

Fig. 6. Cyclic GMP in the spinal cord during and after bilateral ischemia. For details, see Fig. 1. The control level of cyclic GMP in the spinal cord was 0.51 ± 0.06 pmole/mg protein.

DISCUSSION

The changes in the cyclic nucleotides of the cerebral cortex both during and after an ischemic episode may reflect alterations in the functional state of the affected region. The changes in the cyclic nucleotides of the cerebellum and spinal cord during cortical ischemia could be a response to the diminished output from the cerebral cortex; subsequently, in the post-ischemic interval, the changes may reflect the complex restoration of excitability in the cortex. Whether these changes in the non-ischemic regions are neuronally mediated is not immediately obvious. Extra-neural factors such as the integrity of the circulation should be considered. However, several lines of evidence would argue against such a possibility. First, the high-energy phosphate metabolites in both spinal cord and cerebellum were as high if not higher in the experimental gerbils than in the sham-operated controls. When compared to the more than 90 percent depletion of these metabolites in the cerebral cortex, the effect of carotid occlusion on the spinal cord and cerebellum appeared to be negligible. Secondly, the changes in cyclic nucleotides observed in the non-ischemic regions were considerably different from those in the cerebral cortex. The 10-fold increase in cerebellar cyclic GMP and the fall in cyclic AMP in the spinal cord are qualitatively different from events which occurred in the cerebral cortex. While these arguments do not exclude the possibility of extra-neural factors being involved, it does provide indirect evidence that the cause of these changes in the cerebellum and spinal cord is not due to a direct ischemic insult.

The effects on the cerebellum and spinal cord are more subtle than those in the cortex and probably express the loss of cortical influence during ischemia. Support for this view comes from the electrophysiological studies of Stone et al.[7] and Bloom et al.[8]. These investigators have demonstrated that iontophoretically applied cyclic AMP inhibits excitability in the Purkinje cells of the cerebellum and the pyramidal tract neurons of the cerebral cortex; cyclic GMP under similar conditions enhanced the excitability of the pyramidal tract neurons in the cerebral cortex. With respect to cellular excitability, if cyclic AMP is inhibitory and cyclic GMP excitatory, the altered levels of cortical cyclic nucleotides during ischemia would be consistent with a quiescent state. In fact, it is well-established that there is a rapid loss of recordable electrical activity following the onset of ischemia[13-14].

Upon recirculation, both cortical cyclic nucleotides increase to levels above those observed in the cerebral cortex of control gerbils. The elevated levels of cyclic GMP would indicate a hyperactive condition; however, the effect of cyclic GMP might be offset by the 80-fold increase in cyclic AMP. It is interesting to note that the levels of GABA, a putative inhibitory neurotransmitter, are also elevated almost 3-fold during the post-ischemic period (W. D. Lust, unpublished observation).

Further explanations for the changes of cyclic nucleotides in non-ischemic regions come from pharmacological studies on cyclic nucleotides in vivo. CNS depressants and anticonvulsants decrease cerebellar levels of cyclic GMP, whereas convulsants or CNS stimulant increase cyclic GMP levels in both cerebellum and cerebral cortex[17-2] Based on this pharmacological information, the elevated levels of cyclic GMP in the cerebellum in the 20 min ischemia group would suggest that these animals would be more prone to seizures than the other animals. In fact, seizures were only observed in this group of gerbils.

A relationship between cyclic AMP and neuronal activity or excitability is not as apparent, since this cyclic nucleotide appears to be unresponsive to pharmacological manipulation. However, cyclic AMP does increase both in mouse cerebellum and cerebral cortex following maximal electroshock[20,22]. Compared to the persistent large increase in cortical cyclic AMP, the increase of cyclic AMP in the cerebellum is small and of a short duration. Prolonged elevation of cyclic AMP in the cerebellum would tend to reduce its inhibitory output and allow the convulsion to persist. The relatively small fluctuations in cyclic AMP levels suggest that the inhibitory cerebellar influence would be unaffected by the occlusion. However, the greatly increased levels of cyclic GMP favor a abnormal output in the 20 min ischemic group.

There is a paucity of information on the cyclic nucleotides in the spinal cord. This is perhaps the first demonstration of a significant decrease in cyclic AMP in neural tissue. The explanation of these changes is not clear; perhaps the decrease of cyclic AMP during and after the ischemic episode reflects a decreased inhibitory influence.

In summary, there are substantial changes in cyclic nucleotides in the ischemic cerebral cortex. Secondary to these changes, there are changes in the cyclic nucleotides in the cerebellum and spinal cord, areas presumably not made ischemic by the common carotid occlusion. These changes during and after an ischemic episode are qualitatively different with increasing periods of ischemia.

REFERENCES

1   Breckenridge, B. McL., The measurement of cyclic adenylate in tissues, Proc. Nat. Acad. Sci., U.S.A., 52 (1964) 1580-1586.
2   Schmidt, M. J., Schmidt, D. E., and Robison, G. A., Cyclic AMP in the rat brain: microwave irradiation as a means of tissue fixation. In Greengard, P, Paoletti, R., and Robison, G. A. (Editors): Advances in Cyclic Nucleotide Research, Raven Press, New York, 1972, pp 425-434.
3   Kimura, H., Thomas, E., and Murad, F., Effects of decapitation, ether and pentobarbital on guanosine 3',5'-phosphate and adenosine 3',5'-phosphate levels in rat tissues, Biochim. Biophys. Acta, 343 (1974) 519-528.
4   Levine, S., and Payan, H., Effects of ischemia and other procedures on the brain and retina of the gerbil (Meriones unguiculatus), Expl. Neurol., 16 (1966) 255-262.
5   Lust, W. D., Mrsulja, B. B., Mrsulja, B. J., Passonneau, J. V., and Klatzo, I., Putative neurotransmitters and cyclic nucleotides in prolonged ischemia of the cerebral cortex, Brain Res., 98 (1975) 394-399.
6   Mrsulja, B. B., Lust, W. D., Mrsulja, B. J., Passonneau, J. V., and Klatzo, I., Post-ischemic changes in certain metabolites following prolonged ischemia in the gerbil cerebral cortex, J. Neurochem., 26 (1976) 1099-1103.
7   Stone, T. W., Taylor, D. A., and Bloom, F. E., Cyclic AMP and cyclic GMP may mediate opposite neuronal responses in the rat cerebral cortex, Science, 187 (1975) 845-847.
8   Bloom, F. E., Siggins, G. R., Hoffer, B. J., Segal, M., and Oliver, A. P., Cyclic nucleotides in the central synaptic actions of catecholamines. In Drummond, G. I., Greengard, P., and Robison, G. A. (Editors): Advances in Cyclic Nucleotide Research, Raven Press, New York, 1975, vol 5, pp 603-618.
9   Nelson, S. R., Schulz, D. W., Passonneau, J. V., and Lowry, O. H., Control of glycogen levels in brain, J. Neurochem., 15 (1968) 1271-1279.
10 Lowry, O. H., and Passonneau, J. V., In a Flexible System of Enzymatic Analysis, Academic Press, New York, 1972, pp 151-156.
11 Steiner, A. L., Wehmann, R. E., Parker, C. W., and Kipnis, D. M., Radioimmunoassay for the measurement of cyclic nucleotides. In Greengard, P., and Robison, G. A. (Editors): Advances in Cyclic Nucleotide Research, Raven Press, New York, 1972, vol 2, pp 51-61.
12 Lowry, O. H., Rosebrough, N. J., Farr, A. L., and Randall, R. L., Protein measurement with the folin phenol reagent, J. Biol. Chem., 193 (1951) 265-275.
13 Hossmann, K.-A., and Sato, K., Effect of ischemia on the function of the sensorimotor cortex in cat, Electroenceph. Clin. Neurophysiol., 30 (1971) 535-545.
14 Swaab, D. F., and Boer, K., The presence of biologically labile compounds during ischemia and their relationship to the EEG in rat cerebral cortex and hypothalamus, J. Neurochem., 19 (1972)

2843-2853.

15 Ferrendelli, J. A., Steiner, A. L., McDougal, D. B., and
    Kipnis, D. M., The effect of oxotremorine and atropine on cGMP
    and cAMP levels in mouse cerebral cortex and cerebellum, Biochem.
    Biophys. Res. Commun., 41 (1970) 1061-1067.

16 Ferrendelli, J. A., Kinscherf, D. A., and Kipnis, D. M., Effects
    of amphetamine, chlorpromazine and reserpine on cyclic GMP and
    cyclic AMP levels in mouse cerebellum, Biochem. Biophys. Res.
    Commun., 46 (1972) 2114-2120.

17 Lust, W. D., and Passonneau, J. V., Influence of certain drugs on
    cyclic nucleotide levels in mouse brain following electroconvul-
    sive shock, Trans. Am. Soc. Neurochem., 4 (Abstr.) (1973) 115.

18 Mao, C. C., Guidotti, A., and Costa, E., Evidence for an involve-
    ment of GABA in the mediation of the cerebellar cyclic GMP
    decrease and the anticonvulsant action of diazepam, Naunyn-
    Schmiedeberg's Arch. Pharmacol., 289 (1975) 369-378.

19 Lust, W. D., Kupferberg, H. J., Passonneau, J. V., and
    Penry, J. K., On the mechanism of action of sodium valproate:
    the relationship of GABA and cyclic GMP levels to anticonvulsant
    activity. In Legg, N. J. (Editor): Clinical and Pharmacological
    Aspects of Sodium Valproate (Epilim) in the Treatment of
    Epilepsy. Tunbridge Wells, England: MCS Consultants, 1976, pp
    123-129.

20 Lust, W. D., Goldberg, N. D., and Passonneau, J. V., Cyclic
    nucleotides in murine brain: the temporal relationship of changes
    induced in adenosine 3',5'-monophosphate and guanosine 3',5'-
    monophosphate following maximal electroshock or decapitation.
    J. Neurochem., 26 (1976) 5-10.

21 Opmeer, F. A., Gumulka, S. W., Dinnendahl, V., and
    Schonhofer, P. S., Effects of stimulatory and depressant drugs
    on cyclic guanosine 3',5'-monophosphate and adenosine 3',5'-
    monophosphate levels in mouse brain, Naunyn-Schmiedeberg's
    Arch. Pharmacol., 292 (1976) 259-265.

22 Sattin, A., Increase in the content of adenosine 3',5'-
    monophosphate in mouse forebrain during seizures and prevention
    of the increase by methylxanthines, J. Neurochem., 18 (1971)
    1087-1096.

CHANGES IN PO_2 AND ION FLUXES IN CEREBRAL HYPOXIA-ISCHEMIA

Ian A. Silver

Department of Pathology, University of Bristol

The Medical School, Bristol BS8 1TD, England

INTRODUCTION

Brain hypoxia may be produced by a number of pathological conditions ranging from the hyperacute to slow progressive changes over weeks or even years but ultimately leads to shifts in ionic balance. Cellular responses to hypoxic situations vary markedly according to the rate of onset of the condition and if it is complicated by ischemia, metabolic blockade, anemia, circulating toxins, tissue edema or other factors. Another major consideration is the normal activity of the cells which have been rendered hypoxic, their physiological function and their anatomical arrangement, particularly in relation to the microvasculature.

One of the consequences of hypoxia which is an early and important event in all regions of the brain is a change in ionic balance between the intra- and extracellular compartments together probably with alterations between the various intra-cellular locations e.g. from mitochondrial to cytosolic space. A great deal of attention has been paid recently to potassium ion movements in the brain under physiological and seizure conditions [1,2,3,4] and during hypoxia [5,6,7,8].

Cerebral tissue hypoxia may develop in the following conditions:-

(1) Arterial hypoxemia which may be due to inadequate oxygen in the inspired air, to ineffective gaseous diffusion or circulatory perfusion in the lungs or which may be simulated by a deficiency in oxygen carrying capacity of the blood as in anemia or failure to 'unload' oxygen from oxyhemaglobin.

299

(2) Ischemia.   Inadequate blood flow not only leads to sub-
optimal oxygen and substrate delivery but also interferes with
removal of CO_2 and other metabolic products.   It may be sudden and
total as in occlusive embolism, thrombosis or severe vascular spasm;
slowly developing and incomplete as in viral endarteritis or severe
polycythemia, or rapidly progressing, widespread and multi-factorial
as in hypovolemic, septic or other forms of circulatory shock[9].

(3) Metabolic Blockade.   Aerobic metabolic pathways are susceptible
to blocking at many points and this may occur either independently
of, or in conjunction with, changes in blood flow or oxygen
availability.   The metabolic situation in 'blocked' cells is
effectively hypoxic e.g. in carbon monoxide intoxication or
spreading depression [10], whether or not the environment lacks O_2 and
this elicits ion movements which may be those of truly hypoxic cells
[11,12,13].   However in such circumstances the blood flow may or may
not change.   If it increases, in a reflex to compensate the apparent
cellular hypoxia, the tissue becomes hyperoxic; on the other hand,
the reduced metabolic activity may result in a reduction or
redirection of local flow.

Compensatory Mechanisms

(1) Tissue hypoxia leads directly or indirectly, to complex
adjustments of systemic and local circulation which tend to reduce
or eliminate the hypoxic zone.   Such adjustments may be brought
about or maintained at least to some extent by the ion fluxes
resulting from hypoxia.   Hydrogen and potassium ions and other
simple inorganic substances have been implicated in control of
local flow [14,15,16].   These regulatory mechanisms may be strictly
local or they may involve bulk transfer of blood flow from some
organ systems to others which is particularly the case when hypoxia
of an immediately vital organ such as the brain is involved.   Since
these responses are important in determining the nature and degree
of ion fluxes and the rate of accumulation or washout of ions in
hypoxic tissue spaces in addition to the multiple local factors now
recognised at least in potassium homeostasis [1], the increase in
cardiac output, vasoconstriction of peripheral and splanchnic areas
and raised blood pressure that are characteristic of the
sympathetico-adrenal response to hypoxia and asphyxia must be
considered.   The circulatory and other homeostatic mechanisms which
have evolved to protect the organism against environmental or
pathological changes may act to spare some organs the full rigors of
the insult while simultaneously exposing others to further
physiological deprivation.   In most acute situations the body's
reactions are such that some organs can be identified as being
treated as 'essential' while others become, at least temporarily,
'disposable'.   Because biological responses tend to be stereo-
typed and represent a compromise that has proved to be evolutionarily

successful, certain organs or groups of organs, particularly the skin and abdominal viscera may be treated as expendable in terms of blood supply, when the survival of the heart, lungs and brain has to be assured in hypoxic emergency.   While such responses are clearly of survival value in overcoming short term hypoxic episodes, they may actually contribute to the death of the organism in other, slightly more persistent pathological states such as hemorrhagic shock.

(2)   Chronic hypoxia, such as is found in populations at high altitude leads, via the renal and other unidentified erythropoietic mechanism, to increased bone marrow activity and polycythemia [17]. While this gives a greater oxygen capacity to the blood, it may lead to viscosity problems which ultimately reduce capillary flow and produce severe cerebral malfunction and death [18].

MATERIALS AND METHODS

Animals

Experiments on hypoxia were performed on white Wistar-derived rats, half-lop rabbits and cats.

Anesthesia

A variety of anesthetic agents was used which included pentobarbitone (Sagatal, May and Baker Ltd.), fentanyl citrate and fluoranisone (Hypnorm, Janssen S.A., Belgium) Urethane and α-chloralose.   For measurements during hypoxemia, the respiratory movements were paralyzed with gallamine triethiodide (Flaxedil, May and Baker Ltd., U.K.), the animals were respired with a Palmer pump (C.F. Palmer Ltd., London) and the expiratory CO$_2$ level monitored with a Beckman Infra-red CO$_2$ analyser.

Electrode Systems

Microelectrodes were constructed for the measurement of pH, K$^+$, Na$^+$ and Ca^{++} and for oxygen tension, hydrogen clearance and glucose concentration.   Some preliminary observations were made with a lactate sensitive microprobe.

Ion exchanger electrodes sensitive to K$^+$ and Ca^{++} were double or triple barrelled and constructed according to Zeuthen, Hiam and Silver [8] and derived from the designs of Walker [19] and Khuri, Agulian and Kalloghlian [20].   The all glass pH probes (Corning 0150) were either of the designs of Hinke [21] or Thomas [22,23] or were double barrelled, adapted from the method of Zeuthen [24].   All glass Na$^+$ sensitive microelectrodes were of the same designs as those used for pH measurement but with the appropriate sensing glass (Corning

NAS 11-18) [24,25].

Surface electrodes sensitive to K^+ were constructed from 20μm silicone rubber membrane (Siloprene 1000, Wacker, G.M.B.H., F.D.R.) incorporating 3% valinomycin [26] glued to the end of glass capillary tubing (O.D. 0.9 mm; I.D. 0.5 mm) with R.T.V. silicone rubber adhesive and filled with 0.5 M KCl.

Oxygen tension was measured with the platinum-iridium needle electrodes [27] or metal filled micropipettes [28] and glucose with a glucose oxidase coated platinum micro anode incorporating an oxygen supply [29]. Some attempts were made to identify lactate levels with a recessed gold-in-glass microelectrode in which the recess was filled with lactate dehydrogenase and NAD incorporated in agar gel and covered with Rhoplex (Rhom Hass, Philadelphia, Pa). Under favorable circumstances polarographic reduction of the NAD formed in the presence of excess lactate gave a current proportional to the lactate concentration. Such electrodes are as yet in an early stage of development but should prove useful in the study of hypoxic tissue where pyruvate concentrations are low.

Microhydrogen clearance electrodes for measurements of local blood flow were those of Lübbers and Baumgärtl [30] or Heidenreich et al [31]; alternatively the hydrogen generating and detecting system of Stosseck, Lübbers and Cottin [32] was used.

Cell membrane potentials and standing D.C. levels were monitored with the reference barrel of double barrelled electrodes or with a separate micropipette. Silver/silver chloride indifferent electrodes were used in all cases.

Hypoxia was produced (a) by giving the animals gas mixtures to breathe consisting of 10%, 5%, 3% and 0% oxygen in 5% CO_2 in nitrogen, (b) by producing local ischemia through arterial or venous occlusion, (c) by inducing hypovolemic shock; in the rabbit by bleeding to 50 mm Hg mean arterial pressure (M.A.P.) and in the rat by the bleeding to 30-35 mm Hg M.A.P.

RESULTS

(1) Arterial Hypoxia

Table 1 shows ion fluxes and PO_2 changes in response to hypoxemia in the brain. Hypoxemia was always complicated by increased blood flow to the brain, which occurred before there was a detectable change in local pH or pK, although the extent of this response was modified by anesthesia.

TABLE 1   ARTERIAL HYPOXIA (RAT)

Time	0	30 sec.	1 min.	5 min.	8 min.
PO_2 (Torr)	22 ± 12.5	3.8 ± 2.3	0	0	0
K^+ (mM)	3.0 ± 0.01	3.1 ± 0.04	3.15 ± 0.07	27.3 ± 1.3	49.3 ± 6.1
Na^+ (mM)	143 ± 8.0	142.3 ± 9.2	141.9 ± 9.0	50.3 ± 6.4	47.6 ± 4.3
Cl^- (mM)	127.3 ± 6.1	_____	128.7 ± 7.1	47.2 ± 5.1	45.3 ± 4.8
pH	7.39 ± 0.04	7.39 ± 0.04	7.30 ± 0.13	7.05 ± 0.21	6.73 ± 0.34

Extracellular PO_2, K^+ and pH during acute, severe hypoxia (N_2 5% CO_2 breathing) in brain cortex.

The regions most rapidly affected by acute arterial hypoxia were the cerebral cortex and hippocampus (Fig. 1).   With severe hypoxia, spontaneous respiration usually ceased in rats after 0.5 - 5 minutes but if artificial ventilation was maintained the circulation might survive for a further 3-5 minutes in young healthy adults.

Changes in extracellular ion activity were detectable within 15 sec. of the outset of severe arterial hypoxia and initially were often biphasic and of small extent despite major falls of PO_2 which

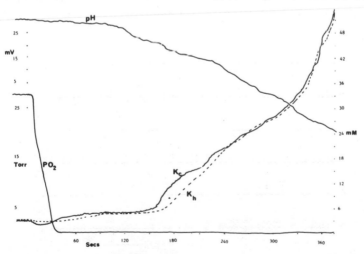

FIG. 1 Simultaneous records in acute hypoxaemia of extracellular potassium concentration in cortex (K_c) and hypothalamus (K_h) together with extracellular cortical pH and PO_2.   Note lag on hypothalamic trace.

occurred within 5 - 8 sec. together with increased blood flow.
Frequently there was an early fall in K^+ concentration of 0.5 mM
which accompanied hyperpolarization of neurones but this was
rapidly followed (by 30 sec.) by an increase of extracellular K^+
activity of 2-5 mV which seemed to be associated with uptake of
water by the brain cells, small falls in intracellular pH and
reduction of the extracellular space which could be detected
immediately by a rise in brain impedance [33] or subsequently from
electromicrographs.   After this small progressive rise which
lasted 2-4 minutes, a new phase of rapidly increasing extracellular
K^+ activity appeared which led to a 10 fold increase in K^+
concentration within a further 2-4 minutes.   This anoxic
depolarization phase was concurrent with a marked fall of intracellular pH and was irreversible once the extracellular K^+
concentration reached about 20 mM.   If no O_2 was provided, the
animal died and intra and extracellular levels of K^+, Cl^- and Na^+
rapidly equilibrated.

       In graded hypoxia, although 5% O_2 induced a generalized
sympathetic discharge, it did not lead to drastic changes in
extracellular K^+ levels in the CNS.   This was despite the fact
that electrical silence in the cortex although not in the
hypothalamus was usual at 5% O_2 in anesthetised animals (Fig. 2).
When O_2 in the inspired air was reduced to 3%, the brain was unable
to maintain normal membrane potentials in the cortical neurones
and there was a slowly accelerating rise in extracellular K^+ until
a critical point was reached (about 17-20 mM) when irreversible
changes appeared and even if O_2 was then supplied at higher
concentrations, many cells were incapable of recovering their
membrane polarization.

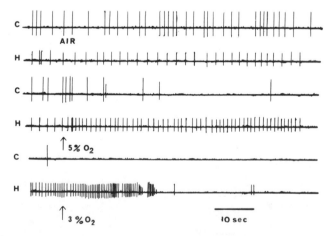

FIG. 2   Simultaneous records of unit activity in cortex (C) and
hypothalamus (H) during graded hypoxia.   Note electrical silence
in cortex with 5% O_2 (inspired) and stimulation of hypothalamic unit.

(2)   Acute Ischemia

Table 2 shows the ion fluxes produced in brain as a result of acute ischemia of a duration comparable to that of the acute hypoxia in Table 1.

TABLE 2   ACUTE ISCHEMIA (RAT)

Time	0	30 sec.	1 min.	4 min.	8 min.
PO$_2$ (Torr)	22 $\pm$12.5	2.1 $\pm$1.0	0	0	0
K$^+$ (mM)	3.0 $\pm$0.01	3.3 $\pm$0.1	4.6 $\pm$1.0	28.5$\pm$2.2	48.1$\pm$4.6
pH	7.39$\pm$0.04	7.37$\pm$0.03	7.25$\pm$0.06	7.0$\pm$0.18	6.85$\pm$0.2

Extracellular PO$_2$, K$^+$ and pH in brain cortex.

Although the changes are somewhat similar between ischemia and hypoxia in the brain, it can be seen that in ischemia the onset of K$^+$ release from the cells occurred sooner, as did the pH changes (Fig. 3), but with increasing time the deleterious effects of total ischemia did not accelerate as fast as those in hypoxia although it might be expected that pH and K$^+$ changes in the absence of a circulation would be more pronounced than they are.   Intracellular measurements of pH in brain cells showed that the changes were greater in the presence of hypoxic circulation and also in severe oligemia than in total ischemia, but this was not reflected immediately in extracellular measurements.

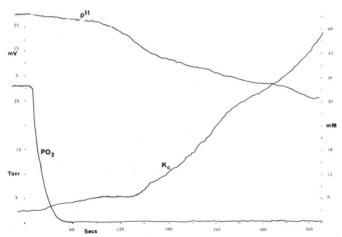

FIG. 3   Simultaneous records of extracellular pH, PO$_2$ and potassium concentration (K$_c$) during acute cerebral ischemia.   Note early pH fall, later arrested.   c.f. Fig. 1.

(3) Hypovolemia

     Hemorrhagic shock affected the different species and regions
more diversely than did either acute hypoxia or ischemia.   In
general the brain was protected initially from the effects of
hypovolemia by circulatory compensation which deprived other organs
of their blood supply.   This situation persisted until the
peripheral capacitance vessels relaxed and true 'shock' developed.
In these circumstances, ion movements were first seen especially in
the 'blood deprived' areas e.g. the gut but developed only later in
heart and brain when blood electrolyte changes were already
apparent.

     Table 3 compares brain and liver ion fluxes in shocked rats
and demonstrates the more rapid change in pH in the liver although
it is clear that loss of K^+ by brain is more closely associated
with pH fall than in the liver.

TABLE 3   HYPOVOLEMIA (RAT) (Bled to MAP 30-35 mm Hg)

Time	0	(Hemorrhage)	1 hr.	(Hemorrhage)	4 hr.
		- - - - - >		- - - - - >	
BRAIN					
PO_2 (Torr)	22 ± 12.5		12.1 ± 6.1		8.3 ± 7.5
K^+ (mM)	3.0 ± 0.01		4.3 ± 1.1		17.9 ± 5.3
pH	7.33 ± 0.10		7.31 ± 0.18		6.7 ± 0.24
LIVER					
PO_2 (mmHg)	18.6 ± 10.1		2.4 ± 2.0		0
K^+ (mM)	3.2 ± 0.07		4.3 ± 0.12		9.7 ± 3.1
pH	7.33 ± 0.10		7.02 ± 0.13		6.6 ± 0.22

Extracellular PO_2, K^+ and pH in brain cortex and liver
during development of hypovolemic shock.

DISCUSSION

Ion fluxes in hypoxia appear to be secondary to a failure of energy metabolism imposed on cells by oxygen deprivation but the presence or absence of blood and cerebrospinal fluid circulation also affects the rate of development and severity of the changes that occur. The nature of the ion movement that is found is associated with the degree of breakdown of oxidative metabolism and of the ATP-linked mechanisms [34,35] that normally maintain membrane potentials, but different cell types vary in their response to insult. Brain cells leak K^+ ions almost immediately they become hypoxic and before there is obvious extracellular pH change, while in other tissues such as liver, there is clear correlation between increased extracellular hydrogen ion concentration and potassium ion release. A third relationship is seen in macrophages [36] which maintain their functional and structural integrity and their motility in hypoxic and acidic environments for long periods, although some of their activities such as bacterial destruction through membrane superoxide production [37] may be impaired in the absence of oxygen.

In brain, in acute hypoxia the general fall in PO_2 was followed by widespread leakage of K^+ which was first detectable in the cortex and hippocampus. Only 10-20 sec. later were similar changes found in the diencephalon and brain-stem. The values shown in Table 1 are for cortex; a similar chart for brain-stem would show slower, but ultimately similar changes (see Fig. 1). However, K^+ diffused very rapidly and K^+ concentrations after about 3-4 minutes became similar in all brain regions. By contrast, in hypovolemic shock local non-perfused areas could be identified in brain (and also in liver) with PO_2 electrodes and these areas acted as foci for early K^+ release. The process built up slowly at first, but terminally led to a suddenly accelerating general K^+ outflow which was irreversible.

The relationship of pH changes and K^+ release in the brain in hypoxia and ischemia requires comment. It appears from the work of Kovach and his colleagues (personal communication) that ultra-structural changes in the brain following total ischemia (decapitation) and mitochondrial damage [38,39] are less severe than those which occur in graded hypoxia or hypovolemia when blood flow is maintained, albeit at a reduced level. Our results suggest that a possible reason for this is that in total ischemia, the pH fall although abrupt does not continue at the same rate once the glucose in the tissue pool has been exhausted (see also Siesjö et al in this publication). Lowry et al [40] have shown that mouse brain rapidly (within 2 sec.) changes to anaerobic glycolysis in acute ischemia and that there is a vastly increased lactate production. This situation leads to a rapid build-up of hydrogen ions to levels incompatible with membrane polarization but the same workers also showed that total substrate reserves were exhausted within one minute. The increase in blood glucose that occurs during the sympathetico-adrenal response to hypoxia may contribute not only to the maintenance of hypoxic tissue energy metabolism, but also to the rapidity of the fall of intracellular pH [41]. Conversely the increase in blood flow may assist in masking the true extent of hydrogen ion production since there is rapid removal of easily diffusible substances.

The enigma which was pointed out by Haldane [42] remains as to why brain cells, which can retain their capacity for energy production in the absence of O_2, should become incapable of regaining their normal function of maintaining their membrane potential and electrical activity after such a short period of O_2 deprivation. This behaviour contrasts markedly with that of other cells, particularly muscle cells, which share with neurones the capacity for rapid discharge of electrical activity that in turn requires the existence of well polarized plasma membranes. The drastic ionic fluxes characteristic of hypoxic damage to brain cells may well merely reflect failure of energy transduction between ATP-ase and the sodium-potassium membrane pump, but equally, they may be ultimately responsible for irreversible damage to the mechanism. From the observations reported here, intracellular pH falls would appear to be one likely cause of irreversible pathological change.

The relationship between intracellular and extracellular hydrogen ion concentration clearly varies from one cell type to another, and presumably reflects not only the intracellular buffering capacity or the ability to segregate dangerous products in membrane bound vesicles, but also the permeability of the plasma membrane. It seems from our rather limited series of observations that an intracellular pH of 6.7 is tolerated by most cells, but that only muscle and macrophages can survive undamaged prolonged intracellular environments of 6.6 or lower.

ACKNOWLEDGEMENT

This work was supported by NINDS Program Project 5 P01-NS-10939-04.

REFERENCES

1.   Katzman, R: Maintenance of a constant brain extracellular potassium. Fed. Proc. 35:1244-1247, 1976.

2.   Lux, H.D., Neher, E: The equilibration time course of $[K^+]_o$ in cat cortex. Exp. Brain. Res. 17:190-205, 1973.

3. Sypert, G.W, Ward, A.A. Jnr: Changes in extracellular potassium activity during neocortical propagated seizures. Exp. Neurol. 45:19-25, 1974.

4. Somjen, G.G, Rosenthal, M, Cordingley, G, LaManna, J, Lothman, E: Potassium, neuroglia and oxidative metabolisms in central grey matter.   Fed. Proc. 35:1266-1271, 1976.

5. Bito, L.Z, Myers, R.E: On the physiological response of the cerebral cortex to acute stress. (Reversible asphyxia). J. Physiol. Lond. 221:349-370, 1972.

6. Dora, E, Zeuthen, T: Brain metabolism and ion movements in the brain cortex of the rat during anoxia.   In Kessler, M. et al (Editors): Ion Selective and Enzyme Electrodes in Biology and Medicine.   Munich, Urban and Schwarzenberg, 1976, pp 294-298.

7. Vyskočil, F, Kris, N, Bures, J: Potassium sensitive micro-electrodes used for measuring the extracellular brain potassium concentration during spreading depression and anoxic depolarization in rats.   Brain Res. 39:255-259, 1972.

8. Zeuthen, T, Hiam, R, Silver, I.A: Recording of ion activities in brain with ion selective microelectrodes.   In Berman, H.J, Herbert, N.C. (Editors): Ion Selective Microelectrodes. New York, Plenum Press, 1974.

9. Kovach, A.G.B, Sandor, P: Cerebral blood flow and brain function during hypotension and shock.   Ann. Rev. Physiol. 38:571-596, 1976.

10. Leão, A.A.P: Further observations on the spreading depression of activity in the cerebral cortex.   J. Neurophysiol. 10: 409-414, 1947.

11. Prince, D.A, Lux, H.D, Neher, E: Measurement of extracellular potassium activity in cat cortex.   Brain Res. 50:489-495, 1973.

12. Mayevsky, A, Zeuthen, T, Chance, B: Measurements of extra-cellular potassium, ECOG and pyridine nucleotide levels during cortical spreading depression in rats.   Brain Res. 76:347-349, 1974.

13. Dora, E, Chance, B, Kovach, A.G.B, Silver, I.A: CO-induced localised toxic anoxia in the rat brain cortex.   J. appl. Physiol. 39:875-878, 1975.

14. Kuschinsky, W, Wahl, M, Bosse, O, Thorau, K: Perivascular
    potassium and pH as determinants of local pial arterial
    diameter in cats.   Circulation Res. 31:240-247, 1972.

15. Haddy, F.J, Scott, J.B: Metabolic factors in peripheral
    circulatory regulation.   Fed. Proc. 34:2006-2011, 1975.

16. Heuser, D, Betz, E: Measurement of potassium ion and hydrogen
    ion activities by means of microelectrodes in brain vascular
    smooth muscle.   In Kessler, M. et al (Editors): Ion Selective
    and Enzyme Electrodes in Biology and Medicine.   Munich,
    Urban and Schwarzenberg, 1976, pp 320-330.

17. Monge, C, Whittembury, J: High altitude adaptations -
    whole animal.   In Bligh, J. et al (Editors): Environmental
    Physiology of Animals.   Oxford, Blackwell Scientific
    Publications, 1976 (in press).

18. Monge, M.C: Chronic mountain sickness.   Physiol. Rev. 23:
    148-165, 1943.

19. Walker, J.L: Ion specific, ion exchanger microelectrodes.
    Anal. Chem. 43:89-93A, 1971.

20. Khuri, R.N, Agulian, S.K, Kalloghlian, A: Intracellular
    potassium in cells of the distal tubule.   Pflügers Arch. ges.
    Physiol. 335:297-308, 1972.

21. Hinke, J.A.M: Glass microelectrodes for measuring intra-
    cellular activities of sodium and potassium.   Nature, Lond.
    184:1257, 1959.

22. Thomas, R.C: A new design of a sodium sensitive glass micro-
    electrode.   J. Physiol. Lond. 210:82-83P, 1970.

23. Thomas, R.C: Intracellular pH of snail neurones measured with
    a new pH sensitive glass microelectrode.   J. Physiol. Lond.
    238:159-180, 1974.

24. Zeuthen, T: A double-barrelled Na$^+$-sensitive electrode.   J.
    Physiol. Lond. 254:8P, 1976.

25. Thomas, R.C: Intracellular sodium activity and the sodium
    pump in snail neurones.   J. Physiol. Lond. 220:55-71, 1972.

26. Pick, J, Toth, K, Pungor, E, Vasak, M, Simon, W: A potassium
    selective silicone-rubber membrane electrode based on a neutral
    carrier.   Anal. Chim. Acta. 64:477-480, 1973.

27. Silver, I.A: Some observations on the cerebral cortex with an ultra-micro-membrane-covered oxygen electrode. Med. Electron Biol. Engng. 3:377-387, 1965.

28. Whalen, W.J, Riley, J, Nair, P: A microelectrode for measuring intracellular PO$_2$. J. appl. Physiol. 23:798-801, 1967.

29. Silver, I.A: Measurement of pH and ionic composition of pericellular sites. Phil. Trans. R. Soc. Lond. B. 271: 261-272, 1975.

30. Lübbers, D.W, Baumgärtl, M: Herstellungstechnick von palladinierten Pt-Stich-elektroden (1-5 μ Aussendruckmesser) zur polarographischen messung des Wasserstoffdruckes fur die Bestimmung der microzirkulation. Pflügers Arch. ges. Physiol. 294:R39, 1967.

31. Heidenreich, J, Erdmann, W, Metzger, H, Thews, G: Local hydrogen clearance and PO$_2$ measurements in micro areas of the rat brain. Experientia 26:257-259, 1970.

32. Stosseck, K, Lübbers, D.W, Cottin, N: Determination of local blood flow (microflow) by electrochemically generated hydrogen. Pflügers Arch. ges. Physiol. 348:225-238, 1974.

33. Van Harreveld, A: The extracellular space in the central nervous system. In Bourne, G.H. (Editor): The Structure and Function of Nervous Tissue. New York, London, Academic Press, 1971, vol. IV, pp 447-511.

34. Skou, J.C: Enzymatic basis for active transport of Na$^+$ and K$^+$ across cell membrane. Physiol. Rev. 45:596-603, 1965.

35. Dahl, J.L, Hokin, L.E: The sodium-potassium adenosinetri-phosphatase. Ann. Rev. Biochem. 43:327-336, 1974.

36. Silver, I.A: The physiology of wound healing. In Hunt, T.K. (Editor): Wound Healing. Minneapolis, 3M Co. 1976 (in press).

37. Webb, L.S, Keele, B.B, Johnston, R.B: Inhibition of phagocytosis-associated chemiluminescence by superoxide dismutase. Infect. Immunity 9:1051-1056, 1974.

38. Schutz, H, Silverstein, P.R, Vapalahti, M, Bruce, D.A, Mela. L, Langfitt, T.W: Brain mitochondrial function after ischemia and hypoxia: I. Ischemia induced by increased intracranial pressure. Arch. Neurol. 29:408-416, 1973a.

39. Schutz, H, Silverstein, P.R, Vapalahti, M, Bruce, D.A, Mela, L,
     Langfitt, T.W: Brain mitochondrial function after ischemia
     and hypoxia: II. Normotensive systemic hypoxemia.   Arch.
     Neurol. 29:417-425, 1973b.

40. Lowry, O.H, Passonneau, J.V, Hasselberger, F.X, Schultz, D.W:
     Effect of ischemia on known substrates and cofactors of the
     glycolytic pathway in brain.   J. Biol. Chem. 239:18-30, 1964.

41. Siesjö, B.K, Zwetnow, N.N: The effect of hypovolemic
     hypotension on extra- and intracellular acid-base parameters
     and on energy metabolites in the rat brain.   Acta. Physiol.
     Scand. 79:114-124, 1970.

42. Haldane, J.B.S: Symptoms, causes and prevention of anoxaemia
     (insufficient oxygen supply to the tissues) and the value of
     oxygen in its treatment.   Brit. Med. J. 2:65-71, 1919.

COMMENTS ON: CHANGES IN PO$_2$ AND ION FLUXES IN CEREBRAL HYPOXIA-

ISCHEMIA

M. O'Connor

Department of Neurosurgery, School of Medicine

University of Pennsylvania, Philadelphia, Pa. 19174

The demonstration of inhomogeneous damage in shock relative to hypoxia is consistent with the hypothesis that inhomogeneous perfusion is present and may be responsible for many of the graded biochemical changes noted in ischemia. In our laboratory we have also noted marked inhomogeneity in ischemic lesions as was mentioned earlier by Dr. Welsh. (Fig. 1b) In hypoxic animals the lesion demonstrated by frozen tissue fluorescence is likely to be more homogeneous as can be seen in Figure 1a. However, even in the hypoxic insult, there is usually evidence of some metabolic inhomogeneity. This is especially evident when there is slight oligemia associated with hypoxia. (Fig. 1c) I think it is important to keep this finding in mind when trying to interpret biochemical changes in either hypoxic or ischemic lesions. That is, when a graded change in one of the metabolic parameters is noted, it may be due to a slight diffuse or to a marked focal variation. This problem has, of course, been recognized at the subcellular level for some time.

In oligemic lesions we have found that not only is there spacial inhomogenity, but also temporal dispersion as Dr. Silver has found. Dr. Welsh has shown the regional abrupt change in the redox state of NADH during the course of ischemia (Fig. 2, Welsh). We also have evidence in support of Dr. Silver's observation of the temporal dispersion of the regional changes in extracellular potassium. When recording both surface potassium with a valinomycin electrode and extracellular potassium with a liquid ion exchange microelectrode we have found in the model described by Dr. Welsh, that there is an early slow rise followed by a more abrupt rise in surface potassium. (Fig. 2a) During the rapid surface increase, there is a much faster increase in potassium recorded with the microelectrode. Since only

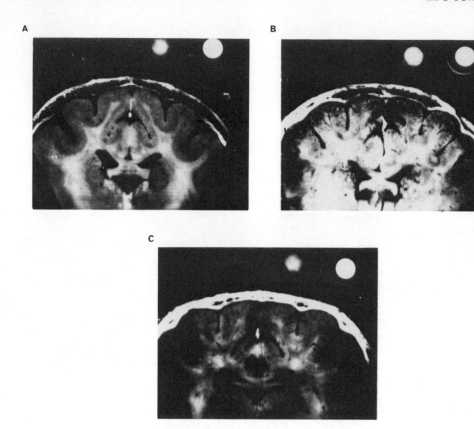

Figure 1

Frozen tissue fluorescence photograph of section of cat brain
during insult.

        A.   Severe Hypoxia
        B.   Ischemia
        C.   Moderate Hypoxia

one microelectrode is used, it cannot be said that the changes
recorded with the microelectrode are regional and temporally dis-
persed. However, if the ischemic insult is reversed and, after
recovery, repeated, then it is found that the synchronization of the
microelectrode change relative to the surface change may be shifted.
(Fig. 2b) Thus, it seems that the surface change might be a summa-
tion of micro-regional changes.

The magnitude of the changes in extracellular potassium are
similar to those noted by Dr. Silver. However, in our oligemia

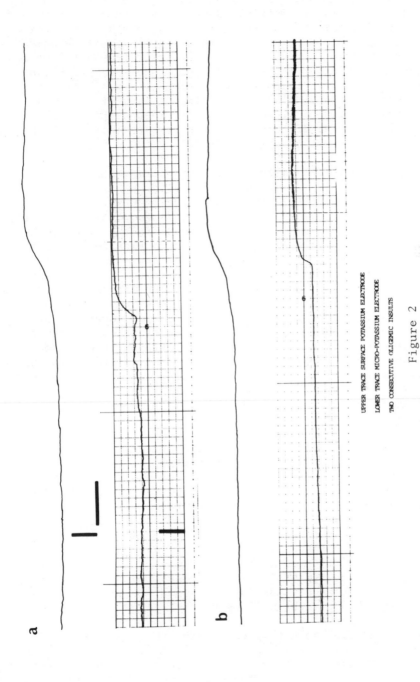

UPPER TRACE SURFACE POTASSIUM ELECTRODE
LOWER TRACE MICRO-POTASSIUM ELECTRODE
TWO CONSECUTIVE OLIGEMIC INSULTS

Figure 2

Surface potassium and microextracellular potassium electrode recordings during two consecutive oligemia insults. Oligemia insult started approximately 8 minutes before calibration marks. Cal: 10 fold change in potassium, 1 minute.

model, what appears to be a rise of 30 meq/liter of potassium in the extracellular space is reversible. Reversible, that is, in the limited sense of return of the surface potassium, EEG, and frozen tissue fluorescence to near normal. The oligemia model in which these changes were found reversible is different from both the acute hypoxia and the prolonged hemorrhagic shock models of Dr. Silver in which these changes were found irreversible. The most striking difference between the models is the relative lack of systemic insult in the oligemia model which was described by Dr. Welsh. Therefore, the apparent difference in the irreversibility of the insult might be a result of the associated systemic insult.

It is thought that a major portion of energy consumption of the brain is expended to maintain ion homeostasis. It is not possible to say with certainty which cellular elements fail during ischemia or hypoxia. However, since the major portion of oxidative metabolism occurs in mitochondria it is possible to say which cellular elements have the highest potential for oxygen consumption. There is some controversy as to whether this potential resides in the neurons or glial cells. This can be resolved by identifying the cellular elements which contain most of the mitochondria. We have done this with serial electron micrographs in a small portion of the cat visual cortex and found that by volume, over 90% of the mitochondria were in neurons or their processes. Most of these were in neuronal processes which were identified by the presence of a synapse or a myelin sheath. If I may generalize from this observation, it would seem that neurons, and not glial cells, are responsible for ion homeostatic mechanisms requiring energy since they are the cells which have the machinery required to support such a highly energetic process.

In the cortex, the neuronal and glial elements are interwoven with spacing much less than the intercapillary distance. Therefore, the supply of substrate and oxygen to each should be the same. This being the case, in conditions such as ischemia and hypoxia where supply is limited, the factor determining failure should be energy demand. Therefore, in the cortex the elements with the highest potential for oxygen consumption, the neurons, should be responsible for failure of ion homeostasis.

When considering regional failure, where the distances being considered are much larger than intercapillary distance, the major determinant of failure might well be supply.

To summarize, I have attempted to make three points.

1. There appears to be spacial and temporal dispersion of metabolic and ionic changes and therefore one must be careful in interpreting graded changes in pooled data.

   2.   What appears to be irreversible changes in ion homeostasis in the brain may be a result of the associated systemic insult.

   3.   The cell type most likely responsible for ion homeostasis and therefore for failure of ion homeostasis is the neuron, since the neurons have the highest potential for oxidative energy metabolism.

EVENTS MARKING IRREVERSIBLE INJURY

JAMES H. HALSEY, Jr.

Department of Neurology

University of Alabama Medical Center, Birmingham, Ala.

Dr. Silver is the world leader in the art of microelectrode construction. He has made important approaches to the question, "When in the course of hypoxia and ischemia does the nerve cell reach the point of irreversible injury?" Clearly this is some time after the arrival of zero PO_2 in a stop flow experiment and is also after the arrest of spontaneous electrical activity which is now known to consist mainly of synaptic potentials, while the critical events probably occur in the cell body. Two of his measurements appear to come close to the critical point. These are the arrival of an intracellular pH of 6.7 and failure of the Na^+- K^+ pump reflected in a high extracellular K^+ of 20-30 mM.

Though it would be nice if these are in fact the irreversible events themselves, this seems too simple. For example, as pointed by Dr. Siesjo, the pathological consequences of hypoglycemia are the same as of hypoxia. Yet no substantial fall in the pH occurs. We ourselves have seen that cerebral infarction made in hypoglycemic gerbils is more severe than in normoglycemic gerbils.

Analogously, if failure to maintain ionic gradients manifested by loss of K^+ to extracellular fluid were critical, then the extracellular K^+ ought to be about the same for irreversible injury by a variety of insults. Instead we hear that the critical point appears to be about twice as high for acute hypoxia as for shock, with graded hypoxia and ischemia in between. It may be that further data will resolve some of these details. An obvious variable is the rate at which the critical point is approached. I think it more likely that these ionic changes will ultimately be found in some circumstances to coincide closely with and sometimes temporally reflect the critical injury but not themselves comprise it. Yet

even if so, these will have been important contributions to the
detailed description of the pathophysiology of ischemia.

I would like to offer some additional descriptive observations
of acute ischemia from our laboratory pertaining to oxygen consumption. When total cerebral ischemia is made by bilateral carotid artery ligation in the gerbil the PO_2 falls almost linearly to
zero within 1-2 seconds. We thought at first that these oxygen
disappearance slopes in this acute stop flow condition would reflect oxygen consumption rate, the sharper the slope, the faster
the O_2 consumption. [1] The problem is more complicated, however.
If a number of these O_2 disappearance rates are plotted against the
local PO_2 at which the occlusion was made a linear relationship
is seen. This linear relation holds even if the tissue PO_2 is
made to change by altering the arterial PO_2 or PCO_2 prior to ligation without changing metabolism. Dr. Reneau, helping us with
interpreting this, thinks the O_2 consumption rate may be given by
extrapolation of this line to PO_2 zero. Experiments are under way
to evaluate this. [1]

Another approach to the estimate of local metabolism has
been to measure both local flow and local PO_2 at the same point,
using an electrode sensitive both to H_2 and to O_2 - the flow being
determined by H_2 clearance rate after inhalation. In a series of
gerbils following ischemic insults we found that in the first few
minutes of reperfusion after ischemia the flow had recovered to
relatively higher levels than the O_2 while the relationship was reversed later. [2] We thought qualitatively that this might indicate
relatively increased O_2 consumption in the early minutes - either
uncoupling of metabolism from ATP synthesis, or stimulation of
metabolism by reparative processes, while later on suppression of
metabolism was suggested.

I should like to mention one other contribution from our laboratory to the description of events which are a consequence of
ischemic injury. This is the progressive alteration by ischemia
of a neuronal enzyme. The Calcium-Magnesium activated vesicular
ATP-ase is located in presynaptic nerve endings in intimate con-
tact with neurotransmitter vesicles, and is thought to be involved
in the process of neurotransmitter release. Dr. Quayle in our
department has shown in the gerbil during total cerebral ischemia
that there is progressive change in substrate binding capacity by
the enzyme and in maximum velocity of the reaction. [3] These abnormalities are evident within 5 minutes of total ischemia and
increase progressively with duration of ischemia. These changes
appear earlier and are much greater than of any other enzyme so
far studied that we know of. This marked apparent sensitivity is
probably mainly because the enzyme is peculiar to neurons. Though
it may mediate an important function it probably is not involved
in the structural integrity of the cell.

In summary, it appears that a number of electrophysiologic events, and now a biochemical one, are being identified which occur around the time of the irreversible injury. The nature of the injury itself, however, remains unknown.

REFERENCES

1. J. Halsey, S. Ganji, W. Erdmann, and H. Mardis: Studies in cerebral ischemia. Microvasc. Res. (in press), 1976.

2. R. Kelly, and J. Halsey: Comparison of local blood flow and oxygen availability at the same locus in the ischemic gerbil brain. STROKE 7:274-278, 1976.

3. E. Quayle, S. Christian, and J. Halsey: Effects of ischemia on the Mg^{++} requiring ATP-ase associated with neuronal synaptic vesicles in gerbil brain. STROKE 7:36-40, 1976.

This investigation was supported in part by NS 08802.

CEREBRAL HEMODYNAMIC AND METABOLIC ALTERATIONS IN STROKE

Martin Reivich, Myron Ginsberg, Robert Slater, Peter G. Tuteur, Herbert I. Goldberg, Neil S. Cherniack and Joel Greenberg

Cerebrovascular Research Center, Department of Neurology, School of Medicine of the University of Pennsylvania, Philadelphia, Pa.

Major alterations in cerebral hemodynamics and metabolism occur in association with strokes. These include abnormalities in the control mechanisms regulating cerebral blood flow as well as disorders of cerebral metabolism.

We have examined the transient cerebral circulatory responses to hypercapnia in a group of patients with cerebrovascular disease, and compared these responses to those measured in a group of normal volunteers.[1] The cerebral blood flow (CBF) response to 5% CO_2 inhalation and its removal were determined in four normal subjects and 18 patients with mild to severe cerebrovascular disease as determined by clinical and angiographic criteria. In the steady state, cerebral blood flow was determined by inert gas techniques using either ^{85}Krypton or ^{133}Xenon. Arterial venous oxygen differences were used to measure the transient cerebral blood flow changes. In the normal subjects, the time course of the increase in cerebral blood flow is similar to that of arterial P_{CO_2}, but an overshoot occurs in the CBF response in the patients with mild cerebrovascular disease which is not present in the arterial P_{CO_2}.

In contrast, in the patients with severe cerebrovascular disease the rate of change of cerebral blood flow is much slower than that of arterial P_{CO_2}. During the off transient, similar results were observed.

In order to more directly compare these responses, the step response for cerebral blood flow was calculated for each group (Fig. 1). The CBF response shows an overshoot in patients with mild cerebrovascular disease compared to the normal subjects, while

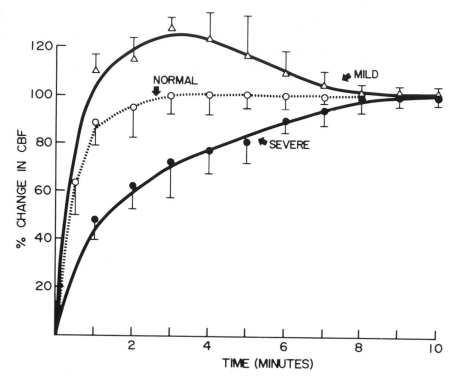

FIG. 1 Average changes in cerebral blood flow with time to a step
increase in Pa_{CO_2} in normal subjects, patients with mild cerebrovascular disease and patients with severe cerebrovascular disease.

in the patients with severe cerebrovascular disease, the cerebral
blood flow response is significantly slower than normal.

The off response of cerebral blood flow to a step change in
arterial Pco_2 shows a small undershoot in the normal volunteers
and a much greater undershoot in the patients with mild cerebrovascular disease (Fig. 2). The patients with severe disease show
no undershoot and a somewhat slower response.

In contrast to these changes in the transient responses of
cerebral blood flow the steady state response was only slightly
decreased in the patients with cerebrovascular disease and there
was no relationship between the blunting of the response and the
clinical severity of the disease.

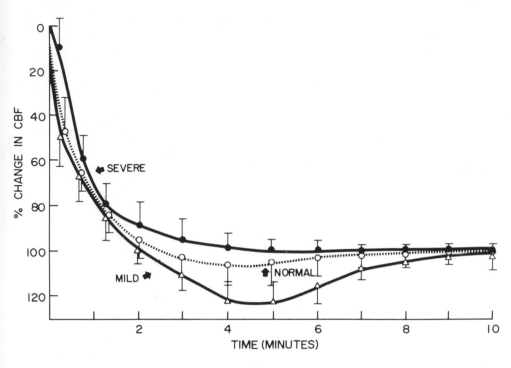

FIG. 2 Average change in cerebral blood flow with time when a step decrease is produced in Pa_{CO_2} in normal subjects, patients with mild cerebrovascular disease and patients with severe cerebrovascular disease.

The differences in the transient CBF response in the patients and normal subjects can be explained in several ways. Blood flow seems to be the highest in those areas of the brain with the greatest metabolic rate; and in the normal brain, the ratio of blood flow to metabolism is nearly the same throughout the brain[2]. If cerebral blood flow is controlled by a single factor such as extracellular fluid (ECF) pH, the increase in the rapidity of the transient CBF response seen in patients with mild cerebrovascular disease could be explained by increasing inhomogeneity in the distribution of blood flow to metabolism in the brain caused by the vascular lesions. Regions of the brain in which the ratio of flow to metabolic rate is high (luxury perfusion) would equilibrate more rapidly with CO_2 because of their higher flow and would have a higher venous O_2 content than would regions where the ratio of flow to metabolism is more uniform. Consequently, these high blood flow regions would contribute disproportionately more to the mixed

cerebral venous blood.[3] Because the blood from regions with a
higher ratio of perfusion to metabolism rates would have a greater
O_2 content, the mixed arterio-venous difference in O_2 content
would narrow more rapidly than it would if flow, metabolic and
hence CO_2 equilibration rates were more uniform.

Apparent overshoots in the CBF response would occur if there
were areas in which CBF responded paradoxically to CO_2 changes;
blood flow decreasing rather than increasing with hypercapnia.
Initially the high flow regions would contribute more to the $(A-V)O_2$
difference and tend to narrow it, while later when the flow areas
were represented more in proportion to their true weight the mean
$(A-V)O_2$ difference would widen. As increasingly severe disease
interfered more extensively with gas exchange across capillaries,
changes in ECF Pco_2 and pH would be uniformly slowed throughout
the brain reducing the speed of the CBF response. Also, with
extensive vascular lesions, the ability of the smooth muscle in
the blood vessel wall to shorten might be affected, further dimin-
ishing the rate with which vascular dilation and contraction occurred with CO_2 changes.

In order to clarify further the factors important for the
regulation of CBF the transient CBF data from the normal subjects
were examined in detail by means of a lumped parameter mathematical
model of this control system.[4] A three component model represent-
ing the intravascular, extracellular and intracellular compartments
was constructed in which the concentrations of molecular CO_2, bicarbonate ion and hydrogen ion were considered in each compartment.
This resulted in a set of nine differential equations which
described the controlled system. The controller, represented by
the vascular smooth muscle response, was assumed to act instantan-
eously with no appreciable time delay. This was felt to be a
reasonable assumption since studies of the major resistance vessels
of the brain showed them to react with a time constant of less than
15 sec. to a change in pH of the extracellular fluid bathing them.
Fig. 3 shows the results from one such set of experiments in which
mock cerebrospinal fluid with a bicarbonate concentration of zero
was placed by means of a micropipette around arterioles 30-200μ in
diameter.

The on and off CBF transients were examined using the model
with either an ECF pH controller or ECF Pco_2 controller. The model
predictions are significantly slower than the experimental data
(Fig. 4). Similar results were obtained for the off transient,
although here the descrepancy was not as great (Fig. 5). These
results suggest that the cerebral circulatory response to hypercapnia is not regulated solely by ECF pH or Pco_2 but may also have
a more rapid component. This rapid component may depend on changes
in arterial Pco_2 or possibly a neural mechanism as suggested by
some recent studies.[5,6,7]

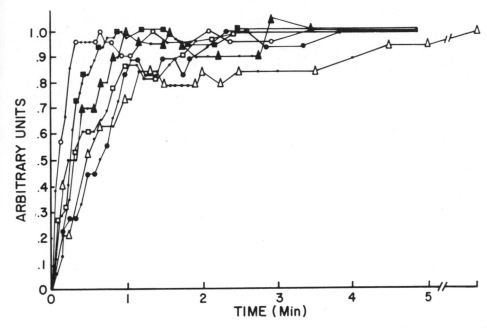

FIG. 3   Vessel diameter reactions to the perivascular injection of a mock CSF with a bicarbonate concentration of 0 mEq/liter.   The diameter changes have been normalized.

This would be compatible with the observations made in the present study which show that CBF in normal subjects responds more rapidly than changes in cerebral venous Pco_2 but more slowly than changes in arterial Pco_2. If the rapidity and the degree of the CBF response to CO_2 depend on changes at two sites, the difference in the transient CBF response in patients with mild or severe cerebrovascular disease could be explained as follows: In mild disease, a decrease in the sensitivity of the vascular response to the slow component, e.g. ECF pH, would tend to accelerate the transient CBF response; but with more severe disease, as shortening of the vascular smooth muscle was mechanically slowed, the rate of the transient response would decrease.

In further studies, we have examined the time course of the cerebral hemodynamic changes occurring in patients with unilateral acute strokes.[8]   A bilateral reduction in blood flow was observed consistent with the phenomenon of diaschisis.   Changes in cerebral blood flow on the side opposite an infarction have been demonstrated

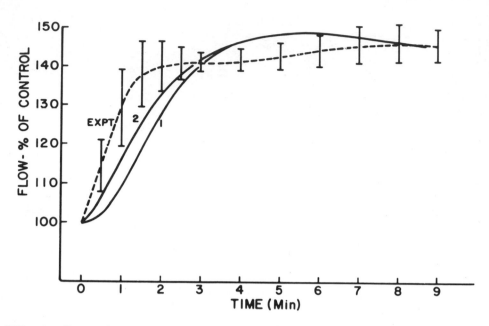

FIG. 4 Comparison of model predictions (solid lines) to the on
cerebral blood flow transient data (dashed line with standard error
bars) from normal subjects: (1) using an ECF pH blood flow controller and (2) using an ECF Pco_2 blood flow controller.

repeatedly since first described by Kempensky et al,[9] in 1961.
Most past observations of this phenomenon have been limited since
the method used to measure cerebral blood flow was invasive.

We have studied a series of 15 patients using the Xenon inhalation method, which has allowed us to make repeated measurements
in the same patient in order to serially study the changes in
cerebral blood flow that occur. In 12 out of the 15 patients, significant blood flow changes (>14%) in the nonishchemic hemisphere
occurred during the period of observation. These data show, contrary to implications from prior studies which did not examine the
first 10 days post stroke in detail, that diaschisis is not a
phenomenon that reaches its peak at the onset of a stroke as the
term suggests, but is a process that continues to evolve during
the first week after stroke. A similar time course of change was
found in the ischemic hemisphere and the flow changes in the two
hemispheres appeared parallel to one another.

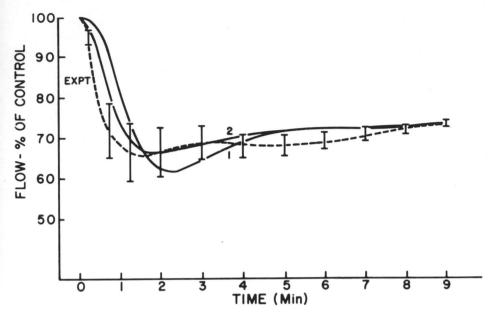

FIG. 5 Comparison of model predictions (solid lines) to the off
cerebral blood flow transient data (dashed line with standard error
bars) from normal subjects: (1) using an ECF pH blood flow controller
and (2) using an ECF Pco_2 blood flow controller.

The fact that the flow changes in the nonischemic hemisphere
were not static, rules out the possibility that the observed flow
reductions were secondary only to pre-existing vascular disease.
This progressive decline in flow in the nonischemic hemisphere has
not previously been recorded. If diaschisis was caused by decreased
metabolic demand secondary to a reduction of neuronal and synaptic
activity a continued decline in blood flow would not be expected,
but only a sudden precipitous drop at the onset of the stroke.
These data do not rule out the possibility that a neural mechanism
plays some role in the phenomenon of diaschisis, but such a mechanism does not appear to be sufficient to explain the progressive
decline in non-ischemic hemisphere flow during the first 10 days.
Previous studies have suggested that vasoactive substances released
from infarcted or ischemic tissue may play a role in the hemodynamic
changes observed following an acute stroke.[10,11,12]

It is likely that multiple causes are responsible for diaschisis and no single hypothesis will explain all the data. The observed phenomenon is likely to be a composite of immediate neuronal effects compounded or masked by loss of autoregulation and modified by the presence of vasoactive substances in the CSF.

In order to more closely examine the cerebral hemodynamic and metabolic alterations occurring in stroke, we have studied various parameters in animal stroke models. Occlusion of the middle cerebral artery in the baboon produces marked focal reductions in flow (Fig. 6) in the cortex and underlying white matter.[13] Mean hemispheric flow is reduced by approximately 29% and remains at this level. In spite of this, although there was a significant fall in the cerebral metabolic rate for oxygen and glucose by 75 minutes after middle cerebral artery occlusion, these values returned toward normal during 4 3/4 hours after occlusion reaching 93% and 94% of their control values by that time. There is a suggestion that anaerobic glycolysis may be increased since the cerebral production of lactate increased from .67 ± .95 to 1.91 ± .26 μM/100 gms/min by 75 minutes after occlusion. This change, however, did not reach the level of significance. The cerebral uptake of oxygen was in excess of that required for glucose oxidation suggesting

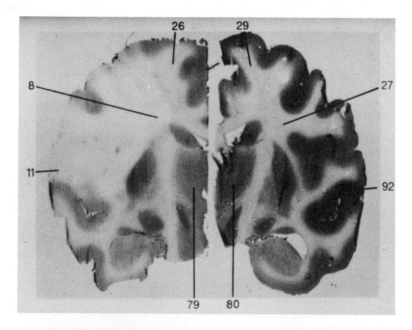

FIG. 6   Autoradiogram of a coronal section through the brain of a baboon following middle cerebral artery occlusion. The numbers represent regional cerebral blood flow values in cc/100gm/min.

that cerebral oxidative metabolism is being supported by substances other than glucose.

In spite of the fact that these metabolic alterations tend to return toward normal, if the animal is allowed to survive, he is left with a marked hemiparesis. Thus there is some irreversible damage produced which is not detected by metabolic studies of the whole brain. The marked focal CBF changes seen by autoradiographic studies also suggest that local metabolic abnormalities are present which go undetected.

In order to investigate this possibility further, we examined the regional metabolic alterations that occur following middle cerebral artery occlusion in the cat. In this model a striking perfusion deficit, as demonstrated by carbon black injection, is present involving the posterior sylvian, middle ectosylvian and posterior ectosylvian gyri.[14] Regional cerebral blood flow (rCBF) was most markedly reduced in the middle and posterior ectosylvian gyri being on the average only 23% and 21% respectively of the values in the non-ischemic hemisphere. The flow reduction in the posterior sylvian and middle suprasylvian gyri was nearly as marked, being 31% and 33% respectively. Other gyri were less affected. Flow in the central white matter was considerably reduced in the ischemic hemisphere being 32% of the non-ischemic hemisphere.

Measurement of cortical redox state in the area of most marked rCBF change revealed a reduction of pyridine nucleotide occurring within 3 to 3.5 seconds of the onset of ischemia and attaining a maximum value 30 to 70 seconds following middle cerebral artery occlusion (Fig. 7). The maximal reduction of pyridine nucleotide on the average was 28% which is somewhat less than that produced by nitrogen anoxia, suggesting that intracellular hypoxia was not total. These data indicate that an abrupt disturbance in cortical oxidative metabolism occurs in association with focal cerebral ischemia. The rapidity of the intracellular NAD+ reduction is incompatible with substrate depletion but rather suggests a marked slowing of mitochondrial respiration.

Following the peak change in pyridine nucleotide fluorescence there was a slow decline starting at about 1 1/2 minutes after middle-cerebral artery occlusion. This may be due to re-entry of circulation into the ischemic zone via collateral channels and a subsequent increase in tissue oxygen levels with reoxidation of NADH. In a study of compression ischemia, it was shown that even a small increase in flow may be sufficient to produce partial reoxidation of NADH.[15]

An alternate explanation for the reoxidation of NADH during ischemia may be a depression of local cerebral metabolism triggered

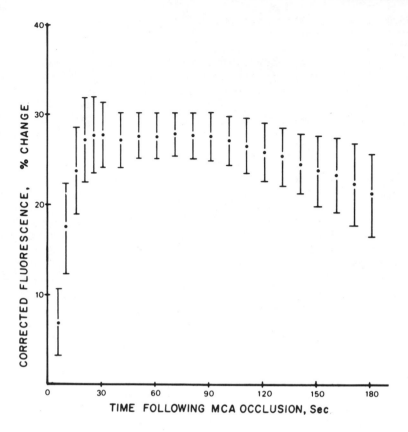

FIG. 7 Time course of change (mean ± S.D.) of pyridine nucleotide fluorescence following middle cerebral artery occlusion in the cat.

by the ischemic insult. In support of this concept are the studies of Waltz[16] and Sundt and Waltz[17] in which focal ischemia was observed to be associated with hyperoxygenation of the local venous blood without an increase in local flow being present. These data imply that the metabolic requirements of the tissue were reduced with a consequent decrease in oxygen extraction from the perfusing blood. Bruce et al[18] have also reported, in compression ischemia, a reduced extraction of oxygen by the brain associated with an increase in glucose utilization when CBF is reduced to 40% of normal. Thus there may be a critical level of cerebral perfusion at which oxygen utilization is inhibited in association with an increase in anaerobic glycolysis.

In order to examine this hypothesis further, studies of local cerebral glucose consumption following middle cerebral artery MCA occlusion were performed in a series of cats using the ^{14}C-deoxy-glucose method.[19] In all animals a striking derangement of meta-bolism was observed within the basal ganglia of the ischemia hemi-sphere which consisted of a central area of decreased glucose utilization surrounded by a zone of increased glucose metabolism.[20] In some animals similar interdigitating areas of hypo- and hyper-metabolism were present in the cerebral cortex. These areas of hypermetabolism most likely represent regions of increased anaerobic glycolysis. These findings lend support to the concept that with reduction of cerebral perfusion below some critical level an enhancement of anaerobic glycolysis occurs possibly in association with a reduction in oxygen utilization.

Information concerning the level of cerebral perfusion at which this enhanced anaerobic glycolysis occurs was obtained in studies in which local flow and glucose metabolism were measured simultaneously by means of ^{3}H-antipyrine and ^{14}C-deoxyglucose re-spectively in a series of cats following middle cerebral artery occlusion. These data suggest that when regional cerebral blood flow is reduced to approximately 40% of normal, an increase in anaerobic glycolysis may occur in that area. This critical level of cerebral perfusion agrees quite well with that reported by Bruce et al[18] in their study of compression ischemia.

In addition to the alterations in glucose metabolism observed on the side of the middle cerebral artery occlusion, there was a small but significant ($P < .025$) reduction in glucose utilization in the contralateral hemisphere when compared to a series of control animals. The average value for glucose utilization in the contra-lateral cerebral cortex in the experimental animals was 4.06 ± 0.45 mg/100gm/min. compared to 5.88 ± 0.71 mg/100 gm/min. in the control animals. This may represent the metabolic correlate of diaschisis and underlie the flow changes observed in the contralateral hemi-sphere following a stroke.

ACKNOWLEDGEMENT

This work was supported by USPHS grant NS-10939.

REFERENCES

1.   Tuteur, P., Reivich, M., Goldberg, H.I., Cooper, E.S., West, J. W., McHenry, L.C., Jr., and Cherniack, N.: Transient responses of cerebral blood flow and ventilation to changes in PaCO$_2$ in normal subjects and patients with cerebrovascular disease. Stroke (in press).

2.   Reivich, M.: Blood flow metabolism couple in brain. In: Brain Dysfunction in Metabolic Disorders. (Ed.) F. Plum. Res. Publ. Assoc. Nerv. Ment. Dis. 53:125-140, 1974.

3.   Cherniack, N. and Longobardo, G.: Oxygen and carbon dioxide
      gas stores of the body. Physiol. Rev. 50:196-243, 1970.

4.   Greenberg, J. H., Noordergraaf, A., and Reivich, M.: The
      control of cerebral blood flow--model and experiments. Pro-
      ceedings of International Conference on Cardiovascular System
      Dynamics. MIT Press, 1976 (in press).

5.   Stone, H.L., Raichle, M.E., and Hernandez, M.: The effect of
      sympathetic denervation on cerebral CO_2 sensitivity. Stroke
      5:13-18, 1974.

6.   Harper, A.M., Deshmukh, V.D., Rowan, J.D., and Jennett, W.B.:
      The influence of sympathetic nervous activity on cerebral
      blood flow. Arch. Neurol. 27:1-6, 1972.

7.   Ponte, J. and Purves, M.J.: The role of the carotid body
      chemoreceptors and carotid sinus baroreceptors in the control
      of cerebral blood flow. J. Physiol. 237:315-340, 1974.

8.   Slater, R., Reivich, M. and Goldberg, H.I.: Cerebral diaschi-
      sis in stroke. Stroke 7:7-8, 1976.

9.   Kempinsky, W.H., Boniface, W.R., Keating, J.B.A. and Morgan,
      P.P.: Serial hemodynamic study of cerebral infarction in man.
      Circ. Res. 9:1051-1058, 1961.

10.   Meyer, J.S., Stoica, E., Pascu, I., Shimorzu, K. and Hartman,
      A.: Catecholamine concentrations in CSF and plasma of patients
      with cerebral infarction and haemorrhage. Brain 96:277-288,
      1973.

11.   Zervas, N.T., Hori, H., Negola, M., Wurtman, R.J., Larin, F.
      and Lavyne, M.H.: Reduction in brain dopamine following ex-
      perimental cerebral ischaemia. Nature 247:283-284, 1974.

12.   Kogure, K., Busto, R., Scheinberg, P., and Reinmuth, O.:Energy
      metabolites and water content in rat brain during the early
      stage of development of cerebral infarction. Brain 97:103-
      114, 1974.

13.   Reivich, M., Kovach, A.G.B., Spitzer, J.J., and Sandor, P.:
      Cerebral blood flow and metabolism in hemorrhagic shock in
      baboons. Advances in Exp. Med. and Biol. 33:19-26, 1973.

14.   Ginsberg, M.D., Reivich, M., Frinak, S. and Harbig, K.:
      Pyridine nucleotide redox state and blood flow of the cerebral
      cortex following middle cerebral artery occlusion in the cat.
      Stroke 7:125-131, 1976.

15. Harbig, K. and Reivich, M.: The effect of ischemia and hypoxia
     on the pyridine nucleotide redox state of the cerebral cortex
     of cats. In: Cerebral Circulation and Metabolism, Sixth
     International CBF Symposium (Ed.) T.W. Langfitt, L.C. McHenry,
     Jr., M. Reivich, and H. Wollman, Springer-Verlag, New York,
     1975, pp. 180-183.

16. Waltz, A.G.: Red venous blood: Occurrence and significance in
     ischemic and nonischemic cerebral cortex. J. Neurosurg. 31:
     141-148, 1969.

17. Sundt, T.M., Jr., and Waltz, A.G.: Cerebral ischemia and
     reactive hyperemia. Circulation Research. 28:426-433, 1971.

18. Bruce, D.A., Schutz, H., Vapalahti, M., Gunby, N. and Langfitt,
     T.: Interactions between cerebral blood flow and cerebral
     metabolism. Surg. Forum 23:417-419, 1972.

19. Reivich, M., Sokoloff, L., Kennedy, C., and Des Rosiers, M.:
     An Autoradiographic method for the measurement of local glucose
     metabolism in the brain. In: The Working Brain. Alfred Ben-
     zon Symposium VIII. (Ed.) D.H. Ingar, and N.A. Lassen, Munks-
     gaard, Copenhagen, 1975, pp. 377-384.

20. Ginsberg, M.D., Reivich, M. and Giandomenico, A.: Alterations
     of regional brain metabolism during focal cerebral ischemia.
     Neurology 26:346, 1976.

CEREBRAL HEMODYNAMIC AND METABOLIC ALTERATIONS IN STROKE: FORMAL

DISCUSSION OF PAPER BY DR. MARTIN REIVICH, ET AL.

Thoralf M. Sundt, Jr.

Department of Neurologic Surgery

Mayo Clinic, Rochester, Minnesota

I am pleased to have the opportunity to discuss this fine paper by Dr. Reivich and colleagues. There is a considerable amount of correlative data between clinical and laboratory studies presented by these investigators that agrees quite closely with some of our work in this field. Time permits only specific comments referable to three aspects of this work: (1) cerebral autoregulation, (2) critical cerebral blood flow, and (3) variations in NADH studies with laboratory preparations.

CEREBRAL AUTOREGULATION

It appears there is indeed a difference between patients with mild and severe cerebral vascular disease in the manner in which CBF responds to changes in Pa_{CO_2}. There is currently considerable interest in the parenchymal system of adrenergic nerves that have been identified by Hartman, et al (1). The question has arisen from a number of investigators whether or not the locus ceruleus has a central role in cerebral autoregulation. Studies in our laboratory by Dr. David Bates have indicated that bilateral destruction of the locus ceruleus stereotactically results in decreased levels of catecholamines in the paraventricular hypothalamic nuclei, anterior ventral nuclei of the thalamus, and parietal cortex of cats (2). This was correlated with a significantly abnormal CBF-Pa_{CO_2} response curve 10 days after the stereotactic procedures in those animals with accurately placed stereotactic lesions. In animals in which the lesions were not located in the locus ceruleus verified histologically, there was no change in catecholamines in the areas of biopsy or in the CBF-Pa_{CO_2} response curve. Although the animals with the accurately placed lesions had abnormalities in the CBF–Pa_{CO_2} response curves, their autoregulatory response to changes in perfusion pressure was preserved.

I wondered if Dr. Reivich had any data relating the ability of the two groups he studied to compensate for variations in mean arterial blood pressure (MABP) as it appears from this work, as well as, of course, from the work of many other investigators, that there is in fact a difference in the ability of brain to respond to variations in Pa_{CO_2} and MABP and the terms autoregulation to Pa_{CO_2} and autoregulation to MABP are becoming popular. Also were the two groups matched for age? I was particularly impressed by the temporal profile of CBF changes in patients with stroke who demonstrated the phenomenon of cerebral diaschisis. Were these changes in CBF correlated with the level of consciousness in these patients? It is a common clinical observation that the greater the cerebral insult, that is, the larger the infarction, the more depression there is in the patient's level of consciousness. This can be observed immediately after a stroke and prior to the time when increasing intracranial pressure, as from cerebral edema, can be invoked as the cause for the stupor.

CRITICAL CEREBRAL BLOOD FLOW

There is a great deal of conflicting data regarding some subjects concerning cerebral blood flow such as the role of the autonomic nervous system. Therefore it is comforting to find one subject that can be agreed upon by a variety of investigators. This is the level which we can refer to as critical cerebral blood flow (3). This term can be used to define that blood flow below which there is a change in physiological function of the brain and which if, allowed to persist for a long enough period of time, will produce cerebral infarction. In humans undergoing carotid endarterectomy under halothane anesthesia at a Pa_{CO_2} of 40, this critical CBF has been found to be in the level of 18 to 20 ml/100g per minute. There is close agreement between our studies in this regard and the Danish group of patients reported by Boysen (4). Below a CBF of 18 ml/100g per minute, the EEG changes and the lower the CBF, the more rapid and severe is the EEG change. These studies are performed with an intraarterial injection of xenon-133 and the indicator arrives in the area predestined for ischemia prior to occlusion of the major vessel. Accordingly these clinical studies are uniquely free of artifacts related to "look through" and Compton scatter (5).

Extrapolation to and correlation with laboratory data reveals this critical blood flow is approximated in most animal preparations by blood flow reduction to approximately 40% of that animal's normal, a figure already referred to by Dr. Reivich. This has been our experience as well.

This is of major importance because the tissue tolerance to ischemia at a CBF of 15 ml/100g per minute approximates several hours and the situation of incomplete focal cerebral ischemia cannot be compared to the setting of total complete ischemia as seen with cardiac arrest where the tissue tolerance to ischemia approximates only 4 minutes. The metabolic changes which take place in focal incomplete ischemia may not always be similar to those seen with anoxia or total cerebral ischemia as seen with cardiac arrest or decapitation. Examples include: the higher levels of NADH in anoxia than in focal incomplete ischemia (our data supports that reported by these workers) and differences in the levels of tissue metabolites. Levels of lactic acid after 1 hour of focal incomplete ischemia are much higher than the levels seen 4 minutes after total circulatory arrest (6).

The differences between the tissue tolerance to ischemia with incomplete ischemia and total ischemia give hope to the clinician and a major challenge to the laboratory investigator.

VARIATIONS IN NADH STUDIES WITH LABORATORY PREPARATIONS

Our experience with NADH levels of fluorescence in areas of focal incomplete ischemia is consistent with that reported by Dr. Reivich and his colleagues but there are some differences. Perhaps this is in large measure related to the differences in the laboratory preparations. We have used the squirrel monkey which has a more severe reduction of blood flow than the cat following middle cerebral artery occlusion. Two illustrations will summarize briefly our work in this regard. The first slide demonstrates the correlation between CBF, ATP, lactic acid, and NADH levels drawn from a number of studies in our laboratory using the model of focal incomplete ischemia in the squirrel monkey produced by MCA occlusion (5-10). In normal brain NADH remains constant throughout a wide range in CBF, Pa_{CO_2}, and MABP. However, with reduction in CBF to approximately 40% of normal, there is a prompt rise in NADH that remains at this elevated level during the period of ischemia. During ischemia NADH levels vary with changes in MABP (fall with rise in MABP and rise with a fall in MABP). There is a steady decline in ATP and rise in lactate levels during the period of ischemia that is reversed with restoration of normal CBF. NADH records only cortical changes and that may be different from the tissue samples of ATP and lactate which have incorporated subcortical areas as well.

One has to be cautious regarding the excitation energy employed when evaluating NADH fluorescence in areas of focal incomplete ischemia. It has been our experience that with too high a level of excitation energy photodecomposition occurs which is particularly noticeable during the period of ischemia, in contrast to a base-

line level prior to the introduction of ischemia, and that this
fall in fluorescent level may not accurately reflect a change in
the metabolic state of the brain or in the microcirculation (9,10).
I agree with Dr. Reivich that in his model of the cat, it is quite
possible that the NADH level does in fact fall as a result of the
improving microcirculatory responses and changes in metabolism that
may not be reflected in the more severe areas of ischemia seen in
the squirrel monkey.

The next slide, drawn from a publication which will soon appear
in the "Journal of Neurochemistry", correlates the EEG and NADH
levels in the parietal cortex of a squirrel monkey following MCA

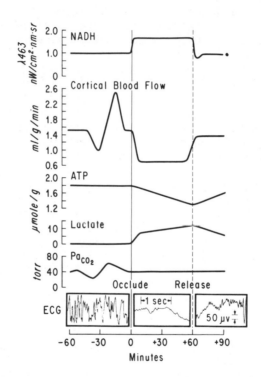

Fig. 1. Correlation of cortical NADH fluorescence, cortical blood
flow, and tissue ATP, and lactate levels at various tensions of
Pa_{CO_2} in normal brain, and at a Pa_{CO_2} of 40 torr in partially
ischemic brain. This figure is a composite of multiple investigations of focal incomplete ischemia in the squirrel monkey (see
text for references). NADH remains at a constant level in normal
brain throughout a wide range in Pa_{CO_2} and CBF, and only rises
after the latter falls below 40% of normal.

occlusion (11). Our work agrees quite closely with Dr. Reivich in
this regard in that the prompt rise in NADH levels following MCA
occlusion occurs within 15 seconds from the time of arterial occlusion and precedes the change in the EEG. This increase in NADH
began within 2 to 5 seconds following MCA occlusion in our animals.
The rise in NADH consistently occurred before the onset of EEG
changes which were not evident until 10 to 17 seconds after MCA
occlusion. This lag time between the rise in NADH fluorescence
in vivo and the change in electrical activity of the brain has been
reported in the past by Dr. Britton Chance using other types of
laboratory models and is therefore consistent with and supportive
of his data. The return to normal levels, with restoration of flow,
of NADH fluorescence in these animals indicates the potential reversibility of this degree of partial ischemia.

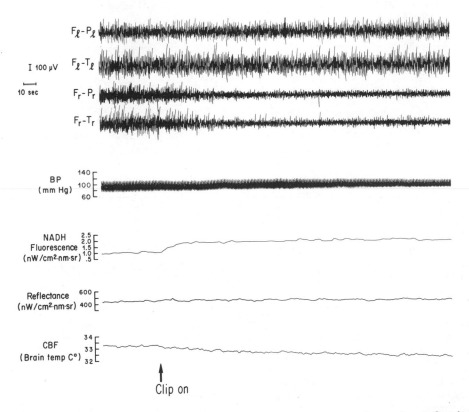

Fig. 2. Photograph of typical animal tracing at time of occlusion
of the middle cerebral artery. NADH rise precedes slightly the
unilateral reduction in EEG activity. Reflectance does not change
during occlusion. A decrease in CBF is indicated by reduction in
cortical temperature.

REFERENCES

1. Hartman BK, Zide D, Udenfriend S: The use of dopamine β-hydroxylase as a marker for the central noradrenergic nervous system in rat brain. Proc Natl Acad Sci USA 69:2722-2726, 1972.

2. Bates D, Weinshilboum RM, Campbell RJ, Sundt TM Jr: The effect of lesions in the locus ceruleus on the physiological responses of the cerebral blood vessels in cats. Circ Res (in press).

3. Sundt TM Jr, Sharbrough FW, Anderson RE, Michenfelder JD: Cerebral blood flow measurements and electroencephalograms during carotid endarterectomy. J Neurosurg 41:310-320, 1974.

4. Boysen G: Cerebral hemodynamics in carotid surgery. Acta Neurol Scand 49 (Suppl 52):1-84, 1973.

5. Hanson EJ Jr, Anderson RE, Sundt TM Jr: Comparison of [85]krypton and [133]xenon cerebral blood flow measurements before, during, and following focal, incomplete ischemia in the squirrel monkey. Circ Res 36:18-26, 1975.

6. Sundt TM Jr, Michenfelder JD: Focal transient cerebral ischemia in squirrel monkey: effect on brain ATP and lactate levels with electrocorticographic and pathologic correlation. Circ Res 30:702-712, 1972.

7. Michenfelder JD, Sundt TM Jr: Cerebral ATP and lactate levels in the squirrel monkey following occlusion of the middle cerebral artery. Stroke 2:319-326, 1971.

8. Michenfelder JD, Sundt TM Jr: The effect of Pa_{CO_2} on the metabolism of ischemic brain in squirrel monkeys. Anesthesiology 38:445-453, 1973.

9. Sundt TM Jr, Anderson RE: Reduced nicotinamide adenine dinucleotide fluorescence and cortical blood flow in ischemic and nonischemic squirrel monkey cortex. 1. Animal preparation, instrumentation, and validity of model. Stroke 6:270-278, 1975.

10. Sundt TM Jr, Anderson RE: Reduced nicotinamide adenine dinucleotide fluorescence and cortical blood flow in ischemic and nonischemic squirrel monkey cortex. 2. Effects of alterations in arterial carbon dioxide tension, blood pressure, and blood volume. Stroke 6:279-283, 1975.

11. Sundt TM Jr, Anderson RE, Sharbrough FW: Effect of hypocapnia, hypercapnia, and blood pressure on NADH fluorescence, electrical activity, and blood flow in normal and partially ischemic monkey cortex. J Neurochem (in press).

CEREBRAL HEMODYNAMIC AND METABOLIC ALTERATIONS IN HYPOVOLEMIC SHOCK

A.G.B. Kovach

Experimental Research Department Semmelweis Medical

University, Budapest, Hungary

Defects in central nervous function following trauma and severe blood loss were clearly recognized in the first classical description of the characteristic symptoms of the condition by Ambroise Paré in 1975. In 1899 Crile suggested on the basis of experimental results that the central nervous system (CNS) played an important role in the development of shock.[1] He thought that impulses originating from the injured areas inhibited the medullary vasometer centers, thus reducing blood pressure and, if long lasting, sufficiently resulted in a specific impairment of the circulation. Later, other theories gained dominance and the interest in CNS changes during shock disappeared. Opinions in the literature are controversial as to the role of somatic and visceral nociceptive afferent impulses in the development of irreversible shock[2,3,4,5,6]. It was generally assumed, that owing to its well developed blood flow autoregulatory mechanisms, the brain's vital functions are protected during hypotension in hypovolemic and other types of shock.

Contrary observations made in our and other laboratories in the last two decades have established that the CNS is in fact vulnerable in prolonged hemorrhagic hypotension and shock.

It has been demonstrated that spontaneous electrocortical activity (EEG)[7] and somatosensory evoked potentials[8,9] disappear during hypovolemia and do not return after reinfusion. Also metabolic[7,8,9,10,11,12] and functional[13,14,15] alterations suggest that the CNS is seriously affected in shock.

Its metabolic characteristics render the brain comparatively

sensitive to reductions in cerebral blood flow (CBF). Nervous
tissue has a high oxygen consumption and, since it contains very
little dissolved oxygen and has relatively small energy reserves
it is highly dependent upon a continuous blood supply. It has been
implied that different hypoxic insults produce states that are
approximately comparable, but this is not strictly true. For
example stagnant ischemic anoxia can be presumed to produce local
hypercapnia, hypoglycemia and build up of metabolic waste products,
which is not the case in arterial hypoxia. The difference in local
chemical environment will produce variations in hemodynamic, metabolic and functional effects.

The primary goal of our studies was to investigate the performance of the regional cerebral circulation and metabolism in
the hypotensive and normovolemic phase of irreversible hemorrhagic
shock, as well as to elucidate possible reasons for the lack of
restitution of brain function in the subsequent normovolemic
period following reinfusion.

CEREBRAL BLOOD FLOW IN SHOCK

The number of reports on cerebral blood flow changes during
shock is relatively small compared to the increasing amount of
data appearing on CBF in hypotension or in hypoxia. It should be
emphasized at this point that shock, due to its complex pathological mechanism, is not comparable to hypoxia, anoxia, hypotension,
or rapid exsanguination. The data obtained from these situations
need special interpretation when applied to changes observed
during shock.

Total CBF decreases in different experimental shock conditions
by 25-44% in anesthetized dogs.[16] Such decrease in total flow
alone would not explain the serious functional defects, because a
comparable degree of arterial hypoxia has no irreversible effects.

Several studies on regional cerebral blood flow (rCBF) changes
in the dog in shock have been reviewed[16] and substantial regional
blood volume differences have been identified by the benzidine
method in both hemorrhagic and in tourniquet shock.[8,17] The most
significant changes were ischemia of the cerebral cortex, disruption
of the normal capillary pattern, the appearance of empty capillaries
and intravascular sludge formation.

Regional blood flow measured by a head conductivity technique
[18,8,12,19,20,21,22] and by the H_2 clearance method[18,8,12,19,20,21,
22] decreased to 70% in the parietal cortex, to 40% in the ventromedial hypothalamus, and to 55% in the hypophysis during the late
phase of hemorrhage in anesthetized dogs.

Blood flow fell to about 40% in the hypothalamus, to 60% in the VPL nucleus of the thalamus, and to 70% in the white matter[23], [24] while vasodilatation of the pial vessels and decreased cortical blood flow was observed during hemolytic shock brought about by transfusion of incompatible blood.[25] Blood flow to the deep nuclei of the brain remained significantly depressed three hours after starting the transfusion despite the return of the MABP to normal.[24]

Experiments were carried out on baboons of both sexes, anesthetized with Sernylan (1 ml/kg). The animals were ventilated artificially and immobilized with Flaxedil (May and Baker Ltd.U.K.) Regional cerebral blood flow (rCBF) was registered by two methods. Repeated measurements were taken by monitoring the cerebral clearance of ^{133}Xe using a multi-channel computer based system.[26] At the end of each experiment local blood flow was also determined by an autoradiographic technique employing ^{14}C-antipyrine.[27] Arterial and cerebral venous pressures, end-tidal CO_2 content of expired air, cortical electric activity and ECG were monitored continuously, while intermittent arterial and cerebral venous (sagittal sinus) blood samples were taken and analyzed for pH, blood gases, hematocrit and metabolites. Cardiac output was determined by the thermal dilution method. In control animals repeated measurements were made of rCBF and metabolism over a period of 5-6 hours. The experimental animals were bled into a pressure -buffered reservoir system. Mean arterial blood pressure (MABP) of these animals was first set at 55-60, then at 35-40 mm Hg. Each hypotensive period lasted for 90 min and at the end of the second bleeding phase the blood in the reservoir was re-infused. Measurements were taken one hour after reinfusion. In another group, experimental animals were sacrificed at the end of the second bleeding before reinfusion in order to obtain autoradiograms during the hypotensive state.

Table I summarizes the hemodynamic data. There was a substantial and significant decrease in cardiac output during hemorrhage. Mean CBF also declined but to a much lesser degree especially in the second bleeding period. Comparison of percentage changes revealed that cardiac output dropped to 27% of its initial level while mean CBF decreased to 56% during bleeding II. Diminution of the brain blood flow could be attributed mainly to the decreased flow in the grey matter as revealed by compartmental analysis, while the slow flow (flow in the white matter) was maintained if not augmented. A marked hemodilution also occurred during hemorrhage. There was a fairly uniform decrease in blood flow due to hemorrhage in all of the brain regions studied with the ^{133}Xe technique.

In the control animals mean CBF did not change significantly during the 5-6 hours of observation. After reinfusion of experimented animals a marked rise in CBF occurred involving both the fast and slow compartments.

Table I

	Control	Bleeding I	Bleeding II	Reinfusion
		90'	90'	60'
MABP /mm Hg/	112 + 9	56 + 1	33 + 1	98 + 15
CO /ml/min/kg/	207 + 13	90 + 5	56 + 7	175 + 34
CBF /ml/100g/min/	39 + 2.1	34 + 1.5	22 + 1.6	78 + 18
FAST FLOW /ml/100g/min/	55 + 2.2	50 + 2.6	35 + 5.7	112 + 32
SLOW FLOW /ml/100g/min/	17 + 1.7	25 + 1.6	17 + 2.6	52 + 19
HTC /per cent/	37 + 2	28 + 2	28 + 2	32 + 2

MABP = mean arterial blood pressure; CO = cardiac output;
CBF = mean cerebral blood flow; HTC = hematocrit
[x] arithmetic mean of stochastic flows recorded from eight brain regions.

There was a slight but significant decrease in cerebral oxygen consumption ($CMRO_2$) from 3.28 ml/100 g/min to 2.74 ml/100 g/min, but it returned to the initial level after reinfusion (3.53 ml/100 g/min). A similar change was seen in the cerebral uptake of glucose.

Cerebral venous Po_2 which is thought to be an important indicator of gross tissue hypoxia did not fall below the critical level of 20 mm Hg.

Mean arterial Pco_2 was maintained between 32 + 3 and 33 + 3 mm Hg during the control and experimental observations by changing the ventilatory rate. A metabolic acidosis developed during bleeding with arterial pH falling significantly from a control value of 7.42 + 0.02 to 7.26 + 0.05 at the end of the first bleeding period and to 7.06 + 0.06 at the end of the second bleeding period. At the same time arterial bicarbonate decreased significantly from a control value of 22.9 ± 0.6 mEq/1 to 15.6 ± 2.6 and 0.1 ± 0.8 mEq/1 at the end of the first and second bleeding period, respectively.

A significant lactic acidosis developed during hemorrhage with arterial lactate concentration rising from a control value of 1.29 ± 0.18 mM to 12.84 ± 2.74 mM at the end of the second bleeding period. There was also a significant increase in arterial pyruvate concentration from 0.05 ± 0.02 to 0.28 ± 0.03 mM by the end of the bleeding periods. Cerebral lactate output (CMR_{lac}) rose from 1.06 ± 3.10 to 10.93 ± 6.98 µM/100 g/min. Cerebral pyruvate output (CMR_{pyr}) decreased from 1.58 ± 0.34 to 0.34 ± 0.56 µM/100 g/min during bleeding but these changes were not significant. In addition arterial glucose concentration increased during bleeding. There was no significant change in cerebral glucose uptake (CMR_{gl}) which remained between 4.4 and 4.8 mg/100 g/min during the study /Reivich et al, 1973/.

Analysis of the autoradiograms revealed an uneven perfusion as a consquence of prolonged hemorrhage (Fig. 1). Besides a reduction of perfusion rates in all brain regions there were also areas without any uptake of the tracer ^{14}C-antipyrine, indicating no flow at all. It was even more striking that ischemic areas persisted after reinfusion when mean CBF was twice as much as before bleeding.

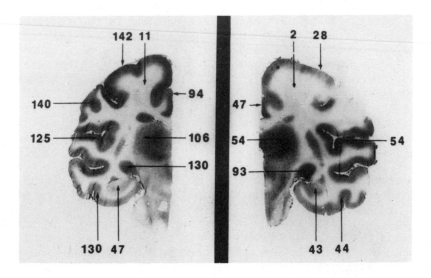

Fig. 1 Coronal section autoradiographs taken from a control (panel A) and experimental animal (panel B) at the end of the second bleeding period (MABP 35 mm Hg). Density of grains is directly related to CBF; darker areas are those with higher CBF. Numbers represent regional CBF values of corresponding areas in ml/100g/ min. Note cortical ischemic zones on the right.

Cortical electrical activity can be correlated with these findings, because the EEG did not show complete recovery in the normovolemic period following profound hypotension.

Local cerebral circulatory, metabolic and functions damage can be induced or affected by:

1/ boundary zone distribution
2/ vasoconstriction /nervous or humoral/
3/ local microvessel sludging /thrombocyte aggregation/
4/ elevated neuronal activity /nociceptive/ not covered by blood flow and oxygen delivery
5/ tissue edema, capillary endothelial change, blood brain barrier damage

To analyze the regional distribution of the non-perfused brain regions in shock and to clarify the microcirculatory vascular architecture alterations and the pathological mechanism of the non reflow phenomenon further experiments were performed on cats. Thirty minutes after reinfusion the brains were perfused with colloid carbon via the carotid arteries. For the detailed morphological study the brains were fixed in 10% formaldehyde solution. Various histological staining techniques were used to show and quantitate the vascular and neuro-glial changes.[28]

Non-perfused brain regions were found in the cerebral cortex in the fronto-parietal paracentral regions and in the temporomedio-basal regions. The circulation of the cerebellum was particularly seriously affected since around 50-70% of the cerebellar surface was unperfused with colloid carbon. Non-perfused regions were also observed in caudate nucleus, globus pallidus, thalamus, hypothalamus, septal regions, dorsal and ventral hypocampus as well as in the mesencephalon. In the majority of experiments there were no unperfused regions in the medulla oblongata. Our histological studies show that these changes can be attributed mostly to intravascular sludging and local vasospasm. Due to the lack of blood-perfusion severe hypoxic neuronal changes developed in laminae 3-5 of the cerebral cortex, in Purkinje cells and in cells of the inferior olive, basal nuclei and reticular formation.

Since the classic studies of Nothnagel and Hurtle[29] in the last century and Chorobsky and Penfield[30] in the early 1930's an increasing number of studies have demonstrated both sympathetic and parasympathetic mechanisms involved in cerebrovascular control. Kovach et al,[31] in 1954 showed that besided sympathetic or parasympathetic nerve stimulation direct stimulation of the pial vessels by catecholamines also caused changes in the cerebral vascular smooth muscle tone. In cross-circulation experiments, in which the brain of the recipient dog was hemodynamically isolated from the trunk and perfused by a donor dog, epinephrine or norepinephrine injection to the recipient's trunk caused a significant increase in its total cerebral blood flow.[31]

Phenoxybenzamine (PBZ) pretreatment is known to have a pronounced protective effect against shock and to inhibit the development of an isoelectric EEG. PBZ produces vasodilatation and a raising of CBF in dogs[12,18,32] and is most effective when given by the intracarotid route.[7,12] In the following studies cerebral blood flow (total and regional) was measured in PBZ pretreated baboons before, and during bleeding and after reinfusion.

PBZ pretreatment significantly influenced CBF during hemorrhagic hypotension. In 6 baboons pretreated with 5 mg/kg PBZ, CBF measured with the ^{133}Xe method did not increase during the first bleeding period at 55 mm Hg MAP; on the contrary, there was a significant rise in flow. During the whole second bleeding period at 55 mm Hg MAP, the CBF remained at control level. After reinfusion it stayed 50% above the pre-bleeding flow level.

Pressure dependent CBF was significantly different after the hemorrhagic shock had developed, and reduction of blood flow through the brain had already started at an MAP of 80-90 mm Hg. Application of PBZ broadened the pressure/flow plateau. In hemorrhagic shock, PBZ pretreatment prevented the pressure dependent decrease in blood flow at MAP levels of 35 mm Hg.

PBZ had a protective effect also against the reduction in rCBF measured with ^{14}C-antipyrine and against the development of focal cortical patchy ischemic areas characteristic of untreated hemorrhagic shock. Neither did the subcortical nuclei, the brainstem and cerebellum show any flow reduction.

The electrocorticogram of the PBZ pretreated shock group did not show significant changes during hypovolemia or after reinfusion. Arterial and cerebral venous pH was significantly less decreased and arterial lactate significantly less raised (6.99 $\pm$ 0.82 mM/l) in PBZ pretreated than in untreated baboons during shock.

The effect of somatic afferent impulses in the regulation of CBF has been much less studied than the role of the vegetative nerves. According to some recent data[33,34] somatic afferent stimulation causes significant changes in the distribution of the lactate and catecholamine content of the brain. In addition to the changes in chemical composition, sciatic nerve stimulation results in functional changes as well, i.e. a specific type of evoked potentials can be recorded in the hypothalamus as shown by Dora et al.[9]

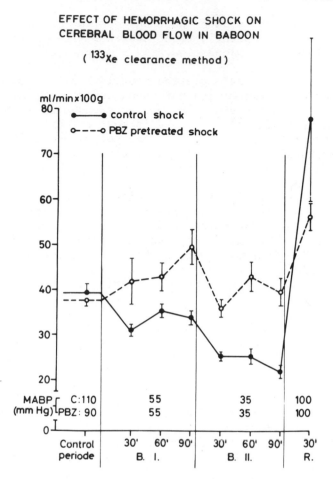

Fig. 2   Cerebral blood flow in the control period, during bleeding
and after reinfusion in control /●———●/ and PBZ pretreated
/O----O/ shock.

In spite of these data one of the most important questions is
still open: does the anatomically abundant innervation of the
dural and pial vessels and of the intracerebral arterioles have any
functional role in the resting tone of the cerebrovascular smooth
muscle and in the autoregulation of CBF?

In addition to the inherent theoretical difficulties, several
methodological considerations present a problem, thus there is a
great deal of contradictory data concerning the effect of nerve
stimulation on CBF.   This may be due in part to the fact that the
experiments were performed under conditions in which cerebral perfusion pressure (i.e. MABP) and arterial Pco_2 were not controlled.
Changes in these parameters occurred during stimulation and the

results are therefore misleading. Any increase in the arterial
pressure or in arterial Pco_2 value can decrease or even totally
blur any vasoconstrictor effect of the stimulation.

The aim of our present work was to study the effect of nociceptive somatic afferent stimulation on the local thalamic and
hypothalamic blood flow and tissue Po_2 in dogs in which arterial
blood pressure, Pco_2 and pH were kept constant.[35]

The experiments were performed on 20 dogs of both sexes
(average weight 8.13 kg) anesthetized with 10 mg/kg i.v. of
chloralose. Combined platinum + gold electrodes were implanted
4-6 days before the experiments, using stereotaxic coordinates, into
the ventral posterolateral nucleus of the thalamus (R:18, L:8,
V:16 mm) and into the ventromedial nucleus of the hypothalamus
(R:19, L:2, V:16 mm) in order to determine regional blood flow and
tissue Po_2 in these areas. The diameter of the double electrode
was 200 μm and it was insulated with Araldite or teflon. The
length of the active surface of the electrode tip was 1.5 mm. Both
tissue Po_2 and regional cerebral blood flow measurements were performed polarographically, the latter by using Aukland's hydrogen gas
clearance technique.[36]

Sciatic nerves were prepared on both sides in order to stimulate somatic afferent C fibers. The parameters of simulation were
20 V, 300 msec, 15 Hz for 3 min. Arterial blood pressure was
stabilized with an Engelking and Willig's modified buffer reservoir
system and was recorded on a polygraph. Heparin was given intra-
venously in a dose of 500 I.U./kg. In order to stabilize arterial
blood Pco_2 and pH levels the dogs were immobilized with Flaxedil
2 mg/kg i.v. and the rate and volume of artificial respiration were
adjusted according to the changes of the Pco_2 level in the expired
air, measured continuously by means of an infrared gas analyzer.
Arterial blood samples were taken from the brachial artery for pH
and Pco_2 analysis in the initial slope period of each flow measurement. Histological identification of the electrode sites was
carried out macroscopically after the experiments using the
methylene blue technique. Ipsilateral sciatic nerve stimulation
caused a 33% contralateral and 27% ipsilateral decrease of the
control thalamic blood flow value of 42 ± 2 ml/100 g/min. Since
arterial blood pressure was kept constant and showed practically
no change, reduced blood flow must be a consequence of the marked
(48% and 40% respectively) increase in peripheral vascular resistance in this area.

Tissue Po_2 in the thalamic VPL nucleus showed a short and
immediate increase 6 sec after the onset of stimulation. This
increase was 14.2% (n=12) in ipsilateral and 11 ± 2% (n=10) in
contralateral stimulation. The duration of this increase was no
longer than 10 sec. (Values are expressed in percentage changes

relative to the control value taken as 100%). This transient
increase was followed by a decline in tissue Po_2 reaching its lowest value around 60 sec (ipsilateral stimulation: 19 ± 2%, n=12,
contralateral stimulation: 16 ± 3%, n=10).

Hypothalamic blood flow decreased by 18% in both cases
(control values: 59 ± 5.0 and 80 ± 7.0 ml/ 100 g/min. respectively).
These changes are statistically significant. At the same time
other measured parameters (MABP, arterial Pco_2 and pH) remained
unaltered.

Cerebrovascular resistance in the ventromedial hypothalamic
area rose by 22% under the effect of ipsilateral and by 23% under
that of contralateral somatic afferent stimulation.

Hypothalamic Po_2 changes were quite similar to those of the
thalamus. The short initial increase (ipsilateral stimulation:
15 ± 1%, n=12, contralateral stimulation 11 ± 2%, n=10) was
followed by a marked decrease during the 45 sec of stimulation
(ipsilateral: 25 ± 2%, n=12, and contralateral stimulation: 19 ±
2%, n=10). After this decline the Po_2 curve tended to return to
its original value.

Blood flow in the white matter decreased by 15% relative to the
initial 21 ± 1.0 ml/100 g/min control value and cerebrovascular
resistance increased by 24% during ipsilateral somatic afferent
stimulation. Contralateral stimulation caused no significant
change in the white matter flow and resistance. MABP, arterial
Pco_2 and pH remained unchanged in both cases.

The parameters of prolonged sciatic nerve stimulation were the
same as those used by Evans.[37] According to his data, one can
stimulate in this way, with careful preparation, the somatic
afferent C fibers carrying nociceptive impulses to the CNS. One
can presume that if C fiber stimulation causes changes in the
regional distribution of CBF, this can also happen in shock conditions where somatic afferentation is increased in painful injuries.

According to the above results, local peripheral resistance
increased and local blood flow decreased in each area studied under
the influence of prolonged ipsilateral sciatic nerve stimulation.
Blood flow decreased more in the thalamic than in the hypothalamic
area, and the smallest changes were observed in the white matter.

It should be emphasized that the results presented here were
obtained in dogs whose blood pressure, arterial Pco_2 and pH were
contolled. In some experiments the continuous control of these
parameters temporarily failed. In those cases a marked increase in
rCBF and tissue Po_2 was noted simultaneously with a significant

elevation of mean arterial pressure during stimulation in each region studied.

Tissue Po_2 decreased in both the thalamic and hypothalamic regions during somatic afferent stimulation. As in the case of local blood flow changes, ipsilateral stimulation was more effective than contralateral. According to our data, the amplitude of Po_2 oscillations in brain tissue decreased significantly during somatic afferent stimulation, while the frequency remained unchanged.[38] Our results corroborate the view of Burgess[39] that oxygen cycles are not random and independent but are coupled from same central source.

CEREBRAL METABOLISM IN SHOCK

Cerebral blood flow, metabolism and electrical activity are tightly coupled processes. Severe decrease in CBF or dysfunction of cerebral tissue metabolism can both lead to the death of neurons. We have shown earlier that brain damage occurring in shock contributes to the irreversibility of this process.[32] To clarify the mechanism of brain injury in shock it would be fundamental to know the sequence of CBF, metabolic and electrical activity changes and furthermore to find out the primary changes initiating neuronal damage. To answer these questions in the following part of the paper four series of experimental results will be discussed.

In the first group of cats regional cerebral glucose metabolism was studied by ^{14}C-deoxyglucose autoradiography.

In the second group of experiments cerebral metabolism and vascular volume were investigated by using modified Chance surface fluororeflectometry.[40,41] In the third and fourth series of experiments the function and the ultrastructure of cerebrocortical mitochondria isolated from ischemic brains and from the brains of animals who had suffered hemorrhagic shock were analyzed.[42,43,44,45]

As we have shown before, using the ^{14}C-antipyrine autoradiographic technique, certain brain regions became unperfused in hemorrhagic shock. In our earlier studies[10,46] the hexokinase activity of the brain from animals in shock was higher than in control rats. To get information on the regional differences in glucose metabolism in shock and to study hexokinase in situ the ^{14}C-deoxyglucose autoradiographic technique was used in cat experiments.[27,47] The cats were anesthetized with 60 mg/kg i.p. α-D-glucochloralose, immobilized with 5 mg/kg Flaxedil and artificially ventilated. The shock model and the recorded parameters were the same as in the baboon experiments.

Normal cerebral metabolic rate of glucose (CMRG) values in cats in 50 structures have been studied in the cerebral and cerebellar cortex, basal ganglia, hypothalamus, midbrain, pons and medulla.

In two experiments out of five the CMRG values did not differ significantly from the controls. The values measured in the cerebral cortex were slightly reduced; usually the tops of the gyri were more affected than the sulci. The EEG, although severely depressed was maintained throughout the experiment.

In two other experiments the autoradiograms showed patchy areas with very small activity. These areas occurred mostly in the cortical structures and basal ganglia. A few appeared in the cerebellar cortex also. The optical density (and the CMRG values) of the surrounding areas sometimes showed high values, comparable to the control ones, in some cases they were even higher. Parts of the caudate nucleus exhibited extremely high optical density (retained capacity for compensatory anaerobic metabolism). The overall picture showed a reduced activity to less than 60% of the control values. Much less affected were the midbrain and brainstem. Towards the end of bleeding the EEG went flat in both cases.

In one experiment, which presumably represents a severe state of shock there was a marked decrease of CMRG. Most of the structures did not show any sign of activity, except some part of the caudate nucleus and the hypothalamus. The midbrain retained some activity, the pons and the medulla seemed to be fairly intact. In this case the EEG ceased early in the bleeding period.

These results show that the regional distribution of decreased cerebral glucose metabolism roughly agrees with the non-perfused brain regions. PBZ pretreatment prevented both the local CBF and glucose metabolism disturbances (Hamar, Kollai, Kovach and Reivich, unpublished).

In the following experiment in vivo optical measurements were performed on cats, anesthetized with 60 mg/kg α-D-glucochloralose, immobilized with 2-4 mg/kg Flaxedil and artificially ventilated. A glass window holding the two stimulating electrodes was implanted into the parietal bone for the surface fluoro-reflectometry. In order to avoid spurious NADH changes caused by cerebrocortical blood content alterations the correction method of Harbig et al,[48] was used.

Hemorrhagic shock was induced by bleeding the animal into a reservoir-buffer system through the femoral artery. Arterial blood pressure was decreased to 30 mm Hg and was maintained at this level by the buffer system until 50-80% of the shed blood was spontaneously taken back by the animal. Following the bleeding period the blood

remained in the reservoir, was reinfused and the animals were kept
alive for a period of one hour. During the experiments the
following tests were applied:

1/   1-2 min electrical stimulation of the brain cortex;
2/   injection of 1 ml physiological saline solution into the
     lingual artery;
3/   1-2 min nitrogen respiration.

In Fig. 3 the effect of electrical stimulation of the cortex
is shown on the cerebrocortical corrected NADH fluorescence and
reflectance. The curves were obtained in a carefully prepared
brain in the control period. The stimulation induced NADH was
calculated by using the correction factor determined at the
plateau phase of the changes.[49,50,51,52,53] The reduction
occurring during stimulation can be ascribed to an increased rate
of aerobic glycolysis and not to tissue hypoxia since Pco_2 increased during electrical stimulation of the cortex.

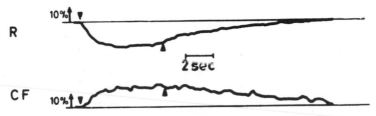

Fig. 3 Reflectance (R) and corrected fluorescence (CF=real NADH)
changes in the cat brain cortex during electrical stimulation of
the cortex in a single experiment. These curves were obtained in
animals with no known damage of the brain. The arrows mark the
start and the end of stimulation. Note: the corrected fluorescence
curve was calculated by using a "k" factor determined at the plateau
phase of the reflectance curve.

The mean values of reflectance, fluorescence and corrected
fluorescence changes obtained during stimulation in controls,
during bleeding and after reinfusion are shown in Fig. 4. As was
demonstrated in the original recording at normal arterial blood
pressure (MABP: 130 mm Hg), electrical stimulation of the cortex
resulted in a reflectance decrease and NADH fluorescence increase
(corrected fluorescence). In the early period of bleeding (B. 30-60)
electrical stimulation of the cortex induced entirely different
vascular and redox changes as compared to the control responses,
i.e. there was a marked NADH oxidation and a small reflectance
decrease during stimulation.[51,54]

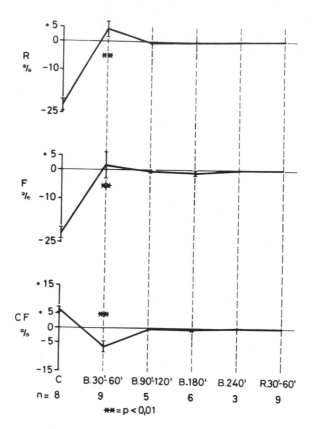

Fig. 4 Mean values of the reflectance (R), fluorescence (F) and corrected fluorescence (CF) changes induced by electrical stimulation of the cortex at normal arterial blood pressure, during bleeding (B) and after reinfusion (R). The vertical bars on the mean values represent the ± SE of mean. Parameters of the stimulation were the following: 10-15 V; 0.5 msec; 15 Hz square wave electric impulses.

According to the in vitro experiments of Chance and Williams[55] NADH oxidation can occur in case of ADP-stimulated respiration or in case of decelerated electron transport because of the lack of substrate. It is hard to explain our NADH oxidation by these in vitro results since at 30 mm Hg MABP the cerebral cortex is hypoxic and the blood glucose level 2 or 3 times higher than at normal arterial pressure. In the later phases of hypotension and after reinfusion of the shed blood, electrical stimulation of the cortex failed to evoke reflectance and responses. The disappearance of these responses may be explained by the maximal dilatation of the cerebrocortical blood vessels or by the severely depressed CBF. Deterioration of the blood perfusion of the brain during bleeding

may be indicated by the anoxic redox and vascular responses. As
seen in Fig. 5 at normal arterial blood pressure N_2 anoxia resulted
in a 28% corrected fluorescence increase and in a considerable
vasodilatation (reflectance decrease). In the early phase of
bleeding (B. 30-60) even though the cerebrocortical blood vessels
were nearly maximally dilated the cortex was hypoxic since N_2-gas
inhalation induced a much slighter vasodilatation (reflectance
decrease) and NAD reduction than in controls. During the later
phases of arterial hypotension the anoxic reflectance and redox
responses continued to decrease and finally vanished.[51,53,56]
After reinfusion, N_2 anoxia produced no reflectance decrease and
the NADH increase was small as compared to the controls. At the
bottom of Fig. 5 the mean values of "k" (correction factor) are
shown. The "k" factor can be determined only when there are
fluorescence and reflectance changes in the cortex during flushing
the lingual artery with physiological saline solution. The de-
clining number of "k" values averaged during bleeding shows that
in those cases where "k" could not be determined the cortical
regions were not perfused with blood. In experiments where the
flush reaction was absent we never obtained redox changes during
N_2 anoxia, indicating that the cortical tissue was already maximally reduced because of the microvascular defect. Reinfusion of
the shed blood did not result in reperfusion of the cortical
regions in the majority of the experiments. In the remaining experiments some minimal blood flow reappeared after reinfusion as
indicated by slight redox changes during anoxia as compared to the
controls. On the other hand, besides the severe CBF disturbances
in shock the brain mitochondrial could also have been irreversibly
damaged since there were no oxido-reduction changes during stimulation even in experiments where some blood flow reappeared after
reinfusion. In Fig. 6 anoxic corrected fluorescence (KF) responses
obtained in a typical experiment are shown. The relatively late
changes in corrected fluorescence during N_2 breathing were due to
the dead space between the animal and the gas tank. In this experiment corrected fluorescence increased by 35% during N_2 anoxia
in the control period but after switching to air, NADH reoxidation
was rapid and complete in 1-2 min. In the course of hypovolemic
hypotension, the amplitude of the anoxic NADH increase diminished
considerably and the kinetics of these curves changed markedly.
Reoxidation was slow and a significant undershoot (oxidation)
appeared in the recovery phase from anoxia in the periods between
B. 30-60 and B. 180. The amplitudes of undershoots varied between
10-20%. The long lasting reoxidation period subsequent to anoxia
at B. 30-60 clearly demonstrates the early disturbance of mitochondrial electron transport. Since the reoxidation time became
gradually slower during the next two periods of hypotension it
seems that the deterioration of mitochondrial electron transport
capacity depends very much on the duration of the hypotensive
period. In the last period of bleeding and after reinfusion no

NADH change occurred during N_2-gas breathing. This indicates
again as was demonstrated in Fig. 5 that the tissue redox level was
already maximally shifted towards reduction before N_2 anoxia was
applied, because of the lack of circulation.

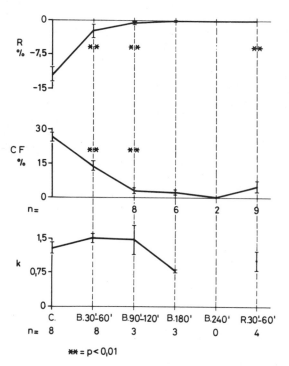

Fig. 5 Mean values of reflectance (R) and corrected fluorescence
(CF) changes induced by nitrogen anoxia at normal arterial blood
pressure (C), during bleeding (B) and after reinfusion (R). At the
bottom of the Figure the mean values of the correction factor (k)
are shown from the same periods but before nitrogen anoxia.
Vertical lines on the mean values represent the ± SE of mean.
Note: The "k" can be determined only when there are fluorescence
and reflectance changes in the brain cortex during flushing of the
lingual artery. The decrease in number of "k" values averaged
during bleeding shows the increasing number of experiments where
the control regions studied became unperfused.

    These in vivo results are in good agreement with our previous
in vitro studies made on isolated mitochondria where we tried to
correlate the severity of shock with the damage to the respiratory
activity of the brain mitochondria.[44,45] The mitochondria were

prepared according to Clark and Nicklas[57] from both hemispheres
of the cat brains after bleeding for various periods of time.
The severity of shock was classified according to the blood volume
retaken by the animals from the shed blood.

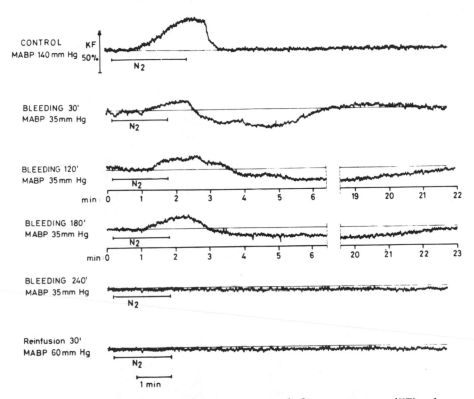

Fig. 6   Anoxic cerebrocortical corrected fluorescence (KF) changes
in a single experiment before and during bleeding and after reinfusion.   The duration of nitrogen anoxia is marked by horizontal
lines, the calibration of corrected fluorescence curves is represented by a vertical arrow at the top of the figure.

On the basis of these criteria the experiments were divided
into 3 groups, namely: control=no bleeding, 0-15% reuptake,
15-50%, and 50-100% reuptake.   Mitochondrial respiration was measured
polarographically in the presence of different substrate couples.
ADP and DNP were added to the medium containing the mitochondria
to stimulate mitochondrial respiration.   The value of the respiratory control ratio (RCR) which is equal to the ADP stimulated
consumption/St4 oxygen consumption was calculated in every case.
In Fig. 7 the St4-ADP- and DNP-stimulated oxygen consumption and

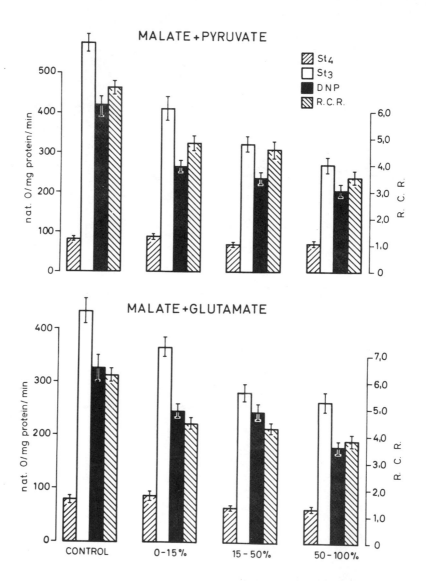

Fig. 7 Effect of spontaneous reinfusion on the oxygen uptake of cat brain mitochondrial incubated with 1 mM Malate+5 mM Pyruvate (upper part) and 5 mM Glutamate+1 mM Malate (lower part). The incubation media contained: 0.01 M triphosphate, 58 mM KCl, 6 mM MgCl$_2$. The pH was 7.4. The St4, St3, and DNP stimulated mitochondrial respiration was measured polarographically at 37°C.

RCR values are demonstrated in the presence of Malate 1 mM+Pyruvate 5 mM as well as of Malate 1 mM+Glutamate 5 mM substrate couples in different degrees of shock. The first group is the control one, in the second group the spontaneous reinfusion was 10%, in the third group it was 34% and finally in the fourth group it was 70%.

As can be seen the ADP and DNP stimulated respiration as well as the RCR values were depressed even in the early shock group and the reduction of these values was most pronounced in the last group. Since the St4 respiration did not change significantly in either of the shock groups as compared to the control value the RCR decrease is due to diminished respiratory capacity. The failure of the mitochondrial energy-linked function in shock has also been demonstrated[58,59,12] in liver, kidney and recently in brain tissue.[60]

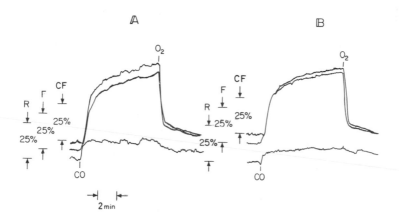

Fig. 8   A typical recording of a CO-O_2 cycle in the same rat brain cortex 10 min (A) and 16 hours (B) after the death of the animal. The cerebrocortical fluorescence (F) and reflectance (R) measurements were performed by using a light pipe fluoro-reflectometer. The perfusion of the cerebral cortex with CO and O_2 gases was made through a teflon chamber attached to the end of the light pipe. The corrected fluorescence (CF) trace was calculated by subtracting the reflectance trace from the fluorescence with a ratio of 1:1.

It seems very interesting that brain mitochondria are much more resistant to pure brain ischemia than to hemorrhagic shock. We have shown that the capability of brain mitochondria to transport electrons is maintained even 24 hours following death.[61] In Fig. 8 cerebrocortical oxido-reduction changes induced by blowing CO and O_2 gases onto the brain surface are shown immediately and 16 hours following the death of the animal. As can be seen in the Figure

the amplitude of the oxido-reduction cycles did not change
appreciably with time. The amplitude of these postmortem oxido-
reduction cycles is comparable to the changes that can be obtained
in vivo by anoxic anoxia.

In another experimental series we have studied the effect of
long lasting brain ischemia on the cerebrocortical mitochondrial
function and ultrastructure.[42,43] The mitochondria were isolated
from rat brains left in the skull at 20-22° for a period of 1, 4
and 12 hours after decapitation. Preparation of the mitochondria
and O_2 consumption measurements were the same as in the shock
experiments. For electron microscopy the mitochondrial fractions
were fixed by adding a few drops of the fraction to Karnovsky's
fixative. After fixation, fractions were pelleted and postfixed
with 1% osmic acid and embedded in Durcupan. Electronmicrographs
were made with a JEOL 100B electron microscope. After one hour
of ischemia neither the respiration nor the morphology of the
mitochondria was obviously altered. There was a strong correlation
between the ultrastructural changes and RCR value of mitochondria,
namely the RCR decreased in proportion to the increasing number of
the so called 'light type' of mitochondria.[43]

SUMMARY

In conclusion our results clearly suggest that vital functions
of the brain, in spite of its well developed autoregulation are
impaired during prolonged hypovolemic conditions.

Regional cerebral blood flow measured by the ^{133}Xe clearance
and ^{14}C-antipyrine autoradiographic techniques demonstrated a
progressive reduction in CBF, with the development of patchy and
circumscribed ischemic areas during hemorrhagic shock which persisted after reinfusion.

In our experience the regional distribution of the underperfused
regions cannot be explained solely in terms of boundary zones
between the main distribution fields of major cerebral arteries.

In our experiments PBZ pretreatment significantly influenced
CBF changes during hemorrhagic hypotension. CBF did not decrease
during bleeding, on the contrary, there was a significant rise in
flow. After reinfusion it was 50 percent above the pre-bleeding
flow level. PBZ had a protective effect also against the reduction
in rCBF measured with ^{14}C-antipyrine and against the development
of focal cortical ischemia characteristic of untreated hemorrhagic
shock. Subcortical nuclei, the brain stem and cerebellum also did
not show flow reduction.

Regional cerebral glucose metabolism, studied by ^{14}C-deoxy-glucose autoradiography decreased or in serious shock involving a flat EEG, was near zero in cortex, while the caudate nucleus and hypothalamus exhibited moderate glucose metabolism, and pons and brain stem were near normal. PBZ had a protective effect also against the reduction in regional glucose metabolism in shock.

All our results suggest the involvement of sympathetic nervous system and catecholamine metabolism in the impairment of cerebral microcirculation during hemorrhagic shock. The formation of sludge in skeletal muscle after hemorrhage is prevented by adrenalectomy and according to the available results, the regional cerebral microcirculatory defect develops through sludge formation. The unevenly distributed local brain damage could be the background of the functional impairment. The focal appearance suggests that, in addition to generalized (blood borne) changes, local factors play an important role in the production of patchy ischemic areas in the brain.

Afferent neural nociceptive input to the brain seems to be elevated during shock. It may be presumed that this leads to increased tissue metabolism and the accumulation of metabolites. The low flow combined with elevated neuronal activity and cellular metabolism produces an imbalance between oxygen delivery and oxygen utilization. The local nature of afferent activation of the CNS can explain the regional impairment in the brain tissue.

Nociceptive afferent stimulation increases while denervation of the carotid sinus or transsection of vagus or spinal afferent pathways decreases, sensitivity to shock. We have presented further evidence that stimulation of the C fibres of the sciatic nerve reduces the cerebral local blood flow and the tissue Po_2 in the n. VPL thalami and V med hypothalami in cardiovasculary restricted (stabilized blood pressure) animals. There is no doubt that hypovolemia is in fact a cardiovascular restriction. According to our results afferent input plays an important role in the regional impairment of the CNS.

The results presented suggest a higher susceptibility of the brain to hemorrhagic shock evoked hypoxia compared to total brain ischemia. The difference may be explained by the following differences. In brain ischemia the electrical activity of the cerebral neurons disappears very rapidly. In contrast to this the cortical electrical activity increases in the early period of bleeding because of the enhanced afferent input and stops only after prolonged bleeding in the last period of hemorrhagic shock.

In total brain ischemia the brain is excluded from the systemic circulation and different toxic substances released or produced in

the brain and even more in other organs cannot reach other regions
and have a much smaller toxic effect compared to hemorrhagic shock.
In hemorrhagic shock the harmful effect of these substances is
probably more pronounced because of the damage to the blood brain
barrier.

Our in vivo fluorometric, reflectometric blood flow results
are in good agreement with the in vitro experiments on isolated
brain mitochondrial function. They both suggest the early damage
to the energy linked function of the brain mitochondria during
hemorrhagic shock. Mitochondria isolated from shocked animals
showed pronounced inhibition of State 3 respiration activity. The
inhibition was more and more pronounced in time during hypotension.
Differences between hypovolemic, ischemic and hypoxic damage in
mitochondrial function suggest that tissue hypoxia alone is not
the factor producing irreversible damage in cerebral mitochondrial
function. PBZ prevented the in vivo monitored fluorometric cortical NAD reduction during hemorrhagic hypotension. Electronmicro-
scopic studies suggest a membrane stabilizing effect of PBZ
treatment in shock.

We can conclude that much basic scientific work needs to be
done to understand the nature of the role of the developing
cerebral dysfunction. There is no doubt that insufficiency
of the cerebrocortical and hypothalamic regulatory mechanisms
can contribute to the development of irreversible shock. In other
words, failure of the body suffering from shock to restore the
homeostatic equilibrium can be attributed to the inadequacy of the
central nervous servocontrol system.

This work was partly supported by NINCDS Grant No. 10939.

REFERENCES

1. Crile, G.W.: An experimental research into surgical shock.
    Philadelphia, Lippincott. p. 160, 1899.

2. Slome, D., O'Shaughnessy, L.: The nervous factor in traumatic
    shock. Brit. J. Surg. 25:900-909, 1938.

3. Overman, R. R., Wang, S. C.: The contributory role of the
    afferent nervous factor in experimental shock: sublethal
    hemorrhagic and sciatic stimulation. Amer. J. Physiol. 148:
    289-295, 1947.

4. Arshavskaya, E. J.: On the mechanism of origin of experimental
    shock in the presence of nocriceptive irritation in different
    age periods (Neuroscien) Fiziol. Us. Moscow, 36:333-341, 1950.

5. Guthrie, C. C.: Experimental shock. J. Amer. Med. Assoc.
    pp.1394-1398, 1917.

6. Popov, L. I.: Shok i krovoposjerya. Tr. Voenno-med. Ord.
    Lenina Akad. S. M. Kirova 102:108-144, 1959.

7. Kovach, A.G.B., Fonyo, A.: Metabolic responses to injury in
    cerebral tissue. In: The Biochemical Response to Injury,(Ed.)
    H. B. Stoner, C. I. Threlfall. Oxford: Blackwell.pp. 129-
    160, 1960.

8. Kovach, A.G.B.: Importance of nervous and metabolic changes
    in the development of irreversibility in experimental shock.
    Part 3, Fed. Proc. 20:122-137, 1961.

9. Dora, E., Kovach, A.G.B., Nyary, I.: Hypothalamic and cortical
    evoked potentials in hemorrhagic shock. In: Neurohumoral
    and Metabolic Aspects of Injury. (Ed.) A.G.B. Kovach, H.B.
    Stoner, J. J. Spitzer, New York and London: Plenum Press,
    pp. 481-487, 1973.

10. Kovach, A.G.B., Fonyo, A., Vittay, T., and Pogatsa,G.: Oxygen
    and glucose consumption and hexokinase activity in vitro of
    brain tissue of rats in traumatic shock. Acta. Physiol.
    Acad. Sci. Hung. 11:173-180, 1957.

11. Kovach, A.G.B., Fonyo, A., Kovach, E.: Cerebral phosphate
    metabolism in traumatic shock. Acta Physiol. Acad. Sci.
    Hung. 16:157-164, 1959.

12. Kovach, A.G.B., Mitsanyi, A., Monos, E., Nyary, I., Sulyok,
    A.: Control of organ blood flow following hemorrhage. Avd.
    Exp. Med. Biol. 33:1-17, 1973.

13. Biro, J., Buki, B., Kovach, A.G.B.: Changes of the higher
    nervous activity following ischemic shock in the rat. Acta
    Physiol. Acad. Sci. Hung. 10:277-289, 1956.

14. Kovach, A.G.B., Rohein, P.S., Iranyi, M., Cserhati, E.,
    Gosztonyi, G., Kovach, E.: Circulation and metabolism in the
    head of the dog in ischemic shock. Acta Physiol. Acad. Sci.
    Hung. 15:217-229, 1959.

15. Williams, L.F., Jr.: Hemorrhagic shock as a source of uncon-
    sciousness. Surgical Clin. N. Am. 48:263-272, 1968.

16. Kovach, A.G.B., Sandor, P.: Cerebral blood flow and brain
    function during hypertension and shock. Ann. Rev. of Physiol.
    39:571-596, 1976.

17. Kovach, A.G.B.: Az idegrendszer schockban. Orvoskepzes 41: 321-
     332, 1966.

18. Kovach, A.G.B.: Circulatory adjustment and its comparative
     physiological aspects after changing blood volume. In:
     Int. Cong. IUPS 24. Wash. DC 6:35-36 (Abstr.), 1968.

19. Nyary, I., Dora, E., Sandor, P., Kovach, A.G.B., Reivich, M.:
     Cerebral blood flow and metabolism in hemorrhagic shock in
     the baboon. In: Third Tbilisi Symp. on Brain Blood Supply,
     Budapest; Akademiai Kiado (In press), 1976.

20. Byary, I. Maklari, E., Kovach, A.G.B.: Hypothalamic blood
     flow in hemorrhagic shock after administration of buffer
     solutions. Acta Physiol. Acad. Sci. Hung. 1976 (In press).

21. Sandor, P. et al: Modifications locales de la circulation
     cerebrale dans diverses regions du cerveau pendant l'emorra-
     gic. In: Regional Congr. Int. Union Phys. Sci. Brasow, Abstr.
     p. 586, 1970.

22. Sandor, P., Kardos, G., Thuroczi, L., Berczi, I. Nyary, I.,
     Sulyok, A., Kovach, A.G.B.: Cortical hypothalamic and
     hypophyseal blood flow during hemorrhagic shock. In: 25th.
     Int. Congr. Physiol. Sci. Munich, p. 49, 1971 (Abstr.).

23. Cantu, R.C., Ames, A., III: Experimental prevention of
     cerebral vascular obstruction introduced by ischemia. J.
     Neurosrug. 30:50-54, 1969.

24. Sandor, P., Tomka, N., Kovach, A.G.B.: Regional cerebral blood
     flow during incompatible blood transfusion. 41st. Ann. Conf.
     Hung. Physiol. Soc. Szeged. Abstr. Acta Physiol. Acad. Sci.
     Hung. (In press).

25. Mchedlishvili, G.I., Garfunkel, M.L., Ormotsadze, L.G.:
     Cerebral circulation under conditions of heterotransfusion
     shock. Pt. Fiziol. Eksp. Ter. 16:25-31.

26. Kassel, N. F., Reivich, M.: On line analysis of cerebral
     blood flow clearance curves. In: Brain and Blood Flow. (Ed.)
     R.W.R. Russel, London: Pitman Medical Publishers, p. 34-38,
     1971.

27. Reivich, M., Jehle, J., Sokoloff, L. et al,: Measurement of
     regional cerebral blood flow with ^{14}C- antipyrine in awake
     cats. J. Appl. Physiol. 27:296-300, 1969.

28. Nagy, A., Dora, E., Kovach, A.G.B.: Selective vulnerability of the brain in hemorrhagic shock. In: Magyar Elettani Tarsasag Vandorgyulese, 42. Eloadaskivonatok, Budapest, p. 187, 1976.

29. Nothnagel, H.: Die vasomotorischen Nerves der Gehirnegefabe. Beitrag zur Lehre von der Epilepsie. Virchows Arch. Pathol. Anat. Physiol. Klin. Med. 1:203-213, 1867.

30. Chorobski, J., and Penfield, W.: Cerebral vasodilator nerves and their pathway from the medulla oblongata. Arch. Neurol. Psychiat. Chicago Arch. Neurol. Psychiat. 28:1257-1289, 1932.

31. Kovach, A.G.B., Menyhart, J., Kiss, S., Erdelyi, A., Kovach, E.: Untersuchungen uber die Ausbildung des irreversiblen Schockes. Acta Physiol. Acad. Sci. Hung. 5:Suppl. 33-34, 1954.

32. Kovach, A.G.B., Rohein, P.S., Iranyi, M., Kiss, S., Antal, J.: Effect of the isolated perfusion of the head on the development of ischaemic and hemorrhagic shock. Acta Physiol. Acad. Sci. Hung. 14:231-238, 1958.

33. Salford, L.G., Duggy, T.E., Plum, F.: Salford, L.G., Duffy, T.E., Plum, F.: Altered cerebral metabolism and blood flow in response to physiological stimulation. Stroke 4:361, 1973.

34. Matrosov, V.D.: The effect of sustained nociceptive stimulation on the adrenaline and noradrenaline contents in different brain areas and in adrenal glands of rats prior to and after removal of the upper cervical sympathetic ganglia. Sechenew Physiol. J. USSR 61:385, 1975.

35. Sandor, P., Demchenko, I.T., Kovach, A.G.B., Moszkalendo, Y.E.: Hypothalamic and thalamic blood flow and pO_2 changes during somatic afferent stimulation on blood pressure and blood gases in stabilized dogs. American J. Physiol. 1976 (In press).

36. Aukland, K. Bower, B.F., Berliner, R.W.: Measurement of Local Blood Flow with Hydrogen Gas. Circulation Research 14:164, 1964.

37. Evans, M.H.: The spinal pathways of the myelinated and the non-myelinated afferent nerve fibres that mediate reflex dilatation of the pupils. J. Physiol. 158:560, 1961.

38. Dmecsenko, I.T., Sandor, P., Moszkalenko, J.E., Kovach, A.G.B.: Izmemenija Krovotoka I Naprjazsenija Kiszlorada V Colovnom Mozge Pro Afferentnoj Szomaticseszkoj Sztimuljacii. Fiziol. Zs. I.M. Szecsenova, 61. pp. 1153-1159, 1975.

39. Burgess, D.W.: Correlation Between Oxygen Cycles in Contra-
     lateral Regions of the Brain, Stroke 3:374, 1973.

40. Chance, B., Mauriello, G. and Aubert, M.:ADP arrival at
     muscle mitochondria following a twitch. In: Muscle as a
     Tissue, (Ed.), K. Rodahl and S. Horvath. New York: McGraw,
     pp. 128-145, 1962.

41. Kovach, A.G.B., Dora, E., Eke, A., Gyulai, L.: Microcircula-
     tory effects on microfluorimetry. FASEB Oxygen Colloquium,
     Anaheim. Submitted to Fed. Proc. Anaheim, 1976.

42. Ikrenyi, K., Dora, E., Hajos, F., Kovach, A.G.B.: Agymitochon-
     driumok Funkcio es morfologiai intergritasanak post mortem
     vizsgalata. Acta Physiol. Acad. Sci. Hung. 1974 (In press).

43. Ikrenyi, I., Dora, E., Hajos, F., Kovach, A.G.B.: Metabolic
     and electron microscopic studies post mortem in brain
     mitochondria. In: Proc. 2nd. Int. Symp. on Oxygen Transport
     to Tissue. (Ed.) H. Bicher, D. Reneau, New York and London:
     Plenum Press, 1976.

44. Ikrenyi, K., Kovach, A., Somogyi, J.: Experimentalis Shockos
     Allatikbol Izolalt Agymitochondriumok Oxidacios Kepessege.
     In: Magyar Elettani Tarsasaga Vandorgyulese 38. Eloadaskivo-
     natok, Budapest, p. 85, 1972.

45. Ikrenyi, K., Kovach, A., Somogyi, J.: Agymitochondriumok
     Oxidacios Kepessegenek Valtozasa Verezteteses Shockban.
     In: Magyar Elettani Tarsasag Vandorgyulese 39. Eloadaski-
     vonatok, Pecs, p. 87, 1973.

46. Kovach, A.G.B., Fedina, L., Mitsanyi, A., Naszlady, A., Biro,
     Z.: Neurophysiological and circulatory changes in hemorrhagic
     shock. Excerpta Med. Int. Congr. Ser. 48:678, 1962.

47. Reivich, M., Kovach, A.G.B., Spitzer, J.J., Sandor, P.:
     Cerebral blood flow and metabolism in hemorrhagic shock in
     baboons. In: Neurohumoral and Metabolic Aspects of Injury.
     (Ed.) A.G.B. Kovach, H. B. Stoner, J.J. Spitzer, Plenum
     Press, New York and London. pp. 19-26, 1973.

48. Harbig, K., Reivich, M., Chance, B., Kovach, A.G.B.: Changes
     in pyridine nucleotide fluorescence in cerebral ischemia.
     In: Cerebral Vascular Diseases: Ninth Conference (Ed.).
     Whisnant and Sandok, New York, Grune & Stratton, pp. 251-
     255, 1975.

49.   Gyulai, L., Dora, E., Eke, A., Kovach, A.G.B.: Microvessel
      reactions and NAD-NADH changes in cat brain cortex during
      cortical stimulation under physiologic and hypercapnic
      conditions. Fed. Proc. 35: 524, 1976.

50.   Gyulai, L., Dora, E., Eke, A., Kovach, A.G.B.: Microvessel
      reactions and NAD-NADH changes in cat brain cortex during
      cortical sitmulation under normo-and hypercapnic conditions.
      In: Proc. 9th. World Conference of the European Microcircu-
      lation Society, Antwerp, 1976 (In press).

51.   Kovach, A.G.B., Dora, E., Gyulai, L., Eke, A.: Oxido-reduction
      state, hemoglobin content and blood flow in cat brain cortex
      during hemorrhagic shock and the effect of phenoxybenzamine
      pretreatment. Fed. Proc. 35:26, 1976.

52.   Kovach, A.G.B., Eke, A., Dora, E., Gyulai, L.: Correlation
      between the redox state, electrical activity and blood flow
      in cat brain cortex during hemorrhagic shock. In: Proc. 2nd.
      Int. Symp. on Oxygen Transport to Tissue. (Ed.) H. Bicher,
      D. Reneau. Plenum Press, New York and London, 1976.

53.   Kovach, A.G.B., Hamar, J., Nyary, I., Sandor, P., Reivich,
      M.: Cerebral blood flow and metabolism in hemorrhagic shock
      in the baboon. In: Abstr. Cerebral Blood Flow and Metabolism.
      Symp. Aviemore, p. 14, 1975.

54.   Dora, E., Chance, B., Kovach, A.G.B.: Locally induced NAD-NADH
      changes post-mortem in the rat brain cortex. Fed. Proc.
      35:829, 1976.

55.   Chance, B., Williams, G.R.: Respiratory enzymes in oxydative
      phosphorylation. J. Biol. Chem. 217:383-427, 1955.

56.   Dora, E., Eke, A., Gyulai, L., Kovach, A.G.B.: Effect of
      hemorrhagic shock on the oxido-reduction state and blood
      content of the cat cerebral cortex. Annual Meeting of the
      Hungarian Physiological Society, Szeged. Acta Physiol. Acad.
      Sci. Hung. 1975 (In press).

57.   Clark, J.B., Nicklas, W.I.: The metabolism of rat brain mito-
      chondria. Preparation and characterization. J. Biol. Chem.
      245:4724-4731, 1970.

58.   Mela, L., Bacalzo, L.V., Miller, L.D.: Defective oxidative
      metabolism of rat liver mitochondria in hemorrhagic and endo-
      toxon shock. Am. J. of Physiol. 220:571, 1971.

57.   Clark, J.B., Nicklas, W.I.: The metabolism of rat brain mito-
       chondria. Preparation and characterization. J. Biol. Chem.
       245:4724-4731, 1970.

58.   Mela, L., Bacalzo, L.V., Miller, L.D.: Defective oxidative
       metabolism of rat liver mitochondria in hemorrhagic and
       endotoxin shock. Am. J. of Physiol. 220:571, 1971.

59.   Mela, L., Crowe, W., Harbig, K., Wrobel-Kuhl, K., Kovach,
       A.G.B.: Inhibition of brain mitochondrial function and
       changes of tissue H+ and K+ concentration in hemorrhagic
       shock. Surg. Forum 26:51-53, 1974.

60.   Mela, L., Harbig, K., Kovach, A.G.B., Reivich, M.: Response
       of Brain mitochondria to hemorrhagic shock. J. Neurochemistry,
       1976 (In press).

61.   Dora, E., Gyulai, L., Eke, A., Kovach, A.G.B.: Redox state
       and blood content changes induced by electrical stimulation
       of the cat brain cortex in hemorrhagic shock. Annual Meeting
       of the Hungarian Physiological Society, Budapest, Acta
       Physiol. Acad. Sci. Hung. 1976 (In press).

ALTERED MITOCHONDRIAL METABOLISM IN CIRCULATORY SHOCK

Leena Mela

Harrison Department of Surgical Research
University of Pennsylvania
Philadelphia, Pennsylvania

Studies of mitochondrial function after circulatory shock, hemorrhagic or endotoxic, have revealed defective oxidative metabolism in several organs, such as the liver, kidney, and the brain (1,2,3). In this comment I would like to emphasize certain important aspects of these findings.

It is now clear, as has been shown by Dr. Kovach and his collaborators (4) as well as by us (3,5), that brain mitochondrial metabolism is not protected against damage and inhibition in circulatory shock. In actuality a significant inhibition of brain mitochondrial function was observed at 1.5 hours of hemorrhagic hypotension at 50 mm Hg mean arterial blood pressure (3,5). This is prior to any significant inhibition of liver or kidney mitochondrial functions. Heart and skeletal muscle mitochondria, on the other hand, are well protected against functional damage in circulatory shock (2,6).

The type of mitochondrial injury induced by circulatory shock has been fairly well characterized. The defect at the mitochondrial level is a failure in the oxidative phosphorylation pathways, not in the electron transfer chain per se. The two enzyme systems contributing to the inhibition are mitochondrial ATPase and adenine nucleotide translocase (1,2). Other energy-linked functions are also disturbed. Particularly Ca^{++} transport activity is inhibited early in shock (7). Thus this parameter constitutes the first indicator of mitochondrial membrane damage in shock.

The cellular etiology of mitochondrial dysfunction is still unresolved. Several contributing factors, however, have been identified. Organ ischemia is presumably an important factor.

Studies of complete ischemia of gerbil brain have shown that the mitochondrial inhibitions induced by circulatory shock and ischemia are very similar (8). Similarly, the fact that mitochondrial inhibition only occurs in organs whose blood flow is significantly reduced during shock indicates that ischemia might be an important etiologic factor. In addition, circulating septic components, such as the recently isolated septic peptides (Clowes, G., personal communication), which seem quite similar to the myocardial depressant factor (9), were shown to have an inhibitory effect on mitochondrial functions during State 3 respiration and Ca^{++} transport (Mela and Clowes, unpublished), thus bearing a close correlation with the type of mitochondrial inhibition seen after circulatory shock. On the other hand, lowered cellular pH, often suggested as one of the factors damaging to the mitochondrial function, can be ruled out at least in the brain. It was shown that before the brain pH dropped significantly, the mitochondrial function was already 60% inhibited (3,5).

Thus, although our knowledge of the various aspects of altered metabolism in shock-induced cellular injury is still limited, certain specifically altered reactions at the mitochondrial level are well characterized. Beyond a certain degree of inhibition these altered mitochondrial energy-linked reactions might form the basis of irreversibility in circulatory shock.

REFERENCES

1. Mela, L., Bacalzo, L. V., and Miller, L. D. Defective oxidative metabolism of rat liver mitochondria in hemorrhagic and endotoxin shock. Am. J. Physiol. 220:571-577, 1971.
2. Mela, L. Mitochondrial metabolic alterations in experimental circulatory shock. In Gram-Negative Bacterial Infections and Mode of Endotoxin Actions (Urbaschek, B., Urbaschek, R., and Neter, E., Eds.), pp. 288-295. Springer-Verlag, Wien, New York, 1975.
3. Mela, L., Crowe, W., Harbig, K., Wrobel-Kuhl, K., and Kovach, A. G. B. Inhibition of brain mitochondrial function and changes of tissue H^+ and K^+ concentration in hemorrhagic shock. Surg. Forum 26:51, 1975.
4. Kovach, A. G. B. Cerebral hemodynamic and metabolic alterations in hypovolemic shock. This volume.
5. Mela, L., Harbig, K., Kovach, A. G. B., and Reivich, M. Response of brain mitochondria to hemorrhagic shock. J. Neurochem., submitted.
6. Mela, L., Hinshaw, L. B., and Coalson, J. J. Correlation of cardiac performance, ultrastructural morphology, and mitochondrial function in endotoxemia in the dog. Circ. Shock 1:265-272, 1974.

7. Nicholas, G. G., Mela, L., and Miller, L. D. Early alterations
   in mitochondrial membrane transport during endotoxemia. J. Surg.
   Res. 16:375, 1974.
8. Ginsberg, M.D., Mela, L., Wrobel-Kuhl, K., and Reivich, M.
   Mitochondrial metabolism following bilateral cerebral ischemia
   in the gerbil. Ann. Neurol., submitted.
9. Lefer, A. M. Role of myocardial depressant factor in the patho-
   genesis of circulatory shock. Fed. Proc. 29:1836-1847, 1970.

DISCUSSION OF PRESENTATION BY A.G.B. KOVACH

James A. Spath, Jr.

Jefferson Medical College

Philadelphia, PA

Autoregulatory mechanisms tend to maintain cerebral blood flow during hemorrhagic shock. Cerebral blood flow is not significantly altered until the perfusion pressure falls below 70 mm Hg during hemorrhage. The mechanism of cerebral autoregulation during hemorrhagic hypotension is unclear, although both metabolic and myogenic components appear to mediate cerebral autoregulation.[1] Investigations by Dr. Kovach and others have observed that although total cerebral blood flow may only be moderately decreased in hemorrhage, areas of severe ischemia may be adjacent to more normally perfused tissue.[2] Such studies define the need for measuring regional cerebral blood flows as well as total cerebral blood flow in hemorrhagic shock. Using hydrogen washout and thermodilution techniques, Kovach et al.[2,3] demonstrated a 60% reduction in hypothalamic flow after hemorrhage to 35 mm Hg. The authors concluded that autoregulation in the hypothalamus during hemorrhage differed from other regions of the brain. In contrast, Slater et al.[4] using radioactive microspheres reported similar patterns of blood flow alterations in cerebellum, gray matter, white matter, and the hypothalamus of conscious dogs subjected to hemorrhage. The percentage of the cardiac output in all areas of the brain was increased three hours after hemorrhage to 50 mm Hg. Thereafter, the percentage of the cardiac output distributed within the brain declined. The development of similar patterns of regional cerebral blood flow with hemorrhage led Slater et al.[4] to suggest the presence of similar mechanisms regulating regional blood flow within the brain. Systemic and cerebral acidosis were implicated in cerebral vasodilation in the face of a maintained arterial P_{O_2} and decreased arterial P_{CO_2}. The decline in the percentage of cardiac output reaching the brain during prolonged hypotension may have been the result of extracerebral vasodilation or increased cerebral vascular resistance during

prolonged shock. From these studies of Kovach et al.[2] and Slater
et al.,[4] it is evident that differing determinations and interpretations of regional autoregulation of cerebral blood flow may be related to (a) the method of measurement, (b) the anesthetic used,
(c) the degree and duration of hypotension, (d) the pattern of bleed-
out and reinfusion and (e) regional differences in cerebral metabolism with developing ischemia.

For example, Marcus et al.[5] recently reported that chloralose
urethan anesthesia produced a 25% decrease in cerebral blood flow
with some redistribution of flow. Normalized to each respective
mean cerebral flow, anesthetized dogs showed greater blood flow to
the cortical white, cerebellum, thalamus and medulla. It is of interest that Marcus et al.[5] found no difference in regional cerebral
blood flows normalized to total cerebral flow in dogs ventilated to
achieve levels of arterial hypoxia or hypercapnia and acidosis greater or equal to those found in hemorrhagic shock. Although cerebral
blood flow increased with acidosis and hypoxia or hypercapnia, the
percentage of flow delivered to the brain stem, cerebellum, cerebral
hemispheres, cortical white and cortical grey areas remained largely
unaltered. However, studies in normovolemic animals are not presumed
to reflect conditions present in hemorrhagic shock. In this regard,
studies conducted by Dr. Kovach and his colleagues provide information concerning the degree and mechanism of redistribution of blood
flow in hemorrhagic shock and the metabolic and functional consequences of cerebral ischemia. Particularly Dr. Kovach and his colleagues have suggested that impaired cerebral blood flow and altered
activity of neurons regulating cardiovascular function may contribute
to circulatory collapse in hemorrhagic shock. In this regard, Fitch
et al.[6] examined the influence of the sympathetic nervous system on
cerebral blood flow in hemorrhaged baboons. The pressure - cerebral
blood flow relationship was studied over a range of 20-100 mm Hg with
10 mm Hg reductions in pressure at twenty minute intervals. Animals
were subjected to one of the following: hemorrhage, hemorrhage and
acute sympathectomy, hemorrhage plus chronic sympathectomy, and
hemorrhage plus phenoxybenzamine. In each case a cerebral autoregulatory response was evoked to hemorrhage. Except in the case of
chronic sympathectomy, the autoregulatory response of the cerebral
vasculature was altered by modification of sympathetic activity.
Acute cervical sympathectomy and phenoxybenzamine decreased the
lower limit of autoregulation from about 65 mm Hg to 40 mm Hg or
less. These results suggested that sympathetic adrenergic innervation limited the autoregulatory response of the cerebral vasculature
to hemorrhage. Furthermore, such results support the dual control
hypothesis of the cerebral response to hemorrhage. Extraparenchymal
or large arterial vessels may constrict with sympathetic activation
during hemorrhage at a time when intraparenchymal vessels are maximally dilated by metabolic or myogenic mechanisms. Thus, activation
of adrenergic innervation may limit the degree of cerebral vasodilation during hemorrhage. Previously Reivich et al.[7] observed that

the cerebral vasculature is not maximally dilated during hemorrhage in the baboon.

The occurrence of cerebral vasoconstriction during shock has recently been reported by Emerson and Parker.[8] Cerebral vascular resistance was increased four hours after administration of endotoxin in dogs. The authors postulate the presence of a vasoconstrictor or plugging of the cerebral vasculature. Thus, limitation of cerebral vasodilation or regional vasoconstriction could promote cerebral ischemic damage during circulatory shock.

Studies by Dr. Kovach and his colleagues have described altered cerebral metabolism and function during hemorrhagic shock. Reivich et al.[9] reported increased lactate, decreased pyruvate output, decreased oxygen consumption and unchanged glucose uptake of brains of baboons following hemorrhage. Again the question of total versus regional alterations in cerebral metabolism during hemorrhage needs to be studied further. Indeed, it seems clear that decreased cerebral blood flow affects the response to hemorrhagic shock, although the involvement of discrete regional ischemia within the brain has been debated. However, the evidence favors differential responses of cerebral vessels to hemorrhage. The mechanism of this differential effect is unclear. Continuing study of cerebral metabolism should provide additional information concerning ischemic metabolism, cellular integrity and cerebral regulation of the cardiovascular system in shock.

References

1. Betz E: Cerebral blood flow: Its measurement and regulation. Physiol. Rev. 52:595-630, 1972.
2. Kovach AGB, Sandor P: Cerebral blood flow and brain function during hypotension and shock. In Knovil E, Sonnerschein RR, Edelman IS (Editors): Annual Review of Physiology. Palo Alto, Annual Reviews Inc, 1976, pp 571-796.
3. Kovach AGB: The function of the central nervous system during hemorrhage. J. Clin. Pathol. 23 Suppl. 4:202-212, 1970.
4. Slater G, Vladeck BC, Bassin R, Brown RS, Shoemaker WC: Sequential changes in cerebral blood flow and distribution of flow within the brain during hemorrhagic shock. Ann. Surg. 181: 1-4, 1975.
5. Marcus ML, Heistad DD, Erhardt JC, Abboud FM: Total and regional cerebral blood flow measurement with 7-10-, 15-, 25-, and 50-μm microspheres. J. Appl. Physiol. 40:501-507, 1976.
6. Fitch W, MacKenzie ET, Harper AM: Effects of decreasing arterial pressure on cerebral blood flow in the baboon. Circ. Res. 37:550-557, 1975.
7. Reivich M: Arterial P_{CO_2} and cerebral hemodynamics. Am. J. Physiol. 206:25-35, 1964.

8. Emerson TE Jr, Parker JL: Cerebral hemodynamics during endo-
    toxin shock in the dog. Circ. Shock 3:21-29, 1976.
9. Reivich M, Kovach AGB, Spitzer JJ, Sandor P: Cerebral blood
    flow and metabolism in hemorrhagic shock in baboons. In
    Kovach AGB, Stoner HB, Spitzer JJ (Editors): Neurohumeral
    and Metabolic Aspects of Injury. New York, Plenum Press,
    1973, pp 19-26.

PARTICIPANTS

R. BERNE, Dept. of Physiology, School of Medicine, Univ. of Virginia, Charlottesville, VA

A. BOVERIS, Institute of Biochemistry, School of Medicine, Univ. of Buenos Aires, Buenos Aires, Argentina

D. BRUCE, Dept. of Neurosurgery, Hospital of the Univ. of Pennsylvania, Philadelphia, PA

N. CHALAZONITIS, Dept. of Biophysique des Neuromembranes Microscopie Electronique, C.N.R.S. Institut de Neurophysiologie et Psychophysiologie, Marseilles, France

B. CHANCE, Johnson Research Foundation, Univ. of Pennsylvania, Philadelphia, PA

R.F. COBURN, Dept. of Physiology, School of Medicine, Univ. of Pennsylvania, Philadelphia, PA

F. COCEANI, The Hospital for Sick Children, Toronto, Ontario, Canada

T. DUFFY, Dept. of Neurology, New York Hospital, Cornell Medical Center, New York, NY

R. ESTABROOK, Dept. of Biochemistry, Southwestern Medical School, Univ. of Texas, Dallas, TX

C. EYZAGUIRRE, Dept. of Physiology, College of Medicine, Univ. of Utah, Salt Lake City, UT

F.S. FAY, Dept. of Physiology, Univ. of Massachusetts Medical Center, Worcester, MA

A. FISHMAN, Cardio-Pulmonary Division, Hospital of the Univ. of Pennsylvania, Philadelphia, PA

R. FITZGERALD, Dept. of Environmental Medicine, Johns Hopkins Univ., Baltimore, MD

R.E. FORSTER, Dept. of Physiology, School of Medicine, Univ. of Pennsylvania, Philadelphia, PA

I. GUNSALUS, Dept. of Biochemistry, School of Chemical Sciences, Univ. of Illinois, Urbana, IL

F. HADDY, Dept. of Physiology, Michigan State Univ., East Lansing, MI

J. HALSEY, Dept. of Neurology, School of Medicine, Univ. of Alabama, Birmingham, AL

A. HESS, Dept. of Anatomy,
Rutgers Medical School,
Piscataway, NJ

F. JOBSIS, Dept. of Physiology,
Duke Univ. Medical School,
Durham, NC

A.G.B. KOVACH, Dept. of Experimental Research, Semmelweis
Medical Univ., Budapest, Hungary

S. LAHIRI, Dept. of Physiology,
Institute for Environmental
Medicine, Univ. of Pennsylvania,
Philadelphia, PA

W. LUST, Laboratory of Neuropathology and Neuroanatomical
Sciences, National Institute of
Neurological and Communicative
Disorders and Stroke, Bethesda,
MD

L. MELA, Harrison Dept. of Surgical Research, Hospital of the
Univ. of Pennsylvania, Philadelphia, PA

M. O'CONNOR, Dept. of Neurosurgery, Hospital of the Univ. of
Pennsylvania, Philadelphia, PA

R. PAUL, Dept. of Physiology,
University College London,
London, England

B. QUISTORFF, Dept. of Biochemistry, Univ. of Copenhagen,
Copenhagen, Denmark

M. REIVICH, Dept. of Neurology,
Hospital of the Univ. of
Pennsylvania, Philadelphia, PA

R. RUBIO, Dept. of Physiology,
School of Medicine, Univ. of
Virginia, Charlottesville, VA

J.W. SEVERINGHAUS, Cardiovascular Research Institute,
Univ. of California, San Francisco, CA

H. SIES, Institut fur Physiologische Chemie, Physikalische
Biochemie und Zellbiologie,
Universitat Munchen, Munich,
West Germany

B. SIESJO, Research Dept.,
University Hospital, Lund,
Sweden

I. SILVER, Dept. of Pathology,
School of Medicine, Univ. of
Bristol, Bristol, England

S. SLIGAR, Dept. of Biochemistry,
School of Chemical Sciences,
Univ. of Illinois, Urbana, IL

L. SOKOLOFF, Laboratory of
Cerebral Metabolism, National
Institutes of Mental Health,
Bethesda, MD

J. SPATH, Dept. of Physiology,
Thomas Jefferson University,
Philadelphia, PA

N. STAUB, Dept. of Physiology,
School of Medicine, Univ. of
California, San Francisco, CA

T. SUNDT, Dept. of Neurosurgery,
Mayo Clinic, Rochester, MN

R.W. TORRANCE, St. John's College, Oxford, England

F. WELSH, Dept. of Neurosurgery, Hospital of the Univ. of Pennsylvania, Philadelphia, PA

M. WILKSTROM, Johnson Research Foundation, Univ. of Pennsylvania, Philadelphia, PA

W.J. WHALEN, St. Vincent Charity Hospital, Cleveland, OH